T0300030

Operative Surgery for Head and Neck Tumours

Operative Surgery for Head and Neck Tumours

Edited By

Jagdeep S. Thakur

Associate Professor, Department of Otolaryngology–Head
and Neck Surgery,
Indira Gandhi Medical College,
Shimla, HP, India

Ripu Daman Arora

Additional Professor, Department of Otolaryngology–Head
and Neck Surgery,
All India Institute of Medical Sciences,
Raipur, Chhattisgarh, India

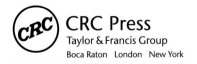

CRC Press
Taylor & Francis Group
Boca Raton   London   New York

CRC Press is an imprint of the
Taylor & Francis Group, an **informa** business

First edition published 2022
by CRC Press
6000 Broken Sound Parkway NW, Suite 300, Boca Raton, FL 33487–2742

and by CRC Press
2 Park Square, Milton Park, Abingdon, Oxon, OX14 4RN

© 2022 Taylor & Francis Group, LLC

CRC Press is an imprint of Taylor & Francis Group, LLC

This book contains information obtained from authentic and highly regarded sources. While all reasonable efforts have been made to publish reliable data and information, neither the author[s] nor the publisher can accept any legal responsibility or liability for any errors or omissions that may be made. The publishers wish to make clear that any views or opinions expressed in this book by individual editors, authors or contributors are personal to them and do not necessarily reflect the views/opinions of the publishers. The information or guidance contained in this book is intended for use by medical, scientific or health-care professionals and is provided strictly as a supplement to the medical or other professional's own judgement, their knowledge of the patient's medical history, relevant manufacturer's instructions and the appropriate best practice guidelines. Because of the rapid advances in medical science, any information or advice on dosages, procedures or diagnoses should be independently verified. The reader is strongly urged to consult the relevant national drug formulary and the drug companies' and device or material manufacturers' printed instructions, and their websites, before administering or utilizing any of the drugs, devices or materials mentioned in this book. This book does not indicate whether a particular treatment is appropriate or suitable for a particular individual. Ultimately it is the sole responsibility of the medical professional to make his or her own professional judgements, so as to advise and treat patients appropriately. The authors and publishers have also attempted to trace the copyright holders of all material reproduced in this publication and apologize to copyright holders if permission to publish in this form has not been obtained. If any copyright material has not been acknowledged please write and let us know so we may rectify in any future reprint.

Except as permitted under U.S. Copyright Law, no part of this book may be reprinted, reproduced, transmitted, or utilized in any form by any electronic, mechanical, or other means, now known or hereafter invented, including photocopying, microfilming, and recording, or in any information storage or retrieval system, without written permission from the publishers.

For permission to photocopy or use material electronically from this work, access www .copyright.com or contact the Copyright Clearance Center, Inc. (CCC), 222 Rosewood Drive, Danvers, MA 01923, 978–750–8400. For works that are not available on CCC please contact mpkbookspermissions@tandf.co.uk

Trademark notice: Product or corporate names may be trademarks or registered trademarks and are used only for identification and explanation without intent to infringe.

Library of Congress Cataloging-in-Publication Data
Names: Thakur, Jagdeep, editor. | Arora, Ripu Daman, editor.
Title: Operative surgery for head and neck tumors / edited by Jagdeep Thakur, Ripu Daman Arora.
Description: First edition. | Boca Raton, FL : CRC Press, 2022. | Includes bibliographical references and index.
Identifiers: LCCN 2021046592 (print) | LCCN 2021046593 (ebook) | ISBN 9780367430122 (hardback) | ISBN 9781032155814 (paperback) | ISBN 9780367430139 (ebook)
Subjects: MESH: Head and Neck Neoplasms—surgery | Surgical Procedures, Operative | Head—surgery | Neck—surgery
Classification: LCC RD521 (print) | LCC RD521 (ebook) | NLM WE 707 | DDC 617.5/1059—dc23
LC record available at https://lccn.loc.gov/2021046592
LC ebook record available at https://lccn.loc.gov/2021046593

ISBN: 978-0-367-43012-2 (hbk)
ISBN: 978-1-032-15581-4 (pbk)
ISBN: 978-0-367-43013-9 (ebk)

DOI: 10.1201/9780367430139

Typeset in Minion Pro
by Apex CoVantage, LLC

To my parents for infusing principles of life
To my teachers and residents for inspiration
To my wife, Anamika, for affection, care and support
My children, Lavanya and Manan, for unconditional love and happiness
—JT

To my parents for all the love and teaching
My brother Gaurav for being always there in tough times
To my wife, Neel, for unconditional love and support
To my twin sons, Ayansh and Anish, and my niece Shamya for bringing happiness in my life
To my teachers, especially my mentor, Prof. Nitin M. Nagarkar, for teaching the art of surgery
And to our patients for believing in us
—RD

Table of Contents

Preface

Surgery always poses a challenge. Surgical training requires direct supervision and theoretical knowledge about anatomy and disease. Besides legal requirements, supervision is always required during training, as the majority of operative surgery books lack minute operative details. This limitation leads to hesitancy among surgeons when they start independent practice.

To overcome this constraint, we present this book, keeping in view the problems faced by residents in learning the surgery. This book emphasises clinical, radiological and laboratory assessment and operative surgery in common head-neck surgeries, providing a systemic and rational operative approach to common surgical procedures rather than complicated and advanced surgical techniques. Giving insight to each aspect of surgery, including surgical tools, this book is especially valuable to trainees, junior consultants and other specialists who are managing head-neck cases.

We would like to thank all the authors who have contributed chapters to this book; Himani Dwivedi and Shivangi Pramanik for their excellent editorial help, support and patience during production, which got delayed due to the Covid-19 pandemic; and the CRC Press, Taylor & Francis, for help at every stage of the publication.

Acknowledgements

We would like to acknowledge our colleagues, associate staff and patients for being the source of knowledge and inspiration.

About the Editors

Jagdeep S Thakur

Dr Jagdeep S Thakur is Associate Professor in the Department of Otolaryngology–Head and Neck Surgery, Indira Gandhi Medical College, Shimla, HP, India. He has more than 18 years of academic and research experience in otolaryngology–head and neck surgery. An editorial member and reviewer of numerous prominent national and international journals, he has numerous national and international research publications and awards. In 2016, he won the best research paper award from the JLO Society and an Indo-American Cancer Association fellowship at MD Anderson Cancer Center, Houston, Texas. He is an active member of philanthropic medical education missions in Asia and Africa. Dr Thakur believes in imparting simple but rigorous post-graduate training so that fellows can deliver the best care to their patients.

Ripu Daman Arora

Dr Ripu Daman Arora presently holds the post of Additional Professor in the department of Otolaryngology–Head & Neck Surgery at All India Institute of Medical Sciences, Raipur, Chhattisgarh, India. He has conducted many head and neck workshops for residents and faculties including the National Conference of Associations of Otolaryngologists in 2015. He was awarded the prestigious Icon of Health, Chhattisgarh, for contributions in the field of ENT and won a foreign travel fellowship from the Indian Society of Otology to University of Cologne, Germany. He has delivered many invited lectures and is reviewer for many journals, and has many publications in national and international journals and chapters in books to his credit.

Contributors

Subinsha A, MBBS, MS
Resident, Department of Otolaryngology–Head and Neck Surgery, All India Institute of Medical Sciences, Raipur, Chhattisgarh, India

Ripu Daman Arora, MBBS, MS, MAMS
Additional Professor, Department of Otolaryngology–Head and Neck Surgery, All India Institute of Medical Sciences, Raipur, Chhattisgarh, India

Vipin Arora, MBBS, MS, FICS
Director Professor, Department of Otolaryngology–Head and Neck Surgery, University College of Medical Sciences and GTB Hospital, Delhi, India

Suvercha Arya, MBBS, MS
Senior Resident, Maulana Azad Medical College and Lok Nayak Hospital, Delhi, India

Avinash Chaitanya S, MBBS, MS, FHNSO
Consultant, Head and Neck Surgical Oncology Care Hospital, Hyderabad, India

Moumita De, MBBS, MS, MCh
Assistant Professor, Department of Burns and Plastic Surgery, All India Institute of Medical Sciences, Raipur, Chhattisgarh, India

Ravi Kant Dogra, MBBS, MD, PDCC (Critical Care)
Associate Professor, Department of Anaesthesia and Intensive Care, Indira Gandhi Medical College, Shimla, HP, India

Nitin Gupta, MBBS, MS
Professor, Department of Otolaryngology–Head and Neck Surgery, Government Medical College, Chandigarh, India

Rajeev Gupta, MBBS, MS, DNB, FISO
Assistant Professor, Shri Aurbindo Medical College, Indore, MP, India

Payal Kamble, MBBS, MS
Clinical Fellow, National Cancer Institute, Nagpur, India

Ravi Meher, MBBS, MS
Professor, Maulana Azad Medical College and Lok Nayak Hospital, Delhi, India

Jiten Kumar Mishra, MBBS, MS, MCh
Assistant Professor, Department of Burns and Plastic Surgery, All India Institute of Medical Sciences, Raipur, Chhattisgarh, India

Nitin M Nagarkar, MBBS, MS, DNB, MNAMS.
Director, All India Institute of Medical Sciences, Raipur, and Professor and Head, Department of Otolaryngology–Head and Neck Surgery, All India Institute of Medical Sciences, Raipur, Chhattisgarh, India

Smriti Panda, MBBS, MS, MCh
Assistant Professor, Department of Otolaryngology-Head and Neck Surgery, All India Institute of Medical Sciences, New Delhi, India

Neel Prabha, MBBS, MD
Assistant Professor, Department of Dermatology,
All India Institute of Medical Sciences, Raipur,
Chhattisgarh, India

Kartik N Rao, MBBS, MS, FHNSO, FACS MCh
Senior Resident, Head and Neck Surgical
Oncology, Department of Otolaryngology–Head
and Neck Surgery, All India Institute of Medical
Sciences, Raipur, Chhattisgarh, India

Shamendra Anand Sahu, MBBS, MS, MCh
Assistant Professor, Department of Burns and
Plastic Surgery, All India Institute of Medical
Sciences, Raipur, Chhattisgarh, India

Dinesh Sharma, MBBS, MS
Assistant Professor, Department of
Otolaryngology–Head and Neck Surgery, Indira
Gandhi Medical College, Shimla, HP, India

Rohit K Sharma, MBBS, MS
Professor and Head, Department of
Otolaryngology–Head and Neck Surgery, SRM
Institute of Medical Sciences, Barrielly, UP, India

Dara Singh, MBBS, MD
Professor, Department of Anaesthesia and
Intensive Care, Indira Gandhi Medical College,
Shimla, HP, India

Kartik Syal, MBBS, MD
Associate Professor, Department of Anaesthesia
and Intensive Care, Indira Gandhi Medical
College, Shimla, HP, India

Anamika Thakur, MBBS, MD
Associate Professor, Department of
Pharmacology, Indira Gandhi Medical College,
Shimla, HP, India

Jagdeep S Thakur, MBBS, MS
Associate Professor, Department of
Otolaryngology–Head and Neck Surgery, Indira
Gandhi Medical College, Shimla, HP, India

Kuldeep Thakur, MBBS, MS, MCh
Assistant Professor, Department of
Otolaryngology–Head and Neck Surgery, Indira
Gandhi Medical College, Shimla, HP, India

Divya Vaid, MBBS, MS
Senior Resident, University College of Medical
Sciences and Guru Teg Bahadur Hospital, Delhi,
India

Saurabh Varshney, MBBS, MS, FACS, FICS
Executive Director and CEO, All India Institute of
Medical Sciences, Deoghar, Jharkhand, India

Hitesh Verma, MBBS, MS, DNB, MBA
Associate Professor, Department of
Otolaryngology–Head and Neck Surgery, All
India Institute of Medical Sciences, New Delhi,
India

Ravneet R Verma, MBBS, MS
Assistant Professor, Department of
Otolaryngology–Head and Neck Surgery,
Government Medical College, Chandigarh, India

The Head and Neck Team

JAGDEEP S THAKUR

THE TEAM

"Alone we can do so little; together we can do wonders."

(Modified from the words of Helen Keller)

The head and neck team consists of more than the surgeon – it's a multidisciplinary team. Typically, the team is led and coordinated by a head and neck surgeon and consists of

- Head and neck surgeon
- Radiation oncologist
- Medical oncologist
- Radiologist
- Pathologist
- Reconstructive surgeon
- Prosthodontist
- Speech therapist
- Oncology nurse
- Physiotherapist
- Nutritional specialist
- Allied specialists: anaesthetist, neurosurgeon, ophthalmologist, psychiatrist, audiologist

However, we consider the patient an important member of the team around whom everything revolves.

To become a **surgeon** one needs to be good anatomist, a lifelong observer and learner and a good communicator. The old saying "It takes a few years to learn how to do surgery, another few years to learn when to do surgery, and a decade to learn when not to do surgery" holds true.

A surgeon should observe and learn from everyone around him/her while in the operating room. One should never hesitate to ask for help from a senior or junior whenever there is a doubt, especially in difficult cases where you need to review anatomy and can ask your assistant or other operating team member for a clue.

You should always have a look at the monitor or talk to the anaesthetist while operating to check the vitals of the patient. A surgeon should be confident but not overconfident. He/she should know the team's capabilities and limitations, and there should be another specialist on hand who can help in case of any complication. It is always better not to start when you cannot finish, and this rule should be strictly followed in oncology cases to avert the need for revision surgery. One should always review the case before surgery and remain calm and confident. Any vascular breach should not be clamped blindly as it will further lead to complication especially neural injury. Digital pressure is the safest method to control haemorrhage, and once proper instruments become available, one should try to use the clamp under direct vision. At the end of surgery, always check cavities for any leftover gauges, needles, or instruments, and check for haemorrhage with raised intrathoracic pressure. Secure the drain at appropriate area with absorbable sutures. Skin closure should always be directly observed if being done by residents. Just before dressing the surgical site, make sure the drain is secured and negative pressure is maintained.

DOI: 10.1201/9780367430139-1

A **subject/patient** is the pivot of the surgical team as treatment planning and outcome directly depends upon him/her. First and foremost, patients should have full information on the disease and its management options. Counselling is an art and the surgeon should have good communication skills and confidence. These skills improve with time, but there are a number of free online modules from various educational institutes. The patient should know that he/she is in good hands. She/he should be told about positive things of surgery first and then about post-operative complications. Once he/she gives consent for surgery, patient should be informed about operative defects, reconstruction and post-operative care, radiotherapy and morbidity. The expected complications or poor outcome must be disclosed when the patient is fully prepared for surgery. This mental preparation will result in better outcome.

The **radiologist** should be specifically requested to evaluate and report on areas of interest if he/she is unaware of surgical approach or resection area. The surgeon should always read the CT and MRI to see the extent of the disease and plan the surgery accordingly, rather than reading the radiologist's report, and whenever in doubt it is better to go to the radiologist who can reconstruct the images according to the surgeon's plan. Further, the radiologist should specifically be requested to comment on the nature of nodes so that cytological diagnosis can be made for further planning of neck dissection. Nowadays, certain benign cysts can be managed by an interventional radiologist and hence surgery may be avoided.

The **pathologist** also must be provided with full clinical and imaging details as sometimes it's difficult for him/her to make a pathological diagnosis. Excised tissue should be marked at the time of surgery as later it becomes difficult to label due to loss of orientation.

The **anaesthetist** needs to be informed on the nature of the surgery and impending complications, if any. In head-neck surgery, the surgeon and the anaesthetist have a common work area, hence coordination and mutual trust are of utmost importance for optimal operative and post-operative outcome.

The **reconstructive surgeon/prosthodontist** should know the surgical plan and expected defect to plan reconstruction. The patient should have full information on defect and reconstruction options. This will help the patient to cope and reduce post-operative morbidity.

The surgeon should discuss the treatment plan with the **radiotherapist**. Many times a tumour may not be resectable and pre-operative chemoradiation can help in such cases. After surgery, the radiotherapist should have full information on operative findings to plan further treatment.

The **speech therapist and physiotherapist** are responsible for helping the patient in reducing post-operative morbidity. They should also know the probable post-operative morbidity so that they can counsel the patient and family members preoperatively. This will improve the patient and family members quality of life.

The oncology nurse is mainly involved during chemotherapy in head and neck tumours. Anticancer drugs have many side effects and carry risk of complications. A well aware oncology nurse brings down these side effects or complications to the minimal.

The allied specialties like pain management, neurosurgeon or ophthalmologist join the head and neck team routinely due to anatomical or physiological need of the disease. The audiologist is required in management of cases involving ear or temporal bone. Patients undergoing chemoradiation usually require evaluation by an audiologist for proper rehabilitation.

Pre-Operative Management

DARA SINGH

INTRODUCTION

Pre-operative preparation of a surgical patient starts with the diagnosis and planning of surgery. In most of surgical centres, the senior resident or most senior resident of the unit is responsible for all the planning, preparation and optimisation of a surgical patient. Assessment and optimisation of patients is important to prevent unnecessary cancellations of surgery, smooth conduct of anaesthesia and surgical procedure, and to avoid perioperative morbidity and mortality.

During the planning for surgery, the following points must be paid special attention:

- Pre-admission planning
- Pre-admission patient education
- Patient screening on OPD basis
- Optimisation of patient in terms of
  - o Head and neck
  - o Cardiovascular system
  - o Respiratory system
  - o Diabetes
  - o Renal and hepatic
  - o Haematology
  - o Drug allergies
- Pre-anaesthetic check-up

PRE-ADMISSION PLANNING

When the patient first consults the surgeon, the pre-admission plan should start in the surgeon's mind. It should include the diagnosis, surgery planned, any radio- or chemotherapy required pre-operatively in malignant cases, any comorbid conditions needing pre-admission optimisation, nature of the surgery (that is, emergent, urgent or planned), any need for removal of tissue or part of it, impact of that removal on patient's day-to-day activities, any loss of skin (if yes, a plan to repair that loss – i.e., flap or graft and type most suitable, e.g., rotational flap and how to raise it, graft split skin, partial or full thickness, etc.).

PRE-ADMISSION EDUCATION

Before talking to patient, imagine you are the patient: what would you like to know about the disease and surgery? Discuss with the patient and family options of treatment, cost of hospital stay, cost expected in post-operative period at home, change in lifestyle after planned treatment, any complications during and after the hospital stay. After discussing all the treatment options and planning the treatment, written informed consent must be obtained from patient. This consent should be written in clear words, in a language most suitable for the patient, explaining the diagnosis, treatment options and plan, along with the possible complications. The consent has to be attested to by one witness to safeguard the treating physician from post-treatment legal issues. When to obtain consent depends on hospital protocol and can vary, from outpatient department (OPD) file preparation to hospital admission to before operative procedure.

DOI: 10.1201/9780367430139-2

SCREENING PRE-ANAESTHETIC CHECK (PAC)

Patient should be screened in anaesthesia OPD on the day of presentation to surgical OPD to ensure that no unnecessary fitness investigations are carried out. This can also decrease the hospital admission days by guiding the fitness of patient for surgery and hence determining the right time to admit the patient for surgery.

OPTIMISATION OF THE PATIENT

While planning for optimisation, one must follow a set sequence (follow hospital protocols) to avoid missing any important organ or system. Organs or systems with more frequent comorbid conditions should be dealt with or screened with special attention, e.g., cardiovascular (hypertension, ischaemic heart diseases), endocrine (diabetes mellitus), respiratory (chronic obstructive pulmonary disease/asthma) and haematological system (anaemia, antiplatelets or anticoagulant treatment). Metastasis and/or any paraneoplastic symptoms should be paid special attention in case of cancer. Second primary malignant tumour or synchronous malignancies are common in certain head-neck cancers, e.g., aerodigestive epithelial cancers and MEN syndrome.

It is also recommended to discuss the following issues with patient:

- Risk prediction due to primary disease and comorbid conditions
- Surgical and anaesthetic implications
- Expectant functional outcome
- Effect on quality of life

In head and neck preparation and optimisation, airway assessment carries utmost importance. A difficult airway at the time of anaesthesia may give rise to unforeseen morbidity or mortality. Airway assessment and investigations should be started before contacting the anaesthesiologist. Any direct or indirect compression or occlusion of airway found on clinical examination and radiological investigations should be documented and investigated thoroughly. Elective tracheostomy should be planned and discussed with the patient and anaesthesia team well in advance. Similarly, post-operative care in case of reconstructive surgery or airway surgery that may require intensive care should be planned.

In case of malignancies of head and neck, a multidisciplinary discussion involving other concerned specialities (e.g., medical oncology, radiation oncology, plastic surgery and anaesthesia) helps the primary treating physician in choosing an appropriate treatment plan.

Functional status of thyroid and parathyroid glands must be looked for in thyroid tumours or swellings. Some malignant tumours involving these glands may also affect their hormonal status, apart from other thyroid swellings. Hypothyroidism requires optimisation for at least 10–15 days, while hyperthyroidism may take longer duration, 4–6 weeks for the same. A euthyroid status should be ensured before planned surgery in patients of a non-emergency nature.

Hypertension is one of the commonest comorbidities in surgical patients across all specialties. It has been observed that nearly half the number of patients undergoing head and neck surgeries suffer from cardiac diseases. Mandatory electrocardiogram (ECG) in patients usually rules out cardiac disease. It is recommended to get an ECG in all the patients above 45 years of age, any patient with history or symptoms of cardiac disease, or in diabetics or hypertensives.

Hypertension and its anticipated sequelae should be evaluated and managed properly before surgery, but rapid or hasty control of blood pressure through over-prescription should be avoided, as it increases risk of complications. Patients with ischaemic heart disease (IHD), recent myocardial infarct (MI) or recent cardiac interventions like stenting must have a consultation with a cardiologist regarding antiplatelet therapy, which increases intraoperative complication. In case of recent MI of less than three months duration, routine surgeries should not be planned.

A comprehensive evaluation of medication being taken by the patient should be done. Certain drugs need to be stopped at different times before surgery, e.g., clopidogrel 5 days before surgery, warfarin 5 days before surgery, ACE inhibitors, anti-hyperglycaemics and diuretics on the day of surgery. Aspirin should be stopped 3–5 days before, if patient is on a therapeutic dose of 150 mg or more. A prophylactic dose (75 mg) can be continued, depending upon the risk-to-benefit ratio. Some drugs need bridge therapy during the perioperative period, e.g., warfarin and clopidogrel with LMWH and oral antihyperglycaemic agents (OHAs) with insulin.

Patients with heart failure, cor pulmonale, pulmonary hypertension and severe valvular lesions carry a higher risk of anaesthetic complications. These patients need special attention and multidisciplinary management. An echocardiogram should always be carried out in such cases.

Head and neck tumours have a strong correlation with smoking, hence associated respiratory disease is routinely anticipated in these patients. In general, a restrictive disease is difficult to optimise as compared to obstructive pathology. Obstructive diseases like chronic obstructive pulmonary disease (COPD) and asthma may improve with bronchodilator therapy. Pulmonary functions should be optimised as normal as possible.

Investigations needed for respiratory diseases are chest X-ray, pulmonary functions and blood gas analysis. Chest X-ray is mandatory in patients with clinical features suggestive of pulmonary disease or metastasis and those older than 55 years. Computed tomogram of the chest is rarely required.

Patients with oral or inhalation steroids (prednisolone 5 mg/day or equivalent) for more than two weeks in the past six months require perioperative intravenous steroid cover to prevent adrenal crisis.

Obstructive sleep apnoea (OSA) and smoking also play an important role in operative management and have adverse peri-operative outcome. Smoking should be stopped at least two weeks before surgery, although 6–8 weeks gives significant advantage in reducing morbidity in the peri-operative period, as this period may allow for restoration of respiratory ciliary function.

Hyperglycaemia is significantly correlated with adverse operative outcome. Poorly controlled glucose levels affect lymphocytic chemotaxis, wound healing, poor collagen synthesis, and cardiac, neurological and renal functions. Therefore, blood glucose should be optimised before surgery. HbA1c is a good indicator of glycaemic control over the past three months. A consultation with a diabetologist 2–3 weeks prior to surgery is advisable.

Oral hypoglycaemics are omitted on the day of surgery and resumed with oral feed. To avoid catabolism, patients on insulin should not miss multiple doses. It is recommended that insulin not be missed more than one missed meal and appropriate replacement started thereafter as IV infusion with neutralised dextrose or DKI (dextrose potassium insulin). These patients should also be monitored for serum potassium.

Kidneys or liver can be affected by primary disease or some other independent pathology. Both organs need functional evaluation before surgery. Hepatic and autoimmune-deficiency viral diseases must be ruled out, especially in case of drug addiction.

Haematological evaluation involves complete blood count. Anaemia is common in head and neck cancer due to bleeding or reduced oral intake. Anaemia requires microscopic examination, diagnosis and treatment accordingly. In anaemias related to malignancies, blood should not be transfused in the immediate pre-operative period. A latent period of 24–48 hours is needed for activation of 2,3-DPG in stored blood.

A written checklist for pre-operative preparation should be available and displayed in the ward to reduce the chances of missing investigations or procedures.

Hygiene of surgical area and adjoining areas (mouth or nasal cavity) needs consideration. Patient should be asked to take a bath with soap and water the night before or on the day of surgery. Sometimes, chlorhexidine gargles are advised in fungating tumours, although disinfection is difficult, especially in oral and nasal surgery, and normal oral flora must be preserved by avoiding unnecessary antibiotics.

Sometime, patients require parenteral antibiotic or blood transfusion. In such cases, peripheral veins on the non-dominant hand should be preferred so as to save large proximal vessels.

Cancer, obesity (BMI >30), age 60 or more, oestrogen intake, immobility (lower limb paraplegia, etc.), prolonged surgical time (>3 hrs), prior venous thrombo-embolism or family history require mechanical or pharmacological prophylaxis for deep vein thrombosis. Low molecular weight heparin is generally used as enoxaparin 40 mg or dalteparin 5000 IU subcutaneously once daily, but unfractionated heparin can also be used for thromboprophylaxis 5000 IU subcutaneously at 12-hour intervals.

PRE-ANAESTHETIC CHECK-UP

A detailed pre-anaesthetic check should precede surgery by a day or two. Evaluation steps should not be bypassed in relatively short surgical procedures. A detailed anaesthesia check prepares the team for various intra-operative and post-operative problems (Figure 2.1). The pre-anaesthetic check involves a detailed history of present and past illness, any

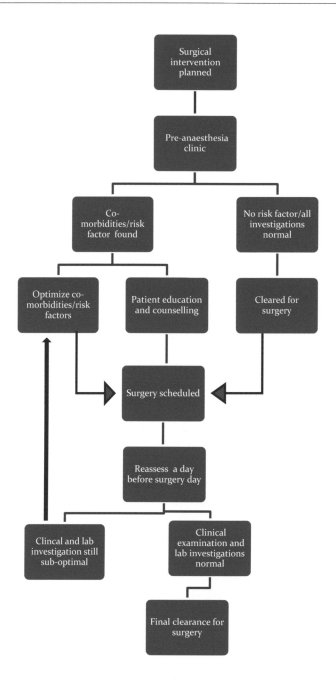

Figure 2.1 Pre-anaesthesia work plan.

treatment, drug intake, comorbidities (asthma, ischemic heart disease, diabetes mellitus, rheumatic heart disease, pregnancy, etc.) and allergies including post-operative nausea and vomiting, etc. It is followed by examination of patient and investigations. Special attention must be paid to airway assessment. Laryngoscopic and CT neck findings help in difficult airway situations, as patient must be counselled for tracheostomy. Naso-tracheal intubation requires decongestion therapy and certain surgeries require elective tracheostomy for post-operative care. These cases require close monitoring, so intensive care team coordination is mandatory.

3

Post-Operative Care

KARTIK SYAL

INTRODUCTION

ENT surgeries are among the most dreaded for anaesthetists due to the commonalities of the two specialities. Among the medical fraternity, airway management is the sole responsibility of anaesthetists and ENT surgeons. Airway management is primarily handled by the anaesthetist in the peri-operative period, and this can be a major point of concern, as ENT surgeries directly and indirectly affect the airway, potentially leading to complications which may even reach to a level of tracheostomy.

Many anaesthesia-related post-operative complications can be mitigated by measures undertaken before and during extubation.

Most of these surgeries involve tissue handling, trauma and dissection around the oro-pharyngo-laryngeal axis, which can lead to airway oedema; this is the most common entity which leads to post-operative complication of respiratory distress per se and even aggravates other reasons for distress. This can be negated by giving steroids. Different steroids are recommended for

use in various doses and routes as well as timing (before extubation surgical incision). Most preferred among them is dexamethasone used in a dose of 0.1–0.25 mg/kg per oral, around 4–6 hours prior to surgery, or by giving injection dexamethasone 0.1–0.2 mg/kg 1–2 hour prior to initiation of surgery. Timing it before surgery would blunt inflammatory oedema from beginning of surgery itself and should be repeated every 6–8 hours for 24–48 hours, depending upon tissue trauma.

Dexamethasone has been the preferred steroid as it has been shown to have maximum effect in preventing significant airway oedema. Also, dexamethasone acts as a pro-analgesic, anti-inflammatory and anti-emetic as well as an anti-tussive, thus benefitting the patient in many ways. (See Table 3.1.)

To further decrease chances of post-operative airway oedema, the correct size of endotracheal tube should be inserted and intubation procedure should be atraumatic. Oversized tube and over-filled cuff generating higher pressures (>25 cm H_2O) and trauma caused due to intubation may

Table 3.1 Doses of Commonly Used Corticosteroids

Drugs	Doses	Timing
dexamethasone	4–10 mg IV	1–4 hours prior to extubation/surgery
hydrocortisone	100 mg IV	1 hour prior to extubation
methylprednisolone	20–60 mg IV	12–24 hours prior to extubation
budesonide	1 mg nebulised	1–4 hours prior to extubation/surgery

DOI: 10.1201/9780367430139-3

also lead to airway oedema aggravated by patient's head movements (for positioning or during surgery). Correct endotracheal cuff pressure should be ensured via cuff manometer or more crudely, by palpation method; this should be checked every 30–45 minutes when nitrous is being used as it may increase pressure due to diffusion.

Careful, planned extubation goes a long way in preventing post-operative complications. This is one surgery where a pre-extubation direct laryngoscopy look is mandatory. Post-thyroid surgery, it is essential that cord movements are seen in laryngoscopy; inadequate cord movements should warn us of impending complications, like chances of aspiration as well as difficulty in breathing. Surgeries involving buccal mucosa, tonsils, etc. are associated with oral bleeding; ensuring there is adequate haemostasis is a shared responsibility of the ENT surgeon and the anaesthetist, and the same has to be checked via pre-extubation laryngoscopy. Any remnant blood or clot should also be suctioned out or removed using a moist gauze with (Magill) forceps. Clot pressure and dislodgement are known to cause complications such as arrhythmias and even sudden death (i.e., coroner's clot, a clot behind the epiglottis causing vagal stimulation), sudden laryngospasm and bronchospasm (dislodgement into airway) leading to post-operative desaturation and even causing and aggravating post-operative retching, nausea and vomiting (gastric irritation). Post-operative bleeding may need interventions in the form of local and systemic tranexamic acid, local application of adrenaline using swab, or even re-exploration of the oral cavity. Any patient having significant bleed to be taken for re-exploration is deemed [to be] a "full stomach" patient, as some amount of blood always reaches the gastric cavity and causes hypersecretion of acidic gastric secretions. Even a small amount of these secretions (e.g., 2.5 ml, at a low pH of around 2.5 ml) trickling into the trachea can cause pneumonitis which may lead to pneumonia. Thus, administration of IV famotidine (20 mg) and IV metoclopramide (0.15 mg/kg) is mandatory, along with taking all other precautions, like rapid sequence induction and cricoid pressure, during intubation.

One important technique during extubation, especially after neck surgeries, is the test to check for leaks around the endotracheal tube. In this test the anaesthetist deflates the endotracheal cuff and checks for leaks around the cuff during positive pressure ventilation. An audible (unaided or through stethoscope) leak alerts us to the possibility of significant tracheal wall oedema, thus negating complication related to the same. Though this test has many false positives and negatives, negative leak detection can alert the anaesthetist to chances of respiratory problems; extubation over intubating bougie may be used in this condition. Also, nebulised adrenaline may be used in this situation, along the tube before and immediately after extubation to decrease airway oedema. Doses of nebulised adrenaline range from 3 to 5 ml of 2.25% racemic mixture to 1 ml of standard adrenaline (1:1000, 0.1%) diluted to make 3–5 ml. Standard practice would be to use 3–5 ml of undiluted easily available adrenaline (1:1000, 0.1%). This is safe even for paediatric use as it is commonly used in cases of post-croup laryngeal oedema. Tracheomalacia will also cause the same negative leak test and will not respond to nebulised adrenaline.

Another factor aggravating post-operative airway complication and especially ENT surgeries is bucking of the patient on the tube during extubation. This leads to higher venous pressures, increases airway irritability and oedema and also causes increased bleeding post ENT surgeries. Extubation should therefore be undertaken smoothly; if need be, small increments of injection propofol 10–20 mg IV may be used, or extubation should be conducted under IV infusion of dexmedetomidine at the rate of 0.2–0.5 mcg/kg/hr.

Tongue oedema can also lead to or aggravate difficulty in breathing in the post-operative period. This may result from reactive oedema to surgical stress or sometimes tongue rotation at the base due to endotracheal tube or even gauze which is placed to prevent aspiration. Anaesthetists and surgeons should be aware of this problem as swollen tongue can lead to significant rise in airway resistance.

Recovery position is of utmost importance in reducing breathing problems post-ENT surgery that may arise due to airway (including tongue) oedema and oozing of blood. For recovery, a 15–20 degree lateral Trendelenburg position with pillow

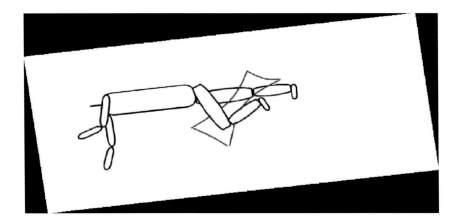

Figure 3.1 15–20 degree lateral Trendelenburg recovery position.

between the knees is warranted, which would take care of bleeding as well as move the tongue away from the central path of airway (Figure 3.1).

Laryngospasm and bronchospasm are two post-operative/extubation anaesthetic complications whose frequency and severity increase in cases involving airway manipulation and other oral cavity surgeries. The most common trigger here is, for obvious reasons, blood oozing into the airway; but surgical manipulation and trauma are another important cause of the same. These can cause hyper-reactivity of the airways that remains for 48–72 hours. It is essential that a predominant entity is established rapidly, as this is an emergency which can lead to catastrophic results, including mortality. Instant decision-making and quick actions are needed. Laryngospasm (Figure 3.2) is associated with rapid desaturation and would be typical of upper airway obstruction where there would be no air exchange despite presence of chest movements. On auscultation, if there is no air entry there is no sound, such as in severe cases, or there might be infrequent high-pitched "crowing" inspiratory stridor sounds. Bronchospasm (Figure 3.3), on the other hand, consists of lower airway pathology, an expiratory wheeze which warrants immediate treatment but is not as catastrophic as most cases of laryngospasm. Negative pressure pulmonary oedema is an entity to be kept in mind during or after (till 24 hours) laryngospasm. It occurs due to vigorous respiratory efforts

against closed glottis. The presence of the same will warrant positive high-pressure ventilation with high FiO2, a propped-up position and further ICU management.

PAIN MANAGEMENT

Efficient pain management follows "preemptive analgesia" and "multimodal analgesia" protocols. In crux, preemptive analgesia means pain management intervention is initiated to blunt peripheral as well as central sensitisation due to incision (initially) and inflammatory (later) reactions. It includes drugs given before surgical stimulus, like injection diclofenac IV (onset of action 15 minutes) given half an hour before surgery so that its effect begins before incision, or regional block/local anaesthesia infiltration done before incision.

The multimodal concept of analgesia in the peri-operative period is based on the fact that multiple interventions (drugs as well as local analgesic-based blocks) with different mechanisms of action are given to utilise their additive and even synergistic beneficial effects on pain relief. Also, this may require smaller doses of each drug for effective analgesia, lessening chances of drug side effects. The combination of non-steroidal anti-inflammatory drugs (NSAIDs) with paracetamol and opioids is a well-established multimodal approach to counter peri-operative pain.

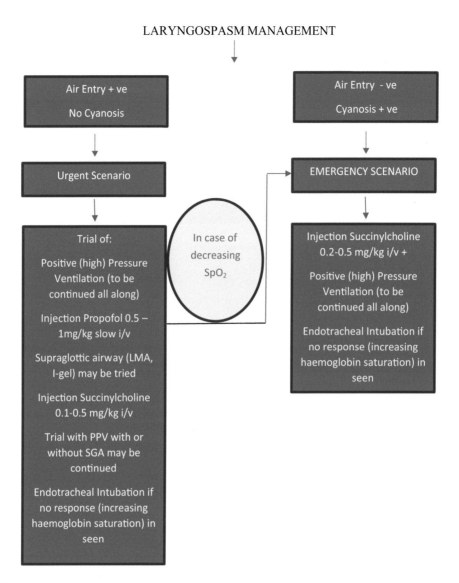

Figure 3.2 Laryngospasm management.

Non-Opioids

NSAIDs are a mainstay of drug-based peri-operative analgesia regimens. These drugs mainly act by inhibiting cyclo-oxygenase enzymes which are present all over the body and are highly activated during tissue trauma, producing pro-inflammatory prostaglandins. Thus, NSAIDs reduce the build-up of prostaglandins and diminish the nociceptive signal transmission. This also justifies the use of these drugs pre-emptively as it would blunt inflammatory response to surgical tissue trauma. There are numerous NSAIDs available, varying slightly in effect and side effects; it's imperative that correct doses are used, which balances effective analgesia and negligible ill effects. Diclofenac is probably the most commonly used NSAID in the peri-operative period due to its highly effective benefit-to-disadvantages ratio. Gastric irritation and renal toxicity are main side effects which must always be considered before prescribing.

BRONCHOSPASM MANAGEMENT MODALITIES

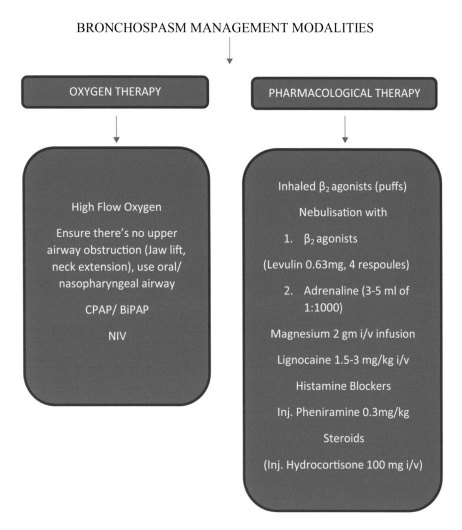

Figure 3.3 Bronchospasm management modalities.

Paracetamol is one of the most widely used analgesics, but its mechanism of action is not clearly understood. It is definitely seen to inhibit prostaglandin synthesis, but only in low levels of inflammation, and it also provides effective analgesia in cases of mild to moderate inflammation. One hypothesis is that paracetamol has both peripheral and central pro-analgesic effects. It has been proven that combination of NSAIDs like diclofenac with paracetamol gives additive analgesic effects without increasing side effects. Paracetamol infusions (10 mg/ml) are popularly used in the peri-operative period for convenience, but ampoules (150 mg/ml, for IV infusion) diluted and administered will give the same result at around one-fifth of the cost.

Opioids

Opioids are an integral part of the peri-operative analgesia protocol, but their isolated use can lead to significant side effects. There are a vast number of opioids having variable analgesic activities along with quite a spectrum of side effects, among them nausea, vomiting, pruritis, constipation, apnoea, etc. There are many options, but injection fentanyl is now the most favoured opioid in the peri-operative period due to its effective analgesic properties along with its superior safety profile when compared with other equipotent doses of opioids. Tramadol and pentazocine are other opioids commonly used in the post-operative period. In order to provide long duration analgesia,

Table 3.2: Doses of Common Opioids and Non-Opioids

Drugs	Intravenous Dose	
Injection diclofenac	1 mg/kg	8 hourly
Injection ketorolac	0.5 mg/kg	6 hourly
Injection paracetamol (slow IV infusion)	7.5 mg/ kg (neonates) 10 mg/ kg (up to 5 years of age) 15 mg/kg	6 hourly
Injection tramadol	1–2 mg/kg	6 hourly
Injection fentanyl	1–2 µg/kg	2–4 hourly
Injection pentazocine	0.2–0.5 mg/kg	4–6 hourly
Injection morphine	0.1 mg/kg	6–8 hourly

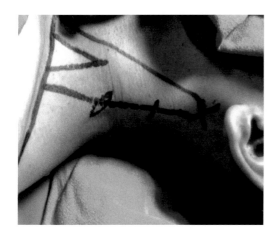

Figure 3.4 Superficial cervical plexus block.

injection morphine may be used, but respiration should be monitored; constipation and pruritis are other side effects which limit its use.

Patient-controlled analgesia (PCA) can also be used, especially after cancer surgeries. Fentanyl and/or morphine via intravenous pumps can deliver continuous infusion along with patient-controlled bolus increments.

Local Anaesthetics

Local anaesthetics have been proven to have a synergistic role in peri-operative analgesia protocols. This can result in effective analgesia leading to patient well-being, and decreases of the need for other analgesics (especially opioids) and thus prevents drug-related side effects. Bupivacaine (0.125–0.25%) is the most commonly used drug, as it provides longer duration of analgesia (2–8 hours, depending on block) compared to another frequently used agent, lignocaine (this may be added to provide quicker analgesia). Administration of local anaesthetics can be done in various ways. Local infiltration is the easiest way to provide additional analgesia; this can even be done before incision, but is generally reserved for post-suturing of incision. There is even a dedicated wound infiltration catheter available, which can be placed below the incision sutures to provide continuous local anaesthetic delivery and hence prolonged analgesia.

Specific nerve blocks can also be undertaken depending on surgery, like infraorbital nerve and sphenopalatine ganglion block for endoscopic sinus surgeries, or greater palatine and maxillary and mandibular nerve block for oral surgeries.

Cervical blocks can be undertaken for neck surgeries' pain. Nerves originating from C_2–C_4 innervate the neck and upper thorax and are amenable for safe blockade using local anaesthetics, thus providing effective long-duration analgesia. Superficial cervical block can be undertaken easily by palpating the posterior border of the sternocleidomastoid, dividing it into three sections from mastoid to insertion, injecting the drug caudally at the upper third mark after getting a pop (muscle fascia) inside the skin (Figure 3.4). Various other ways and deeper injections have been described but need more precision and expert hands; sonographic imaging is also helpful in ensuring a higher rate of success. A good block using bupivacaine (0.25%, 7–10 ml bilaterally) can lead to effective analgesia of 4–8 hours.

Cervical epidural is another modality which can provide effective analgesia to neck pain, but at the risk of complications like quadriparesis, etc.; hence its mention here is mostly to provide a theoretical completion of modalities.

4

Fluid Management in Head and Neck Surgery

RAVI KANT DOGRA

INTRODUCTION

Fluid management during surgery is the key determinant of success of surgery, but it requires special consideration because of extremity of ages, underlying pathophysiology, diversity in procedures, long duration of surgery and variability in blood loss. Surgeries can range anywhere from skull base up to mediastinum. Free tissue transfer, flap reconstruction and oncological surgeries are often long and complex procedures. Restricted peri-operative fluid administration may lead to post-operative complications like tissue hypoxia and dysfunction of vital organs due to decreased cardiac output and limited oxygen delivery causing prolonged hospital stays, increased morbidity and mortality. On the other hand, traditional infusion of fluid during surgery leads to positive fluid balance which in turn leads to increased post-operative complications like cardiac failure or excessive interstitial oedema causing poor surgical outcome, especially in cases of reconstructive surgeries.

TYPES OF FLUID USED IN PERI-OPERATIVE PERIOD

Body water accounts for 60% body weight where 60% is intracellular fluid (ICF) and 30% is extracellular fluid (ECF) (25% intravascular and 75% interstitial). (see Figure 4.1.)

Intravenous fluids are divided in two categories: crystalloids and colloids. These can be isotonic,

hypotonic or hypertonic. Isotonic fluids replace ECF depletion and hypotonic replace both ECF and ICF.

1. **Crystalloids:** Commonly used are D5W (5%, 10%), NaCl (0.45%, 0.9%), Ringer's lactate (RL), Plasma-Lyte A (Ringer's acetate) and hypertonic fluids (3% NS). Crystalloids are primarily used as replacement and maintenance fluid. The concept is to replenish the fluid deficit of milieu interieur and provide the most physiologic solvent.
   a. Normal saline (0.9%) is isotonic, expands intravascular volume by 20% and remains in vascular space for approximately 30 minutes, but it has high sodium and very high chloride, thus causes hyperchloremic metabolic acidosis when used in large volume.
   b. Hypertonic fluid (3% NS) is used to reduce brain water and intracranial pressure (ICP) during neurosurgery.
   c. Balanced electrolyte solutions are RL and Ringer's acetate, also called physiological saline. Lactate and acetate are converted to bicarbonate in the liver. They also contain potassium and calcium.
2. **Colloids** Albumin, synthetic colloid (hydroxyethyl starch, dextran and gelatin), and blood products (whole blood, packed red blood cells (PRBC), fresh frozen plasma (FFP), cryoprecipitate, platelets). Albumin 20% stays in the vascular compartment for 16 hours. Synthetic

DOI: 10.1201/9780367430139-4

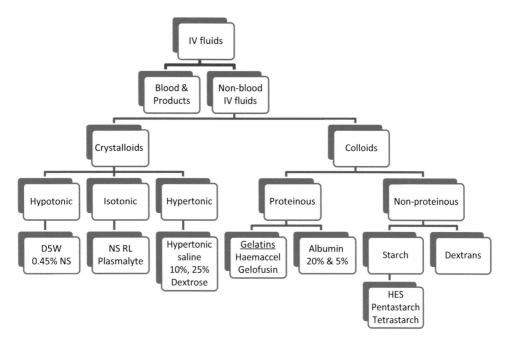

Figure 4.1 Intravenous fluid classification.

colloids have an intravascular half-life of 3–6 hours and are linked to increased mortality and morbidity like coagulopathy, pruritus, nephrotoxicity and acute kidney injury in critically ill patients. Colloids should not be used for routine purposes. They are typically reserved for situations of emergency where intravascular volume is difficult to maintain (unanticipated blood loss is the most common scenario). While semisynthetic colloids definitely provide an edge over crystalloids in resuscitation, they can prove detrimental in the long term, causing situations like acute kidney injury.

EVALUATION OF PRE-OPERATIVE VOLUME STATUS

It is not routinely possible to regularly assess fluid compartments. Therefore, estimation of the patient's pre-operative fluid status relies on indirect indicators and the anaesthetist's assessment. Invasive monitors, such as central venous catheters (CVP) and pulmonary artery catheters (PAC), have their limitations in routine assessments of volume status and they pose their own risks and morbidities. Thus, a proper patient history, a clinical examination with understanding of pathophysiology, is crucial to ensure euvolemic status is achieved

by the patient when they are taken for surgery. Tachycardia, the most sensitive change manifested during hypovolemia, is the least specific way to determine fluid status; therefore, a complete clinical examination should include monitoring of blood pressure (BP), mucosal hydration, skin turgor and urine output. Laboratory investigations are also used as indirect indicators in determination of fluid status. Blood electrolytes, renal function tests, urinary-specific gravity and osmolality, blood lactate and base deficits are important parameters to keep in mind. Volume status can be of significance in patients posted for head and neck surgery as often a mass, tumour or inflamed lymph node can cause difficulty in deglutition, resulting in chronic dehydration. Multiple ENT surgeries are carried out with neoadjuvant chemo-radiotherapy, which alters the haemodynamic, electrolyte status and cardiac contractility and thus requires special attention from anaesthesiologists.

PERI-OPERATIVE FLUID STATUS AND MANAGEMENT

The goals in the intraoperative period of any major surgery are:

1. To maintain effective aerobic metabolism at cellular level with control over hypoperfusion-

related inflammation and neurohumoral responses. This can be achieved by manipulating circulating volume, cardiac output and vascular resistance.

2. Maintaining euvolemia by avoiding iatrogenic side effects of fluid administration like volume overload, electrolyte imbalance and oedema.

The anaesthesiologist can control intravascular volume status while extracellular/ redistributed fluid varies on other factors. So, the factors that determine adequacy of fluid include:

1. Vasodilating property of anaesthetic drugs: most of the inducing agents, opioids and inhalational agents have direct vasodilatory properties causing decrease in preload, afterload and sometimes myocardial depression to varying degrees.
2. Sympathetic blockade: by central neuraxial depression.
3. Microcirculatory dysfunction: inflammatory responses created due to surgical stress cause endothelial dysfunction.
4. Surgical blood loss: associated with direct loss of intravascular volume.
5. Insensible loss: of less importance in head-neck surgery but can be significant in paediatric patients or in surgery of longer duration.
6. Inflammatory redistribution: typically manifests in post-operative phase.
7. Renal output: surgical stress can positively feed back the hypothalamo-pituitary axis, causing overproduction of antidiuretic hormone, suppression of atrial natriuretic peptide and activation of renin–angiotensin–aldosterone system resulting in fluid overload which can manifest both intra- and post-operatively.

Assessment of Quantity of Fluid

Surgeons as well as anaesthetists do underestimate blood loss by assessing blood on surgical gauze pads (4x4 inch hold 10 ml and lap sponges 100–150 ml blood), suction containers, pooled blood on floor and accumulated blood on surgical field. In most surgical patients, conventional clinical assessment is adequate for intravascular volume status, but for high-risk patients, goal-directed therapy (GDT) with haemodynamic management is superior. In conventional clinical assessment,

hypovolemia is assessed on the basis of physical signs like heart rate (HR), blood pressure (NIBP), urine output, arterial oxygenation and pH. In severe hypovolemia, direct arterial pressure measurement is more accurate than NIBP (indirect). Arterial cannulation provides good access for getting blood samples like arterial blood gas (ABG) and assessing pulse pressure variation (PPV) on a ventilated patient.

Administration of intravenous fluids is done mainly in two ways:

1. Calculating requirement based on body weight, modality of anaesthesia, duration and phase of surgery and ongoing blood loss.
2. Goal-directed therapy, i.e., minimal amount of fluid to achieve optimum physiologic variables.

Targeting Overall Fluid Balance

Holliday-Segar formula (4:2:1) is the most traditional calculation (based on body weight and fasting duration) used to maintain fluid dynamics; often challenged in the literature, it is still the most widely used. During fasting, the patient can acquire a fluid and electrolyte deficit due to continuous and uninterrupted renal and gastrointestinal water excretion, and insensible loss from skin and lung. This deficit is calculated as maintenance fluid required per hour using 4:2:1 formula (for first 10 kg, 4 ml/kg/hr; next 10 kg, 2 ml/kg/hr, and for each kg above 20, add 1 mg/kg/hr). This deficit is multiplied by hours of fasting and should be replaced during pre-operative and intraoperative periods. Deficits due to third-space loss and insensible losses must also be calculated for more invasive surgeries.

In case of significant blood loss, crystalloid is used to replenish at a ratio three times that of blood loss until a point when danger of dilutional anaemia overrides the risk of transfusion. Transfusions are to be avoided until haematocrit falls to 24% or haemoglobin less than 8 g/dl, and can be given when there is loss of 10–20% of blood volume (blood volume in men is 75 ml/kg and in women 65 ml/kg).

Goal-Directed Therapy (GDT)

This is a novel approach to achieve optimum tissue perfusion and clinical outcome by measuring different physiological variables related to cardiac output and/or global O_2 delivery. The target is to not exceed sufficient fluid load, and it may be necessary to frequently administer inotropes, vasopressors, vasodilators or packed PRBC.

GDT needs various tools to measure physiologic responses, like PAC, arterial pressure and waveform analysis, VP, echocardiography and serum lactate.

A more accurate assessment of intravascular volume may be performed using direct invasive monitoring and using dynamic parameters like stroke volume variation (SVV), pulse pressure variation (PPV) and cardiac output (CO), rather than static parameters like CVP or PAC as they have a poor relationship with blood volume in predicting the haemodynamic effect of a fluid challenge.

Volume status and perfusion of vital organs can easily be assessed using monitoring of urine output, which should not be less than 0.5–1.0 mL/kg/h. It is especially useful in invasive and/or lengthy procedures where blood loss and fluid replacement are anticipated and intentional hypotension is employed to reduce blood loss, such as in maxillofacial trauma, maxillary orthognathic surgery, radical neck dissection and head and neck microvascular flap surgery.

Appropriate Fluid Selection

The most rational choice of fluid should be safe, efficient intravascular volume expander, isotonic to plasma, with a similar distribution of electrolytes without altering the acid-base balance. The ideal fluid should not derange physiological balance like electrolytes or precipitate peripheral or pulmonary oedema, coagulopathies or renal dysfunction. No single fluid product has all these properties, which keeps the controversy between crystalloids and colloids alive. The plasma volume expansion property of colloid is much better than that of crystalloid.

In absence of robust evidence, administration of fluid remains a clinician's choice, however, isotonic balanced crystalloids like normal saline, Ringer's lactate or Ringer's acetate are considered the fluids of choice for head and neck surgery where only minor blood loss is anticipated. Crystalloids do not generally maintain the oncotic pressure, and equilibrate through extra-cellular fluid (ECF) with only 20% (current study—up to 50% after 30

minutes) remaining in the intravascular compartment. Patients posted for surgery generally have ECF deficit along with intravascular fluid deficit. Therefore, crystalloid effectively replaces losses in both compartments. For most office-based dental and oral surgery, insensible and urinary losses are negligible.

Colloids have no place in office-based minor procedures and may have utility only in long and/or invasive maxillofacial surgical procedures where significant blood loss is anticipated and advanced monitoring of blood pressure and/or urinary output is available.

INTERACTION WITH ANAESTHETIC AGENTS

Perioperative fluid therapy is influenced by haemodynamic effects of anaesthetic agents too. Anaesthetic induction with intravenous agents may be accompanied by haemodynamic changes. Propofol has cardiodepressant properties manifested as hypotension, bradycardia due to loss of systemic vascular resistance, preload and myocardial contractility. On the other hand, ketamine has sympathomimetic effects, resulting in increased heart rate, blood pressure and cardiac output, and is useful in acute hypovolemic shock. Etomidate, with the best haemodynamic stability, is a desirable induction agent in hypovolemia and blood loss due to trauma. Benzodiazepines and opioids should not produce significant haemodynamic changes, particularly if titrated carefully for an intended depth of moderate sedation.

Inhalational agents reduce systemic vascular resistance, causing vasodilation and a decrease in blood pressure. These depressant effects may become apparent in severe hypovolemia and coronary artery disease, potentially leading to hypotension, which may result in myocardial ischaemia. Additionally, positive pressure ventilation in hypovolemic patients will reduce preload and blood pressure.

Healthy patients with normal intravascular volume can tolerate this haemodynamic change easily. Studies have demonstrated that hypotension on induction is most appropriately treated by vasopressor therapy and administration of intravenous fluids. Judicious use of crystalloid solutions (e.g., 200–300 mL bolus in adults) is, however, frequently appropriate for managing hypotension in office-based ENT/dental surgery, realising that large fluid volumes will not be tolerated by patients without placement of a urinary catheter.

FLUID THERAPY FOR HEAD AND NECK SURGERY

An appropriate volume of fluid should be administered to a patient based on different variables: the patient's pre-operative medical and fluid status, surgical procedure, blood loss and anaesthetic technique. Medical conditions such as hypertension commonly result is a decreased intravascular volume that is unmasked under the vasodilating effects of anaesthetic agents. Careful judgement should be employed for management of resistant hypotension, with vasopressors due to anaesthetic drugs in patients receiving angiotensin-converting enzyme inhibitors (ACEIs) and angiotensin receptor blockers (ARBs).

In patients posted for short procedures in dental or oral surgery, isotonic solution of 1000 mL or less is commonly administered. Rehydrating the fluid-deficient patient if due to NPO status is based on the 4:2:1 rule and has shown to improve quality of recovery following oral surgery procedures.

The role of hypotonic solution is limited and dextrose 5% (D5) can be used as maintenance fluid till patient is fasting. However, nowadays early oral feeding has become common, initiated with sugar-containing liquids. Patients with diabetes mellitus may be administered dextrose-containing solutions neutralised with or without insulin based on their early morning or pre-operative blood glucose levels in order to avoid hypoglycaemia.

Anaesthetic challenge increases with complexity and invasiveness of surgery; however, the goal is to maintain sufficient intravascular volume to achieve tissue perfusion and to do so in the face of increased surgical blood loss and inflammatory changes leading to third-spacing, while avoiding pulmonary and peripheral oedema.

POST-OPERATIVE MANAGEMENT

After every major surgery, assessment of fluid status should be done, which includes clinical examination, monitoring of urine output and measurement of other physiological parameters like lactate, central/mixed venous O2 saturation (SCVO2) and cardiac output. The target should be early initiation of oral fluid intake while maintaining a euvolemic

state. Some routine monitoring should be carried out in patients receiving IV fluids. Electrolytes should be checked at least daily. If any electrolyte imbalance is corrected, electrolytes might need to be checked every few hours.

Post-operative fluid administration is mostly based on the following three categories.

1. Pure maintenance requirements: a balance salt solutions (ringer lactate/ringer acetate) is beneficial and should be given at a rate of 1.0–1.2 ml/kg/hr (50–100 ml/hr) to replace the insensible loss in the body. Additionally, 50–100 mEq of Na+ and 40–80 mEq of K+ should be given in 24 hours.
2. Replacement of ongoing losses: any post-operative slow ongoing loss by the gastrointestinal tract or third-space loss should be replenished using isotonic or balanced solution. Blood loss is best replenished using blood or plasma in the post-operative period. Other semisynthetic colloids have failed to show beneficial effect in post-op critical care management.
3. Resuscitation requirements: development of a significant hypovolemic condition like acute haemorrhage or sepsis should be managed by using isotonic solution aggressively.

Anaesthesiologists must take care to prevent of intraoperative and post-operative oliguria, and it should be assessed in view of evidence of hypovolemia and lack of tissue perfusion. Large-volume fluid administration should be avoided to prevent fluid overload in this scenario if hypovolemia is not the reason. A furosemide challenge test can be done to see the renal response in oliguria. Drugs which are renal safe should be used and avoidance of nephrotoxic drugs like NSAIDs and aminoglycosides should be considered.

Head and neck surgery involve significant amounts of pain which causes activation of sympathetic pathway and rennin angiotensin aldosterone system (RAAS). One should plan adequate pain management to prevent RAAS-activated fluid overload.

To conclude, both negative and positive fluid balance can cause serious harm, effecting insufficient tissue perfusion or oedema. This is why goal-directed fluid therapy (GDT) emerges over traditional fluid therapy to optimise the outcome.

Over time the conscience regarding fluid management has evolved from an empirical protocol-based formula of 4:2:1 to individual customised therapy. Choice of fluid has been shifted from most isotonic normal saline to more physiological balanced saline. The ability of each individual to deal with circulating fluid varies differently with respect to age, sex and ongoing stress. Therefore, administration of fluid is very much dependent upon response to routine fluid management and dynamics of ongoing procedure. Moreover, anaesthesiologists are concerned about post-surgical outcome where fluid shift can reverse between compartments, making a euvolemic state turn into a hypervolemic state. Altogether the science of fluid management must be performed like an art.

FURTHER SUGGESTED READINGS

1. Saraghi M. Intraoperative fluids and fluid management for ambulatory dental sedation and general anesthesia. *Anesth Prog.* 2015 Dec;62(4):168–77.

2. Pereira CM, Figueiredo ME, Carvalho R, Catre D, Assuncao JP. Anesthesia and surgical microvascular flaps. *Rev Bras Anestesiol.* 2012;62(4):563–79.

3. Reddi AS. *Fluid, Electrolyte and Acid-base Disorders: Clinical Evaluation and Management.* 2nd ed. Switzerland: Springer Nature; 2018. Chapter 4: Intravenous fluids: Composition and indications. pp. 35–49.

4. Butterworth JF, Mackey DC, Wasnick JD. *Morgan and Mikhail's Clinical Anesthesiology.* 5th ed. McGraw-Hill Education; 2018. Chapter 51: Fluid management and blood component therapy. pp. 1161–81.

5. Edwards MR, Grocott MPW. Perioperative fluid and electrolyte therapy. In: Gropper MA, Cohen NH, Eriksson LI, Fleisher LA, Leslie K, Wiener-Kronish JP, editors. *Miller's Anesthesia.* 9th ed. Philadelphia, PA: Elsevier; 2020. pp. 1480–523.

6. Amin P. Nutrition support. In: Chawla R, Todi S, editors. *ICU Protocols: A Stepwise Approach,* Vol I. 2nd ed. Singapore: Springer; 2020. pp. 443–54.

5

Drugs in Head and Neck Surgery

ANAMIKA THAKUR

INTRODUCTION

Modern drugs have improved the health status of mankind. They play an important role in treatment of all diseases. Although surgery corrects the anatomical disorder, its final outcome depends upon drugs for control of pain, vomiting or infection.

Head and neck surgery carries the risk of pain and infection due to rich sensory supply and bacterial flora. The surgeon should have good pharmacological knowledge of commonly used drugs. This chapter discusses various drugs used in head and neck surgery.

ANTIMICROBIAL AGENTS/ ANTIBIOTICS

Development of antimicrobial agents (AMA) has proved to be one of the most important milestones in the therapeutics. AMA not only cures serious infections but also helps in the prevention and treatment of complications. However, over-prescription of AMAs and their availability even without prescription have facilitated the development of resistance, reducing therapeutic options in the treatment of life-threatening infections.

Antimicrobials are used in prophylaxis to reduce surgical site infection with minimal adverse effects and alteration of normal microbial flora. The majority of head and neck surgical procedures are clean, but surgeries involving the aerodigestive tract fall in the clean-contaminated category as per the surgical wound classification given by Centers for Disease Control and Prevention (CDC), in Atlanta, Georgia, USA.

Strict infection control measures like sterile instruments, clean operative field and good surgical techniques with minimum tissue damage reduce the need of antibiotics.

AMA prophylaxis is not required for clean wounds except in patients at special risk, e.g., diabetics, immunocompromised, infants, elderly or malnourished, or those using corticosteroids, or with excessive handling of tissue/use of electrocautery. The prophylactic antibiotic is to be timed such that peak blood level occurs during the formation of the clot in the surgical wound, and it should remain there throughout the procedure. Prophylactic oral drugs are generally given 1 hour before incision and IV prophylaxis is given just before/after anaesthesia. Single-dose prophylaxis is effective for most procedures and results in decreased toxicity and antimicrobial resistance. Once the clot is formed and is older than three hours, most AMAs do not penetrate it, so there is no purpose to late AMA prophylaxis. AMA may be repeated IV during the procedure in prolonged surgery. Post-operative AMA after four hours of wound closure is recommended in contaminated and dirty surgery.

Cefazolin is the prophylactic agent of choice for head and neck clean procedures. Local wound infection patterns should be considered when selecting antimicrobial prophylaxis. The selection of vancomycin over cefazolin may be necessary in hospitals with high rates of methicillin-resistant

DOI: 10.1201/9780367430139-5

Staphylococcus aureus or *Streptococcus epidermidis* infections.

Nonsurgical prophylaxis is indicated in individuals who are at high risk for temporary exposure to selected virulent pathogens and in patients who are at increased risk for developing infection because of underlying disease (e.g., immunocompromised hosts). Prophylaxis is most effective when directed against organisms that are predictably susceptible to antimicrobial agents.

The following sections will help readers to understand the basic pharmacology of commonly used AMAs, especially their side effects and interaction with other drugs.

Cotrimoxazole

Cotrimoxazole is a combination of trimethoprim-sulfamethoxazole. Its common adverse effects are nausea, vomiting, stomatitis, headache and rashes. Megaloblastic anaemia occurs occasionally in patients with marginal folate levels. Blood dyscrasias occur rarely. As trimethoprim is an antifolate drug, it is contraindicated in pregnancy. When given to treat *Pneumocystis jiroveci* infection in AIDS patients, a high incidence of fever, rash, leukopenia, diarrhoea, elevations of hepatic aminotransferases, hyperkalaemia, hyponatraemia and bone marrow hypoplasia are reported. Risk of bone marrow toxicity is more in elderly.

When given concurrently with phenytoin, cotrimoxazole increases phenytoin level and may result in nystagmus and ataxia. Increased international normalised ratio, bleeding with warfarin and increased antifolate activity with methotrexate may occur. It has renal clearance and half-life of 8–10 hours. Dose should be reduced in patients with moderately severe renal impairment as uremia is reported in them. It is formulated as a single strength tab of trimethoprim 80 mg + sulfamethoxazole 400 mg tab and double strength (DS) tab of 160 mg trimethoprim + 800 mg sulfamethoxazole. Usual dose is 2.5–5 mg/kg IV or per oral 6 hourly.

Ciprofloxacin and Other Fluoroquinolones

Ciprofloxacin and other fluoroquinolones (FQs) are generally well tolerated with recommended doses (Table 5.1). Common but mild adverse effects are nausea, vomiting and diarrhoea. Dizziness, headache, restlessness, anxiety, insomnia, impairment of concentration, bad taste and anorexia may occur. Users should exercise caution while driving. Tremor and seizures occur rarely at higher doses. Rash, pruritus, photosensitivity, urticaria, swelling of lips may occur but serious cutaneous reactions are rare. Abnormal liver function tests may occur occasionally. Tendinitis and tendon rupture have been reported, risk of which increases with advancing age, renal insufficiency and with concurrent use of steroids. FQs should be used cautiously in children as a few reports of cartilage damage have been noted. FQs have also been associated with peripheral neuropathy. Lomefloxacin and pefloxacin may produce phototoxicity. Prolongation of the QTc interval may occur with levofloxacin, gemifloxacin and moxifloxacin. FQs are contraindicated during pregnancy.

As FQs are enzyme inhibitors, they increase the plasma concentration of theophylline, caffeine and warfarin. CNS toxicity may occur when NSAIDs are used concurrently. Gastrointestinal absorption of FQs is inhibited when antacids, sucralfate and iron salts are given together. Levofloxacin, gemifloxacin and moxifloxacin are to be avoided or cautiously used in patients with known prolonged

Table 5.1 Doses of Fluoroquinolones

	Oral dose (mg)	Parenteral dose (mg)
Ciprofloxacin	250–750 BD	100–200
Norfloxacin	400 BD	----
Pefloxacin	400 BD	400
Ofloxacin	200–400 BD	200
Levofloxacin	500–750 OD	500
Moxifloxacin	400 OD	400

QTc interval or uncorrected hypokalaemia and in patients on antiarrhythmics class 1A (quinidine or procainamide) or class 3 (sotalol, ibutilide, amiodarone) and other drugs which increase QTc interval (erythromycin, tricyclic antidepressants). Primary mode of elimination is renal.

Antipseudomonal penicillins include carbenicillin, ticarcillin and piperacillin. Their primary mode of elimination is renal.

Carbenicillin

This antipseudomonal penicillin has t ½ of 1 hour. It is used as sodium salt in a dose of 1–2 g IM or 1–5 g IV every 4–6 hours. At higher doses, sodium may lead to fluid retention and CHF in patients with borderline renal or cardiac function. High doses may interfere with platelet function and cause bleeding.

Ticarcillin

This is more active and produces fewer adverse effects than carbenicillin. Common adverse effects are drug fever, rash and thrombophlebitis at IV site. Serum sickness and anaphylactic reactions may occur. Dose-dependent inhibition of platelet aggregation has been reported. Increased INR with warfarin may occur. Usual dose is 3 g IM/IV 6 hourly.

Piperacillin

This antipseudomonal penicillin is more active than carbenicillin. Its elimination t½ is 1 hour. It is combined with tazobactam to cover β-lactamase producing strains. Drug fever, rash, leukopenia, haemolytic anaemia, thrombocytopenia or anaphylactic reactions may occur. Dose is 100–150 mg/kg/day in three divided doses (max 16 g/day) IM or IV. When > 2 g is to be injected, generally the IV route is preferred.

BETA-LACTAMASE INHIBITORS

Clavulanic acid, sulbactam and tazobactam are used only in combination with specific penicillins or cephalosporins.

Clavulanic Acid

Clavulanate is eliminated mainly by glomerular filtration and its elimination t½ is 1 hour. Adverse effects are similar to that of amoxicillin alone, but it has poor gastrointestinal tolerance. Rashes and candida stomatitis/vaginitis may also occur. Hepatic injury has also been reported. There is an increased risk of rashes when used concurrently with allopurinol.

The usual oral dose of amoxicillin/clavulanic acid is 500/125 mg orally 8 hourly or 875/125 mg orally 12 hourly for severe infections. Inject amoxicillin 1 g /0.5 g + clavulanic acid 0.2 g /0.1 g deep IM or IV 6–8 hourly for severe infections.

Sulbactam

Sulbactam has been combined with ampicillin, cefoperazone and ceftriaxone. Rash, diarrhoea, pain at injection site and thrombophlebitis of injected vein may occur.

It is available as a 375 mg tab and ampicillin 1 g + sulbactam 0.5 g per vial injection; 1–2 vials deep IM or IV injection 6–8 hourly.

Tazobactam

Tazobactam has been combined with piperacillin and ceftriaxone. The primary mode of elimination is renal. Dose is 0.5 g tazobactam combined with piperacillin 4 g injected IV over 30 minutes 8 hourly. Common adverse effects are nausea, vomiting and diarrhoea. Insomnia, headache, drug fever/rash may occur.

CEPHALOSPORIN

Diarrhoea is more common with orally administered cephalexin, cefixime and parenteral cefoperazone. Pain after intramuscular injection and thrombophlebitis after intravenous injection may occur. Rashes are common but anaphylaxis, angiooedema may also occur. Cephalosporine should be avoided in patients with a history of immediate reactions to penicillin. Nephrotoxicity including interstitial nephritis and tubular necrosis may occur with some cephalosporine, chances of which may increase with preexisting renal disease, concurrent administration of an aminoglycoside or loop diuretic. Cephalosporins that contain a methylthiotetrazole group (cefoperazone, cefamandole, cefmetazole, ceftriaxone) can cause hypoprothrombinemia and bleeding disorders, which can be prevented by giving Vitamin K orally in a dose of 10 mg twice weekly. Neutropenia and thrombocytopenia have been reported with ceftazidime and few others. A disulfiram-like interaction with alcohol may occur with cefoperazone, so alcohol and alcohol-containing medications should be avoided.

AZTREONAM

As this monobactam lacks cross-sensitivity with other β-lactam antibiotics (except ceftazidime), it is preferred in penicillin/cephalosporin-allergic patients. Injection site pain, neutropenia, rashes and rise in serum aminotransferases are the common adverse effects. Increased creatinine, thrombocytosis or eosinophilia may also occur. It is eliminated unchanged in urine and has t½ of 1.8 hours, which is prolonged in renal failure. Drug interactions are not much noticed. Dose: 0.5–2 g IM or IV 6–12 hourly.

Carbapenams include imipenem meropenem, feropenam, doripenam and ertapenem. All carbapenams are renally cleared and their dose must be reduced in patients with renal insufficiency.

Imipenem

This carbapenem is combined with cilastatin, which is a reversible inhibitor of dehydropeptidase-I and protects it from rapid hydrolysis. Imipenem can induce seizures at higher doses and in predisposed patients. Increased risk of seizures with ganciclovir and valproic acid has been reported. Diarrhoea, vomiting, phlebitis, skin rashes and other hypersensitivity reactions may occur. Dose: Imipenem-cilastatin 0.5 g IV 6 hourly (max 4 g/day) infused over 40–60 minutes.

Meropenem

This newer carbapenem does not need to be protected by cilastatin as it is not hydrolysed by renal peptidase. It has less propensity to induce seizures, so it is preferred over the imipenem-cilastatin combination. Other side effects are similar to imipenem. Dose: 0.5–2.0 g (10–40 mg/kg) by slow IV injection 8 hourly.

Faropenem

This orally active carbapenem may produce diarrhoea, abdominal pain, nausea and rashes as adverse effects. Dose: 150–300 mg oral TDS.

Doripenem

This carbapenem may cause nausea, diarrhoea, superinfections and phlebitis of the injected vein as adverse effects. Seizures are rare. Dose: 500 mg by slow IV infusion over one hour, every 8 hours.

Ertapenem

It is given as single daily IV infusion as it has long t½ of 4 hours. Adverse effects are headache, confusion, diarrhoea and thrombophlebitis of injected vein. Seizures occur rarely. Dose: 1.0 g infused IV over 60 minutes daily for 7–14 days.

TIGECYCLINE

The primary mode of elimination of this synthetic tetracycline analogue (glycylcyclines) is biliary, so dose adjustment is not needed in renal insufficiency. It has long duration of action as its elimination t½ is 36–60 hours. Only low concentrations are attained in urine, thus it is not suitable for urinary tract infection. It is not given in children and pregnancy.

The most common adverse effects are nausea and vomiting. Epigastric distress, diarrhoea, dizziness, skin reactions, photosensitivity, injection site complications and superinfections may also occur. If given along with warfarin, it increases INR. Dose: 100 mg loading dose, followed by 50 mg 12 hourly by IV infusion over 30–60 min for 5–14 days.

AMINOGLYCOSIDES

All aminoglycosides are ototoxic and nephrotoxic. Their toxic effects increase with increase in dose and duration of exposure of drug, in elderly and in renal insufficiency. Ototoxicity may manifest as either auditory/cochlear damage or vestibular damage. Cochlear damage results in tinnitus and high-frequency hearing loss initially. Kanamycin and amikacin produce greater cochlear damage. Vestibular damage results in headache, nausea, vomiting, dizziness, nystagmus, vertigo, ataxia and loss of balance. Streptomycin and gentamicin produce more vestibular than cochlear toxicity. Aminoglycoside ear drops instillation is contraindicated in patients with perforated eardrum as it can cause ototoxicity. Nephrotoxicity results in increased serum creatinine levels or reduction in creatinine clearance and manifests as tubular damage resulting in loss of urinary concentrating power, low GFR, nitrogen retention, albuminuria and casts. Streptomycin is the least nephrotoxic, whereas neomycin, tobramycin and gentamicin are the most nephrotoxic. Aminoglycosides can produce a curare-like effect with neuromuscular blockade at very high doses, resulting in respiratory paralysis which may result in apnoea and fatalities. This can be usually reversed by prompt IV injection of calcium gluconate or by neostigmine. Myasthenic weakness is accentuated by these drugs. Hypersensitivity occurs rarely.

Aminoglycosides are to be avoided during pregnancy as they can cause hearing loss in the offspring. Concurrent use of drugs like loop diuretics (furosemide) or other nephrotoxic drugs (NSAIDs, amphotericin B, vancomycin, cyclosporine and cisplatin) should be avoided as they potentiate nephrotoxicity. They should be cautiously used with other potentially ototoxic drugs (vancomycin, minocycline and furosemide). Do not mix aminoglycoside with any drug in the same syringe/infusion bottle. They are to be cautiously used in patients over 60 years and in patients with renal damage.

The plasma t½ of aminoglycosides is 2–4 hours and its clearance parallels creatinine clearance at approximately two-thirds. The t½ may be prolonged up to 24 hours and accumulation occurs in elderly, patients with renal insufficiency and in neonates who have low GFR. In these situations dose reduction is needed or dose interval is to be increased (Table 5.2). As they have a low safety margin, their daily dose is to be calculated as per body weight and renal function levels. A single total daily dose regimen for patients with normal renal function (CLcr > 70 ml/min) is recommended over daily doses divided into three equal parts and then injecting IM or slow IV over 60 minutes every 8 hours (Table 5.3)

AZITHROMYCIN

This macrolide has long terminal t½ of >50 hour as it is slowly released from the intracellular sites. It is largely excreted unchanged in bile. Adverse effects include nausea, mild gastric upset, diarrhoea, abdominal pain, headache and dizziness. It may prolong QT interval and cause torsades de pointes

Table 5.2 Dose Adjustment of Gentamicin in Renal Insufficiency

CLcr (ml/min)	% of Daily Dose
70	70% daily
50	50% daily
30	30% daily
20–30	80% alternate days
10–20	60% alternate days
<10	40% alternate days

Table 5.3 Doses and Common Side Effects of Gentamicin and Amikacin

Drug	Dose	Toxicity
Gentamicin	3–5 mg/kg/day IM or IV over 30–60 minutes	vestibular toxicity cochlear toxicity nephrotoxicity
Amikacin	7.5–15 mg/kg/day IM	vestibular toxicity cochlear toxicity nephrotoxicity

arrhythmia. Azithromycin does not affect hepatic CYP3A4 enzyme. It is less likely to have interaction with theophylline, carbamazepine, warfarin, terfenadine and cisapride, but caution may be appropriate. Dose: 500 mg once daily 1 hour before or 2 hours after food (10 mg/kg/day in children older than 6 months) for three days.

CLINDAMYCIN

This lincosamide antibiotic has t½ of 3 hours and its primary mode of elimination is hepatic. Common adverse effects are rashes, nausea, vomiting, diarrhoea, urticaria and abdominal pain. Diarrhoea and pseudomembranous enterocolitis due to *Clostridium difficile* superinfection may occur, in which case this drug has to be promptly stopped and oral metronidazole or vancomycin is to be started. Impaired liver function and neutropenia may occur. Thrombophlebitis of the injected vein may occur. Clindamycin slightly potentiates neuromuscular blockers. Dose: 150–300 mg (children 3–6 mg/kg) QID oral; 200–600 mg IV 8 hourly.

VANCOMYCIN

This glycopeptide antibiotic has t½ of 6 hours and its primary mode of elimination is renal. Nephrotoxicity is a frequent adverse effect. Ototoxicity may also occur rarely. Phlebitis and fall in BP during IV injection may occur. Rapid IV injection has caused chills, fever, urticaria and intense flushing called 'red man syndrome' as it releases histamine from mast cells. It can be largely prevented by prolonging the infusion period to 1–2 hours or pretreatment with an antihistamine (diphenhydramine). Nausea, vomiting and hypokalaemia are the side effects generally seen with oral formulations.

Other nephrotoxic drugs (aminoglycosides, amphotericin B, polymyxin B) when given along with vancomycin can increase nephrotoxicity. Dose: 125–500 mg 6 hourly orally or 1 g 12 hourly infused IV over 1 hour.

LINEZOLID

This oxazolidinone has plasma t½ of 5 hours and the primary mode of elimination is hepatic. Common adverse effects are mild abdominal pain, nausea, taste disturbance and diarrhoea. Rashes, pruritus and headache occur rarely. Its main toxicity is haematologic. Thrombocytopenia, neutropenia and anaemia (mild and reversible on stoppage) occur when linezolid is given for more than two weeks. Optic and peripheral neuropathy and lactic acidosis may develop after more than four weeks of use.

As linezolid is a weak MAO inhibitor, serotonin syndrome (fever, delirium, hypertension, tremor/clonus, hyperreflexia) can occur when it is given along with serotonergic drugs like selective serotonin reuptake inhibitors (SSRIs). Increased hypertensive crisis is possible with pseudoephedrine and tyramine-containing food. Cytochrome P450 enzyme-related interactions have not been reported. Dose: 600 mg BD orally or IV.

MUPIROCIN

This topically used antibiotic is active mainly against gram-positive bacteria, including *S. pyogenes*, *S. aureus* and MRSA. It is indicated in furunculosis, folliculitis, impetigo, infected insect bites and small wounds. Intranasal ointment for eliminating nasal carriage of *S. aureus* may cause irritation of mucous membranes. After topical application to intact skin, it is not appreciably absorbed systemically. Local itching, irritation and redness may occur.

FUSIDIC ACID

This is a narrow-spectrum steroidal antibiotic active against penicillinase producing *Staphylococci* and few other gram-positive bacteria. It is used only topically for boils, folliculitis, sycosis barbae and other cutaneous infections.

POLYMYXIN B AND COLISTIN

These are polypeptide bactericidal antibiotics. They are not used systemically due to neuro- and nephrotoxicity and neuromuscular blockade (respiratory paralysis). When given orally, occasional nausea, vomiting and diarrhoea occur. Applied topically, systemic effect or sensitisation does not occur. Rashes may occur rarely.

When given along with other nephrotoxic drugs (amphotericin B, amikacin, gentamicin, tobramycin, vancomycin), they increase the chance of nephrotoxicity. Avoid intraperitoneal infusion due to risk of NM blockade. Dose: Polymyxin B: 1–1.25 mg/kg IV 12 hourly; colistin sulfate: 25–100 mg TDS oral, 2.5 mg/kg IV 12 hourly.

ANTIEMETICS

Vomiting occurs due to stimulation of the emetic centre situated in the medulla oblongata. The act of vomiting is coordinated by the emetic centre, the chemoreceptor trigger zone (CTZ) and the nucleus tractus solitarius (NTS). It is a manifestation of many conditions, among them CNS infections, increased intracranial pressure, vestibular dysfunction, hepatobiliary disorders, gastrointestinal obstruction or infection, peritonitis, pregnancy, adverse effects of some drugs, chemotherapy and/or radiotherapy, etc. Vomiting as a symptom is treated by appropriate antiemetics. Commonly used antiemetics are discussed below.

Metoclopramide

Promethazine, diphenhydramine, diazepam or lorazepam injected IV enhances its antiemetic action and reduces dystonic reactions. Dexamethasone IV also augments its antiemetic effect. As it accelerates gastric emptying, it can be used to empty the stomach within four hours of food intake for emergency surgery under general anaesthesia and to relieve gastric stasis associated with vagotomy and diabetic gastroparesis. Symptomatic relief in dyspepsia and milder cases of gastroesophageal reflux may can also be obtained. Dose is 10 mg (children 0.2–0.5 mg/kg) TDS orally or intramuscularly, while chemotherapy-induced nausea and vomiting requires 0.3–2 mg/kg slow IV/intramuscularly. Common side effects are restlessness, drowsiness, insomnia, anxiety, agitation, dizziness and loose stools. Muscle dystonia may occur, especially in children, but is reversed on discontinuation of drug and can be rapidly reversed by using a drug having central anticholinergic action (anticholinergic antiparkinsonian drugs, promethazine) or by a central muscle relaxant (diazepam). Long-term use can cause parkinsonism, galactorrhoea and gynaecomastia. It is safe in pregnancy but when used in lactating mothers, the suckling infant may develop loose stools, dystonia or myoclonus.

Ondansetron

It is the prototype agent used for chemotherapy/radiotherapy-induced vomiting, post-operative nausea and vomiting and disease/drug-induced vomiting. It is less effective in motion sickness. Its t ½ is 3–5 hours and duration of action is 8–12 hours. For post-operative nausea and vomiting, 4–8 mg IV is given before induction of anaesthesia which is repeated 8 hourly. For less emetogenic drugs and radiotherapy, 8 mg orally 1–2 hours prior to procedure is given and repeated twice 8 hourly. Although ondansetron is effective as single agent, its efficacy can be enhanced by combining with corticosteroid (dexamethasone). It is generally well tolerated. Common side effects are headache, dizziness, mild constipation and abdomen discomfort. Hypotension, bradycardia, chest pain and allergic reactions may develop after IV injection.

Granisetron

It is more potent and more effective than ondansetron and especially indicated in repeated cycles of chemotherapy. It is given only twice on the day of chemotherapy because of longer t ½ (8–12 hours).

Side effects are similar to those of ondansetron. For post-operative nausea and vomiting, 1 mg diluted in 5 ml to be injected IV over 30 seconds before starting anaesthesia or 1 mg orally every 12 hours.

Palonosetron

It has greater affinity for 5-HT_3 receptors with longer duration of action (elimination t ½ is 40 hours). Hence, it is more effective in suppressing delayed chemotherapy-induced nausea vomiting. Rapid IV injection may cause blurred vision. It may cause additive QT prolongation when given along with moxifloxacin, erythromycin, antipsychotics, antidepressants, etc. For post-operative nausea and vomiting, 75 µg IV is given as single injection just before induction of anaesthesia.

Ramosetron

It is a potent 5-HT_3 antagonist. It was developed in Japan and marketed only in few Southeast Asian countries. For post-operative nausea and vomiting, 0.3 mg IV injection is given before induction of anaesthesia.

Levosulpiride

It blocks central and peripheral D2 receptors. It has atypical antipsychotic, prokinetic and antiemetic properties. It is used in a dose of 25 mg TDS to 75 mg BD as sustained release (SR) tablet for several functional gastrointestinal disorders, e.g., dyspepsia, nausea, bloating, gastroesophageal reflux disease and irritable bowel syndrome.

KEY FACTS

- 5-HT_3 antagonists (e.g., ondansetron) are first-line drugs in chemotherapy/radiotherapy-induced vomiting. They are also used in post-operative nausea and vomiting and disease- or drug-induced vomiting.
- Metoclopramide accelerates gastric emptying and can be used in emergency surgery to empty stomach within four hours of meals.
- Muscle dystonia especially in children is seen with metoclopramide.
- Corticosteroid (dexamethasone) enhances antiemetic effect of ondansetron and metoclopramide.

Table 5.4 Comparative Features of Lignocaine and Bupivacaine

| Drug | Surface Anaesthesia | Nerve Block | | | | | |
		Concentration	Relative Potency	Maximum dose (mg)	Onset	Duration (min)	Cardiotoxicity
Lignocaine	+	0.5–2%	1	300	Fast	60–120	Minimal
Bupivacaine	N/A	0.25–0.5%	4–5	150	Intermediate	120–360	Significant

Table 5.5 Summarised Pharmacology of Common Local Anaesthetics

Drug	Clinical Application	Pharmacokinetics, Toxicity
Lignocaine	Short-duration procedures topical (mucosal), intravenous, infiltration, spinal, epidural, minor and major peripheral blocks	Parenteral Duration 1–2 hrs and 2–4 hrs with epinephrine Toxicity: CNS excitation (high-volume blocks) and local neurotoxicity
Bupivacaine	Longer-duration procedures (but not used topically or intravenously)	Parenteral Duration 3–6 hrs Toxicity: CNS excitation and cardiovascular collapse (high-volume blocks)

LOCAL ANAESTHETICS

Local anaesthetics (LAs) are the drugs which cause reversible loss of sensory perception, especially pain, in a restricted area of the body upon topical application or local injection. When applied to a mixed nerve, they interrupt sensory as well as motor impulses, resulting in loss of autonomic control and muscular paralysis.

They act by blocking nerve conduction by reducing the entry of Na^+ ions during upstroke of action potential. The rate of rise of action potential and maximum depolarisation decreases when their concentration is increased, resulting in slowing of conduction. Conduction block ensues when local depolarisation fails to reach the threshold potential. Thus, Na^+ permeability fails to increase in response to an impulse or stimulus. Generally, orderly evolution of block components occurs, starting with sympathetic transmission and progressing to temperature, pain, light touch and finally motor block.

Addition of a vasoconstrictor, e.g., adrenaline (I: 50,000 to I: 200,000) prolongs duration of action of LAs by reducing their rate of removal from the local site into the circulation. It enhances the intensity of nerve block. It also provides a more bloodless field for surgery. Rate of absorption of LA is reduced and metabolism keeps the plasma concentration lower, thereby reducing its systemic toxicity. Thus, addition of adrenaline enables adequate anaesthesia for more prolonged procedures and extended duration of post-operative pain control and lowers total anaesthetic requirement. A disadvantage of adding adrenaline to LA is that it may increase the chances of subsequent local tissue oedema and necrosis and delay wound healing. Vasoconstrictors should not be added for ring block of hands, feet, fingers, toes or penis and in pinna. Adrenaline containing LA may raise BP and promote arrhythmia and should be avoided in patients with ischaemic heart disease, cardiac arrhythmia, thyrotoxicosis and uncontrolled hypertension, and those receiving β blockers (rise in BP can occur due to unopposed α action) or tricyclic antidepressants (uptake blockade and potentiation of adrenaline).

In the presence of inflammation, LAs often fail to be effective. As pH of the tissue is decreased by inflammation, more fraction of the LA in the ionised form, thereby hindering its diffusion into the axolemma. As there is increased blood flow to the inflamed area, LAs are removed more rapidly from the site. Action of LA may also be opposed by inflammatory products. Effectiveness of adrenaline injected with the LA is reduced at the inflamed site.

Systemic effects follow inadvertent intravascular injection or absorption of the local anaesthetic from the site of administration. At safe clinical doses, LAs produce few apparent CNS effects. Early symptoms of local anaesthetic toxicity are circumoral and tongue numbness and a metallic taste. At higher concentrations, nystagmus, tinnitus and dizziness occur, followed by drowsiness, dysphoria and lethargy. Still higher doses produce excitation, restlessness, agitation, muscle twitching, seizures and finally unconsciousness. No significant effects on the heart are observed at conventional doses. At high doses or on inadvertent IV injection, LAs act as cardiac depressants by decreasing automaticity, excitability, contractility, conductivity and prolonging effective refractory period (ERP). They have a quinidine-like antiarrhythmic action. At high plasma concentrations of LAs, the QTc interval may be prolonged and they can themselves induce cardiac arrhythmias. LAs tend to produce a fall in BP.

CNS adverse effects of LAs are light-headedness, dizziness, auditory and visual disturbances, mental confusion, disorientation, shivering, twitching, involuntary movements and finally convulsions and respiratory arrest. These can be prevented and treated by diazepam/midazolam (0.03–0.06 mg/kg). If seizures still occur, it is critical to prevent hypoxemia and acidosis, which potentiate anaesthetic toxicity. Rapid tracheal intubation can facilitate adequate ventilation and oxygenation and is essential to prevent pulmonary aspiration of gastric contents in patients at risk. Cardiovascular toxicity of LAs is manifested as bradycardia, hypotension, cardiac arrhythmias, asystole and vascular collapse. Injection of LAs may be painful and may sometimes delay wound healing. Addition of adrenaline worsens local tissue damage and may result in necrosis. Allergic reactions are rare with lidocaine. Methylparaben (a preservative in certain LA solutions) is often responsible for the allergic reaction.

Certain precautions are to be taken while administering LAs – for example, aspirate lightly before injecting the LA to avoid intravascular injection, inject the LA slowly and take care not to exceed the maximum safe dose, especially in children. By reducing hepatic blood flow, propranolol (and other β blockers) decreases metabolism of lidocaine (and other amide LAs).

Common Local Anaesthetics

Lidocaine (Lignocaine)

It is currently the most widely used LA. Being versatile, it is good for both surface application and injection. Injected around a nerve, it blocks conduction within three minutes. It is used for surface application, infiltration, nerve block, epidural, spinal and intravenous regional block anaesthesia. A transdermal patch for application over the affected skin for relief of burning pain due to postherpetic neuralgia is also available.

Lidocaine has little effect on contractility and conductivity; it abbreviates ERP and has minimal proarrhythmic potential. It is used as an antiarrhythmic. The early central effects of lidocaine are depressant, i.e., drowsiness, mental clouding, dysphoria, altered taste and tinnitus. Overdose causes muscle twitching, convulsions, cardiac arrhythmias, fall in BP, coma and respiratory arrest.

Bupivacaine

It is a more lipophilic and more potent long-acting amide-linked LA. It is used for infiltration, nerve block, epidural and spinal anaesthesia of long duration. Relatively low concentrations (≤ 0.25%) are used to achieve prolonged peripheral anaesthesia, analgesia for post-operative pain control, labour analgesia and when anaesthetic infiltration is used to control pain from a surgical incision.

Bupivacaine has the highest local tissue irritancy. Bupivacaine is relatively more vasodilatory than lidocaine and may produce fall in BP. It is more cardiotoxic and can prolong QTc interval and induce ventricular tachycardia or cause cardiac depression (Table 5.4). Toxic doses of LAs produce cardiovascular collapse. Recently, IV infusion of lipid emulsion has been used to reverse bupivacaine cardiotoxicity by extracting lipophilic bupivacaine from plasma and cardiac tissues. Use of 0.75% bupivacaine in obstetrics is banned, as it has caused a few fatalities due to cardiac arrest. Bupivacaine is often avoided for techniques that demand high volumes of concentrated anaesthetic, e.g., epidural or peripheral nerve blocks performed for surgical anaesthesia. Because of slow onset of action, it is not preferred for peripheral nerve block. Spinal bupivacaine is not well suited for outpatient or ambulatory surgery because its relatively long duration of action can delay recovery, resulting in a longer hospital stay prior to discharge to home.

The strength of bupivacaine solution for different types of blocks is as follows: peripheral nerve block: 0.25–0.5%; spinal anaesthesia: 0.5% (hyperbaric); epidural anaesthesia: 0.25–0.5%; continuous epidural analgesia: 0.125%.

Levobupivacaine

It is the S-enantiomer of bupivacaine is equally potent but less cardiotoxic and less prone to cause seizures (after inadvertent intravascular injection) than racemic bupivacaine. It is being used as a single enantiomer preparation in some countries.

NONSTEROIDAL ANTI-INFLAMMATORY DRUGS

The nonsteroidal anti-inflammatory drugs (NSAIDs) have different measures of analgesic, antipyretic and anti-inflammatory actions. They are also called nonnarcotic, nonopioid or aspirin-like analgesics. In contrast to opioids, they do not depress CNS, do not produce physical dependence and have no abuse liability.

The anti-inflammatory activity of NSAIDs is mediated mainly through inhibition of prostaglandin biosynthesis. They act primarily on peripheral pain mechanisms, but also in the CNS to raise pain threshold. Various NSAIDs have additional mechanisms of action which includes inhibition of chemotaxis, down-regulation of IL-1 production, decreased production of free radicals and superoxide and interference with calcium-mediated intracellular events. Aspirin irreversibly acetylates and blocks platelet cyclooxygenase (COX) while other NSAIDs are reversible inhibitors of COX.

Topical NSAIDs

Many topical NSAID preparations for application over painful muscles or joints are on the market. They are used for osteoarthritis, sprains, sports injuries, tenosynovitis, backache, spondylitis, etc. Their systemic absorption is low, minimising their adverse effects and making them safe. The strong placebo effect of local application, massaging and the presence of counter-irritants like menthol, methyl salicylate, etc., must also be taken into account while determining their efficacy. They have better response in musculoskeletal pain occurring for short period of time. Topical NSAIDs are also recommended in mild to moderate osteoarthritis of knee and hand. Concentration attained in muscles and joints shows marked variation depending on the type of formulation and distance/depth from site of application.

Preparations are diclofenac 1% gel, ibuprofen 10% gel, naproxen 10% gel, ketoprofen 2.5% gel, flurbiprofen 5% gel, nimesulide 1% gel, piroxicam 0.5% gel.

Choice of NSAID

The choice of a NSAID depends on efficacy, safety and cost-effectiveness. Selection of the analgesic is governed by cause and nature of pain (mild, moderate or severe; acute or chronic; ratio of pain to inflammation) and personal factors of the patient (age, concurrent disease, drug therapy, history of allergy, acceptability and individual preference). One drug cannot be labelled as superior to all others for every patient.

Most of the NSAIDs are almost equally efficacious and they tend to be differentiated on the basis of the adverse effects they produced. Indomethacin is associated with greater gastrointestinal and CNS side effects than are aspirin and ibuprofen. GI and renal side effects limit the use of ketorolac. Diclofenac is associated with more liver function test abnormalities than are other NSAIDs. Nonacetylated salicylates are preferred in patients with renal insufficiency.

Paracetamol or low-dose ibuprofen is preferred in mild to moderate pain with little inflammation. For acute but short-duration pain (post-operative), injectable ketorolac or diclofenac or oral ibuprofen/nimesulide is the choice. For dental pain, fractures, renal colic, acute gout, acute back pain and other grievous trauma, a parenteral NSAID may be given. Ketorolac, diclofenac and parecoxib are available for IM/IV use. Paracetamol can be given by slow IV infusion.

When there is gastric intolerance to traditional NSAIDs, a selective COX-2 inhibitor or paracetamol may be preferred. The selective COX-2 inhibitor celecoxib is probably safest for patients at high risk for GI bleeding but may have a higher risk of cardiovascular toxicity. Ibuprofen or aspirin may be used at the lowest dose for the shortest

Table 5.6 Doses and Pharmacokinetics of Common NSAIDs

Drug	Plasma t½	Dosage
Ibuprofen	2–4 hrs	400–600 mg (5–10 mg/kg) TDS
Diclofenac sodium	~2 hrs	50–75 mg TDS, then BD oral 75 mg deep IM
Aceclofenac	4 hours (approximately)	100 mg BD
Paracetamol	2–3 hrs	325–650 mg 3–4 times a day 10–15 mg/kg
Celecoxib	~11 hrs	100–200 mg BD

period in patients with hypertension or other risk factors for heart attack /stroke when selective COX-2 inhibitors are to be avoided. Nimesulide or COX-2 inhibitors are preferred in patients with history of asthma or anaphylactoid reaction to aspirin or other NSAIDs

Fast-acting drug formulation is suitable for fever, headache and other short-lasting pain, while longer-acting drugs/sustained release formulations are appropriate for chronic arthritic pain. Paracetamol, ibuprofen and naproxen are preferred in children. Due to risk of Reye's syndrome, aspirin should be avoided in children. A low dose of the chosen NSAID is to be given in elderly patients. Paracetamol is the safest in pregnancy. Possibility of drug interaction with NSAIDs should be considered in hypertensive, diabetic, ischaemic heart disease, epileptic and other patients receiving long-term regular medication.

ANALGESIC COMBINATIONS

The combination of codeine (an opioid analgesic) with aspirin or paracetamol provides additional analgesia beyond the ceiling effect of aspirin/ paracetamol. These two classes of drugs act by different mechanisms of pain relief. When pain is refractory to a single agent, such combination is considered. The combination of paracetamol with other NSAIDs as superior to a single agent is not supported by convincing evidence. The fixed dose combinations of analgesics with hypnotics, sedatives and anxiolytics is banned in India to decrease misuse and chance of producing dependence.

6

Surgical Tools

JAGDEEP S THAKUR, RIPU DAMAN ARORA AND DINESH SHARMA

INTRODUCTION

No surgery, simple or difficult, can be performed without proper tools and instruments. Head and neck surgery requires fine instruments and surgical material that can manage any untoward complication (especially neurovascular). It is prudent for a surgical team to ensure the availability of proper and adequate surgical instruments for a particular surgery. Further, any new instruments should be tried in simple case(s) first, otherwise there may be frustration and complications in a difficult case.

Head and neck surgery involves a number of basic and advanced surgical tools which can be divided as follows:.

1. Basic
   - Electrosurgery
   - Power drill and saw
   - Microscope
   - Endoscopic system
   - Microdebrider

2. Advanced
   - Co-ablation system
   - Laser
   - Harmonic scalpel/system
   - Nerve monitoring system
   - Robotic system
   - Transoral ultrasonic surgery (TOUSS)
   - Image guide system

Besides surgical tools, the surgical team should also have basic knowledge of associated instruments and devices – for example, anaesthetic devices – that help during surgery. This chapter discusses important surgical devices used in head and neck surgery which a beginner must understand. However, beginners are strongly advised to read the relevant manuals of the devices and undergo training before using any new tool.

ELECTROSURGERY

The electrosurgery unit is commonly called the electrocautery unit in operating room. However, these two devices differ in functions and use. Direct electric current flows through two heated electrodes in electrocautery, whereas alternating current flows through the human body in the electrosurgery unit.

Physics

The electrosurgery unit works by increasing electric current frequency from 60 Hz to 200 kHz and above. Normal electric current has a frequency of 60 Hz. Delivering the current at this frequency will stimulate neurons and electrocute the patient. However, the human body becomes insensitive to electric current with frequencies of 200 kHz or more. This is achieved through a generator which alters current flow and voltage, thereby delivering energy to the tissue. The current circuit is maintained through active and return electrodes. Patient, operating table and operating team can also be part of this circuit.

The electrosurgery unit has two circuits, namely bipolar and monopolar. As human tissue creates

DOI: 10.1201/9780367430139-6

impedance in the flow of current, it generates heat, producing the desired effects during surgery.

Current flows through tissue between two electrodes of bipolar forceps, and thereby energy is delivered to tissue held between tongs only. However, this current flows between the active electrode and return electrode through the patient's body in a monopolar circuit.

The monopolar circuit has three functions, namely cutting, blend and coagulation. These functions depend upon voltage generated. Low voltage generation leads to cutting by generating heat rapidly, while coagulation occurs with high voltage where heat is produced slowly. Blend functions through modification of the current cycle. Coagulation mode leads to coagulation and charring while vaporisation of tissue leads to tissue cutting. However, cut mode can also be used for coagulation if the tong is held in contact with tissue, as heat will be generated slowly and tissue will coagulate.

Electric current has the inherent property of following the path of least resistance and hence any instrument or material can complete the circuit and lead to complications (burns) at an undesirable area. It is therefore important to hold the return electrode firmly in maximum contact with a flat, vascular and muscular area preferably near the operative field. Further, any conducting material, e.g., instrument or wires, should be away from the monopolar tongs.

Modern electrosurgical units have an 'isolated generator system' and 'patient return electrode monitoring technology' which ensure the generator doesn't produce current if there is a break in circuit. However, one should follow precautions mentioned earlier.

Clinical Application

Electrosurgery is the basic device required in any head-neck surgery. It decreases blood loss and operative time. Monopolar mode should be preferred for making incision and raising sub-platysmal flap, whereas bipolar mode is preferred afterwards. However, one should be careful not to char the skin, which leads to poor scar outcome. One should avoid monopolar electrocautery after flaps have been raised, as it increases risk of facial palsy, even above parotid tissue. Hence, bipolar is preferred for dissection near any neural tissue.

Bipolar mode delivers the energy to tissue held between the tongs. However, in practice, this is not possible as a break in insulation or a high power setting will deliver the energy to adjoining tissue too. Therefore, its output should be kept minimal when you are working near nerves, otherwise nerve palsy is inevitable. The golden rule for monopolar or bipolar mode is to keep the optimum output so as to deliver energy only in the desired tissue. The optimum energy output varies according to the manufacturer of the unit and experience of the surgeon. While using bipolar, keep irrigating the tongs to decrease deposition of eschar. Tongs should be cleaned with a wet wipe or gauge to clear eschar and never scraped with sharp or rough instrument, as this will remove the silicon or PTFE coat, leading to more eschar formation. Another precaution requires use of smoke evacuators as viruses have been found in electrosurgical smoke. A simple, economical method is to use a suction tip during electrosurgery if separate or built-in smoke evacuators are not available.

SURGICAL NAVIGATION SYSTEM

Skull base surgery is quite difficult and requires precise knowledge of anatomy and surgical expertise, as neurovascular structures are embedded or closely adherent to the skull base. A minor surgical breach can have significant complications. The endoscopic approach has completely overtaken open/microscopic skull base surgery. However, this often means limited access and a risk of complications. The invention of the surgical navigation system or image guidance surgery (IGS) has revolutionised endoscopic skull base surgery as it provides real-time anatomical navigation to the surgeon. the basic mechanism of this system works like the global positioning system (GPS) used in mobiles or vehicles for route guidance and navigation. In GPS, a satellite tracks the position of the device and guides/navigates while correlating with its prefilled geographical data. The IGS system has a similar tracking and navigation mechanism. It can be understood with three simple statements.

- Every point in the patient's sinuses/surface landmarks has an x, y, z co-ordinate (real co-ordinates).
- The patient's CT/MRI scan image will have corresponding x, y, z co-ordinates (virtual co-ordinates).

- IGS works by matching and correlating the real and virtual co-ordinates.
- IGS produces three-dimensional localisation information for navigation during surgery.

Clinical Applications of IGS

- Skull base surgeries
  o Trans sphenoidal, trans nasal endoscopic hypophysectomy
  o Trans-sellar surgery
  o Cavernous surgery
  o Trans-pterygoid surgery
- Endoscopic sinus surgeries, especially revision sinus surgeries with un-recognisable anatomical landmarks
- Draf II and III: to localise frontal recess
- Localising lesions of petrous apex and tumours in internal auditory meatus, e.g., meningiomas, schwannomas

Components of IGS

- Head-mounted universal tracker
- Overhead optical tracking camera
- Optical LEDs placed on universal tracker, navigation pointer and other navigation devices
- Monitor
- Software: simultaneous view of axial, coronal and sagittal sections

Steps in IGS

- Get pre-operative high-resolution CT/MRI scan
- Place patient under general anaesthesia
- Attach head mount universal tracker onto patient
- Perform registration and validation
- Check accuracy of registration
- Proceed with IGS

IGS works on two fundamental processes, outlined as follows.

1. Registration:
It relates the patient in the operating room to the pre-operative acquired image data sets and establishes the relation between the two co-ordinate systems. This is achieved through three different landmarks:

- Anatomical landmarks
- Visible on patient and image data; e.g., tragus, outer canthus, inner canthus, nasion
- Position of tip of probe is identified by tracking device and co-ordinates are fed back to navigation software
- Fiducial markers (fixed lines or markers applied to patient before scanning and in operating room)
- Using masks and laser scanning tools

2. Tracking:
Tracking the position of instruments in relation to the patient/operative field provides dynamic positional information for which the tracking system must be:

- Precise
- Consistently accurate
- Fast enough to provide >25 readings per second
- Insensitive to changes in air temperature
- Unaffected by metal objects

Tracking systems are based on:

- Magnetic field (cheap and effective)
- Infra-red light sensors (most commonly used; finds infra-red light via LED attached to patient or location probe)
- Inertial trackers
- Accurate tracking hardware is pole-mounted.

Limitation of IGS: Every instrument has limitations that further restrict its applicability. Current IGS systems have a target registration error range of 1.5–2 mm in detecting instrument position in the operative field, which is affected by other factors too. This minimal error makes the IGS a perfect instrument in skull base surgery, but it can also create overconfidence in the inexperienced surgeon leading to complications.

LASERS

Introduction

Laser is an acronym for "light amplification by stimulated emission of radiation". Lasers are electromagnetic radiations with specific wavelengths depending on the laser medium that produces an intense beam by amplifying light. Laser is a surgical scalpel with the capability of cutting as well as coagulation.

Principle

Normally the atom is stable, with an equal number of electrons and photons revolving around the nucleus in a fixed orbit. When an external source energises an electron to an excited state, the atom soon releases absorbed energy spontaneously (spontaneous emission) and returns to its original state. Alternately, this emission can be induced by a forced interaction between one photon and an excited electron to release a new photon (stimulated emission). These photons move back and forth between two parallel mirrors and trigger a chain reaction to produce an intense beam (light amplification). One mirror is partially silvered and allows exit or leak of laser light.

Properties of Lasers

A beam of laser light is a unique form of electromagnetic energy that can be described as follows.

- Coherent – waves are phase-locked both temporally and spatially
- Monochromatic – one wavelength or colour
- Collimated – parallel waves travelling in one direction

Laser Components

There are three main components of a laser.

- Active medium– to supply a source of stimulated atoms. It may be a solid (Nd:YAG, Ruby, KTP and diode lasers), liquid (inorganic dye) or gaseous (CO_2, argon and helium-neon laser) state
- Laser pump or power source – a stimulation mechanism to activate the medium
- Optical chamber – contains the active medium, directs the output and provides feedback from amplification and collimation

Other components are a cooling system, a delivery system, a control unit and a remote control.

Energy Delivery Modes

There are three operational modes that deliver energy.

- Continuous wave – continue constant and stable energy for > 0.1 second. Used in solid lesions for deeper penetration
- Pulsed wave – intermittently activated for a short time, < 0.1 seconds, when less penetration is required, allowing tissue to cool off between pulses (decreasing thermal damage)
- Q-switched mode – very short but high intensity pulses (<1 μsec.)

Laser Tissue Interaction

Interaction is of four types.

1. Absorption
2. Reflection
3. Scattering
4. Transmission

Interaction depends on the wavelength of the laser beam, laser operation mode, amount of energy applied and tissue characteristics. Electromagnetic (EM) wavelength is the single most important factor that determines its absorption by water, collagen or bone.

Tissue reactions by lasers include the following.

- Photoablative
- Photomechanical
- Photochemical
- Photothermal – the most common reaction used in ENT. Most soft tissues contain 50–75% water intracellularly and laser ablation occurs when intracellular water is heated to boiling, thus exploding the cell, vaporising and coagulating the tissue.

Tissue heat changes are denaturation, coagulation, vaporisation, carbonisation and incandescence as the temperature varies.

Secondary thermal effects are seen in surrounding tissues – haemostasis by coagulation (varies with wavelength of laser, rate of energy applied, fluence and nature of tissue).

Visible spectrum lasers include argon laser (514 nm) and KTP laser (532 nm). Infrared spectrum lasers include CO_2 laser (10,600 nm) and erbium YAG laser (1060 nm).

Visible lasers are delivered to microscope-mounted micromanipulators or a handheld probe through fibre optic cable. A micromanipulator can fix the beam down to 0.05 mm spot size at 250 mm focal length.

The infrared CO_2 laser is a workhorse for ENT surgery. It uses a He-Ne laser for aiming a beam. It can't be transmitted by optical fibres, so it is delivered by a lasing console to a microscope-mounted micromanipulator by a series of 13 mirrors and lenses called a flexing arm. It can seal blood vessels up to < 0.5 mm in diameter.

The optical fibre focuses the smallest light spot, having the highest concentration of energy very close to the fibre tip. Intensity decreases as the distance increases.

Fibre in contact is used for incision/cutting tissue. At 2–4 mm distance (near contact), it vaporises tissue. Non-contact of fibre (>4 mm) is used for coagulation.

Clinical Applications in ENT

- In otology-stapedectomy, small A-malformations, vaporising small acoustic neuromas and small glomus tumours and in some tympanomastoid surgeries.
- In rhinology-papilloma, fibroma, synechiae, inferior turbinate hypertrophy, choanal atresia, telangiectasia, epistaxis, residual polyp.
- In oral cavity-mucosal cyst, leukoplakia fibroma papilloma, haemangioma, epulis, benign tumours, ranula, Ca (lip, buccal mucosa, tongue, tonsil, uvula, soft palate) laser tonsillectomy, uvulopalatopharyngoplasty for OSA.
- In larynx, laryngeal web, cyst, nodule, polyp, haemangioma, leukoplakia, laryngomalacia, recurrent respiratory papillomas, benign tumours, laser partial arytenoidectomy for bilateral VC palsy, subglottic stenosis, laryngeal Ca in situ, T1 and T2 lesions of glottis and supraglottis and in some subglottic tumours.

- Photodynamic Therapy (PDT) – tumouricidal effects of PDT are based on laser activation of a photosensitiser which has been selectively taken up and retained by tumour cells.

Advantages

- Precision
- Haemostasis
- Less soft tissue damage as there is less manipulation of surrounding tissues
- Minimal adhesions
- Minimal post-operative oedema, pain, scarring and fibrosis
- Early mobilisation and minimal hospitalisation
- Preservation of function (vs. open surgery)
- Single-sitting procedure helps in pathological staging of disease (vs. radiotherapy)

Limitations

- Laser beam cannot seal blood vessels >0.5 mm in diameter
- Expensive equipment
- Specific training of surgeon, anaesthetist and staff required
- Fire hazard

Laser Safety Rules

- All operating theatre staff should be trained in laser-use safety measures. (See Table 6.1.)
- Signage warning of laser use should be posted at all entrances.

CONCLUSION

Laser-based therapies represent an area of huge potential. Lasers are commonly employed in various medical disciplines: dermatology, eye surgery, neurosurgery, cardiology, dentistry, ENT, etc. as they have advantage in terms of precision, minimal blood loss and post-operative oedema, excellent haemostasis, improved healing process and short hospital stay. Nevertheless, they require thorough staff training and are not free of complications.

Table 6.1 Biohazards of Lasers and Their Management

Eye protection	• A primary concern of unsafe laser use is eye injury (corneal or retinal burn). Wear approved wavelength-matching laser safety glasses. • The patient should wear same eyewear, moistened sterile cotton eye pads or metallic eye protectors. • Operating room windows must be covered with an opaque material at the wavelength of laser used.
Plume hazards	• Plume content biohazard relates to direct toxic effects of the smoke, so continuous or frequent smoke evacuation is advisable. Viral DNA has been recovered from the plume, so personnel are advised to wear N95 or N100 respirators. Be more cautious in handling tissues infected with HPV.
Protection of other exposed areas	• Exposed skin and mucous membrane surrounding the surgical field should be covered by saline-soaked towels or sponges to protect from overshoot or stray laser strikes.
Coaxial alignment	• Confirm correct alignment of aiming and treatment beams before each procedure by checking beam on moistened wooden tongue blade.
Blackening of instruments	• Endoscopic and microsurgical equipment should be blackened to reduce accidental reflective laser strikes.
Precautions in anaesthetic procedures	• Laser-resistant cuffed endotracheal (ET) tubes must be used, as fire hazard is the most dreaded complication. • ET tubes made of silicone with an outer coating of metal are more resistant to lasers than are PVC and red rubber tubes. The cuff of these tubes is filled with saline diluted in methylene blue so as to identify leaks immediately due to bluish seepage of saline. • New flexometallic tubes are non-combustible, easily sterilised, gas-tight and non-reactive with human tissue. Their limitation is the large external diameter, precluding use in younger patients. • If normal PVC ET tubes are used, self-adhesive reflective metallic foil is wrapped around the tubes. • The cuff is protected by filling with saline and placing saline-soaked cottonoids around it. • A closed ventilator system is preferred for less chance of a gas leak. • Ventilation with high concentration of O_2 and N_2O is to be avoided. Only non-inflammable gases like halothane or enflurane are used. • Jet ventilation is often necessary for glottic and subglottic lesions. • In case of airway fire, immediately extubate the patient, remove supplemental O_2, apply saline into airway and reintubate the patient. Thereafter, perform bronchoscopy to remove large foreign bodies and visualise small airways. Provide a high-humidity environment and positive end expiratory pressure ventilation and give IV steroids.

7

Skin Cancer

NEEL PRABHA AND MOUMITA DE

INTRODUCTION

Commonly encountered head and neck skin cancers include non-melanoma skin cancers (NMSCs) and melanoma. NMSCs are basal cell carcinoma (BCC) and squamous cell carcinoma (SCC). Majority of skin cancers of the head and neck are NMSCs.

BASAL CELL CARCINOMA

It is the most common tumour of skin. It is a locally invasive epidermal tumour made of cells similar to basal cells. It shows slow progressive extension and rarely metastasises.

Epidemiology

- **Age of Onset:** older than 40 years
- **Sex:** males > females
- **Race:** In white-skinned persons it is the commonest tumour.

Etiology and Predisposing Factors

- Ultraviolet radiation mainly in UVB spectrum (290–320 nm), induces mutations in suppressor genes
- Skin phototypes I and II and albinos are highly susceptible to develop BCC with prolonged sun exposure
- Multiple BCC occurs after several years of arsenic intake (as a contaminant in water or as a medicine)

Clinical Features

Five clinical types are described: nodular, ulcerating, pigmented, sclerosing and superficial.

- **Nodular BCC:** Commonest subtype and usually presents on the head and neck. Well defined, firm, translucent/pearly/skin colored/erythematous papule/nodule with smooth surface and telangiectasia.
- **Ulcerating BCC ("rodent ulcer"):** Ulcer with rolled edge and adherent crust in centre.
- **Sclerosing BCC:** Appears as ill-defined yellowish or ivory-white lesion resembling a scar or morphea. On palpation, margins extend in an irregular fashion beyond the visible margins.
- **Superficial BCC:** Seen mainly on trunk. Well defined, thin scaly/non-scaly erythematous plaques with fine, thread-like margins.
- **Pigmented BCC:** Variant of nodular BCC showing brown/blue/black pigmentation.

Sites of Predilection

Approximately 80% of all BCCs occur on the head and neck. All variants of BCC except superficial BCC (trunk and limbs) occur on face. Common sites on face are inner canthus, eyelids and behind the ear.

DOI: 10.1201/9780367430139-7

Course

BCC is a slowly progressive, locally invasive tumour that can involve underlying structures like cartilage or bone, if left untreated.

Diagnosis

Diagnosis is made clinically and confirmed by biopsy.
Various clinical diagnostic points are:

- Thread-like margins, rolled telangiectatic edge
- Slow growth
- Characteristic involvement of site
- Absence of lymph node involvement

Histopathology findings: Epidermis is thin over the tumour mass. Tumour extends into the dermis. The tumour is composed of islands and lobules of basaloid cells in a palisading arrangement. Basaloid cells resemble basal cells and show large, oval or elongated darkly staining nuclei and very small amount of cytoplasm. There is mucinous stroma with artificial cleft between the epithelial island and the stroma.

SQUAMOUS CELL CARCINOMA

Squamous cell carcinoma is the second most common skin cancer after BCC. SCC is a malignant tumour arising from epidermal keratinocytes or their appendages. SCC has a low rate of local, regional and distant spread.

Epidemiology

- **Age of onset:** Incidence of SCC increases with age
- **Sex:** Males > females
- **Race:** Persons with white (skin phototypes I and II)
- **Occupation:** Persons working outdoors

Etiology and Predisposing Factors

SCC develops usually in damaged skin. The most frequent cause, especially in white-skinned patients, is sun damage due to prolonged sun exposure. The cumulative dose of UV radiation received over time is a significant risk factor. SCC may also arise from epithelial precancerous lesions like actinic keratosis and Bowen disease. SCC occurs at site of scars, dermatitis (radiodermatitis, friction dermatitis), chronic granuloma (lupus vulgaris) and leukoplakia. Head and neck SCCs are found to have frequent association with HPV-16. Chronic immunosuppression (organ transplant, AIDS) is associated with an increased incidence of SCC.

Clinical Features

Most SCCs develop on the light-exposed areas of the head and neck. Common sites of head and neck are upper part of face, lower lip and pinna. The first clinical evidence of SCC is induration. The lesions feels firm on palpation and induration extends beyond the visible margin of the lesion. SCCs are often papulonodular, but can be plaque-like, papillomatous or exophytic. Some lesions are hyperkeratotic and others show secondary changes like crusting, erosions and ulcerations. Other physical findings are regional lymphadenopathy due to metastases.

SCC of Oral Cavity

Cigarette smoking, tobacco chewing and alcohol intake are important predisposing factors. It is associated with high morbidity and mortality. The high-risk sites are floor of mouth, ventrolateral aspects of tongue and soft palate. It may present as persistent plaque with rough or granular velvety surface. Later on, it may become firm or nodular.

Oral Verrucous Carcinoma
It is associated with oncogenic HPV types 16 and 18. It appears as extensive hyperkeratotic white leukoplakia. It metastasises late but can be locally destructive.

SCC of Lower Lip

SCC of the lips develops on leukoplakia or actinic cheilitis. In 90% of cases they are found on the lower lip. The presenting sign may be a fissure or small erosion or ulcer which fails to heal and bleeds recurrently. Persistent lip chapping and atrophic vermilion border are important clues for diagnosis. It may appear as a rough papule which slowly progresses into a tumour nodule.

SCCs occurring on the lower lip metastasise in 10–15% of cases.

Course and Prognosis

SCC causes local tissue destruction and has a potential for metastases. Metastases are directed to regional lymph nodes and appear 1–3 years after initial diagnosis. In-transit metastases occur. Squamous cell carcinoma has a low rate of metastasis of about 5%. Low-grade tumours carry an excellent prognosis but the risk of developing metastasis increases significantly in SCCs displaying high-risk features. High-risk features are as follows: diameter >2 cm, perineural involvement, poorly differentiated or undifferentiated tumour, involvement beyond fat involvement of sites such as the external ear or lip, tumour arising from a previous scar and occurrence in immunosuppressed patients.

Histopathology

Shows irregular masses of epidermal keratinocytes that proliferate downward into the dermis. The tumour masses consist of varying proportions of atypical squamous cells and normal squamous cells. Tumour cells vary from large, well-differentiated cells with vesicular nuclei, prominent nucleoli and abundant cytoplasm to completely anaplastic cells. Well-differentiated tumours show foci of keratinisation in the form of horny pearls. The poorly differentiated tumour shows decreased keratin formation.

EVALUATION OF NON-MELANOMA SKIN CANCER

A chronic non-healing, enlarging or ulcerating skin lesion should be suspected as a skin cancer and should be biopsied to prove the diagnosis. BCC rarely spreads to the cervical lymphatics, whereas regional spread is common in patients with SCC. High-resolution axial and coronal imaging is necessary for the complete staging of disease in the patient with NMSC. CT helps in evaluation of primary tumour, status of lymph nodes and bony invasion. MRI detects perineural spread or dural invasion. To rule out distant metastasis, especially in patients with bulky lymph nodes, CT scan of chest is required. Fine-needle aspiration of lymph nodes can also be done for the pathologic confirmation of neck node metastasis.

MALIGNANT MELANOMA

It is a less common malignant tumour arising from epidermal melanocytes. It has significant potential for regional and distant lethal metastasis.

Etiology

The etiology and pathogenesis of cutaneous melanoma are unknown. A role for genetic predisposition and sun exposure in melanoma development has been suggested. The mutation in familial melanoma is the most common in cyclin-dependent kinase inhibitor 2A (*CDKN2A*) gene. Cutaneous melanoma is a greater problem in light-skinned whites (skin types I and II), and sunburns during childhood and intermittent burning exposure in fair skin seem to have a higher impact than cumulative UV exposure over time. Other predisposing and risk factors are the presence of precursor lesions (dysplastic melanocytic nevi and congenital NMN) and a family history of melanoma in parents, children or siblings.

- **Course:** Most MM grow in two phases.
- **Phase of radial growth:** Lesion expands superficially and neoplastic melanocytes remain confined to the epidermis.
- **Phase of vertical growth:** Malignant cells invade dermis and deeper tissues.
- **Clinical subtypes and presentation:** The superficial spreading melanoma (SSM) is the most common melanoma (70%) type in persons with white skin. It begins as an asymptomatic brown to black macule with color variations and irregular, notched borders. SSM can arise *de novo* or in a pre-existing nevus. After a slow radical-growth phase, a more rapid vertical growth occurs which is clinically seen as a papule or nodule.

Nodular Melanoma

Nodular melanoma is the second most common type (15% to 30%) of cutaneous melanoma in fair-skinned individuals. It is most frequently diagnosed in the sixth decade of life. It is mostly seen on trunk, head and neck, and is clinically seen as blue to black nodules which may be ulcerated or bleed.

The following melanomas have poorer prognosis.

- **Lentigo maligna melanoma (LMM):** It represents a minority of cutaneous melanomas (~10%). It develops within chronically sun-damaged skin. Most common site on the face is nose and cheek. Clinically it appears as a slow-growing, asymmetric, brown to black macule with colour variation and irregular border.
- **Mucosal melanoma:** It is a rare clinical variant. It is seen as extensive irregular macular pigmented lesion in oral cavity.

Diagnosis

Clinical diagnosis can be made by the specific character of malignant melanoma lesion, memorised as the ABCDE of malignant melanoma:

- Asymmetrical pigmented lesion
- Border irregularity
- Colour variability
- Diameter >0.5 cm
- Elevation irregularity

INVESTIGATIONS

- **Biopsy:** It is advisable to undergo excisional biopsy. In case of large lesion, an incisional full-thickness biopsy should be taken from the most elevated or most hyper-pigmented part. In epidermis and in dermis cytologically malignant melanocytes are seen. Histological staging can be done by Clark's method or Breslow's method.
- **Fine-needle aspiration cytology (FNAC):** FNAC of enlarged lymph node should be done for confirmation of metastasis.
- **Sentinel lymph node biopsy:** In this method, occult micro metastasis is detected by taking biopsy of non-palpable regional lymph nodes.
- **Imaging:** CT scan, MRI and chest X-ray to detect distant metastasis.

TREATMENT OF SKIN TUMOURS OF HEAD AND NECK

Treatment of BCC

Management of head and neck cutaneous malignancies is aimed at complete removal of the tumour with optimal preservation of the function and cosmesis. The management options can be classified

Table 7.1 Categorisation of Local BCC for Management and Prognosis

Serial Number	Characteristic	Low Risk	High Risk
1	Location	Trunk, extremities <2 cm) Cheek, forehead, scalp, neck (<10 mm)	Trunk, extremities ≥ 2 cm Cheek, forehead, scalp, neck, "mask areas" of face (central face, eyelids, eyebrows, periorbital, nose, lips [cutaneous and vermilion], chin, mandible, preauricular and postauricular skin/sulci, temple, and ear), genitalia, hands, and feet and pretibia any size
2	Borders	Well defined	Poorly defined
3	Primary vs. recurrent	Primary	Recurrent
4	Immunosuppression	No	Yes
5	Prior radiotherapy	No	Yes
6	Subtype	Nodular, Superficial	Aggressive growth pattern
7	Perineural involvement	No	Yes

into ablative modality and excisional modality (surgical excision and Mohs surgery). Surgical approach is the most effective and efficient means. The management depends upon the characteristic of the lesion (see Table 7.1).

Ablative modalities are usually reserved for low-risk, superficial and small basal cell carcinomas and selective cases of squamous cell carcinoma. A major drawback of ablative modality is that depth of the lesion cannot be assessed, which leads to higher relapse rates. Ablative modality involves the use of various chemical, bio-active and mechanical agents to destroy the lesions. The ablative agents used are

electrosurgery, 5-fluorouracil, topical imiquimod, interferon alpha, radiofrequency, photodynamic therapy and radiotherapy. Various ablative methods are summarised in Table 7.2.

SURGICAL MANAGEMENT OF BCC

Surgery provides definitive management of malignancies of the head and neck region. In cases of BCC, ensuring a clear margin is of paramount importance and gives a success rate of more than 95%. Adequate margin of excision depends upon the anatomic location, clinical features and depth

Table 7.2 Ablative Management of BCC

	Modality	Indication	Advantages	Disadvantages	Special Comments
1.	Curettage and electro dissection	Superficial, localised primary tumour of size 2–4 mm	Technically easy	Difficult to define depth in large tumours, no histological control, hypertrophic scarring, dyspigmentation	Relapse Up to 15% (< 2 mm) Relapse 50% (>3 mm)
2.	Cryosurgery	Small, well-defined primary lesion Patients who are poor candidates for surgery	Spares normal tissue	Difficult to define depth in large tumours No specimen available for histology Cosmetically undesirable result due to pigmentary changes	Cure rate >95% (<2 mm)
3.	5-fluorouracil	Limited use in nodulo-ulcerative and superficial BCC	Non-invasive	High degree of relapse Depth cannot be assessed	FDA approved
4.	Imiquimod 5%	Solitary primary superficial BCC (<2 cm)	Non-invasive	Cannot be used on eyes, nose, lips or cochlea Depth cannot be assessed	Variable cure rate
5.	Intralesional Interferon alpha	Superficial and nodular BCC	Pro-inflammatory agent	Frequent painful injections	Obsolete method
6.	Photodynamic therapy	Superficial/morpheaform BCC	Non-invasive	Photosensitisation of patient Limited penetration	Variable cure rate Not FDA approved
7.	Radiotherapy	Option when surgery is contraindicated For palliation		Chronic radiation dermatitis, alopecia, radiation-induced cutaneous malignancies	Five-year recurrence rates of 8.7% and 10% after RT on primary and recurrent BCC. RT reserved for patients >60 yrs due to long-term sequelae

Table 7.3 Categorisation of Cutaneous SCC to Determine Treatment, Recurrence, Metastasis and Prognosis Based on Risk Factors

		Low risk	High risk	Very High Risk
1	Location/size	Trunk, extremities < 2 cm	Trunk, extremities 2 cm–4 cm Head, neck, hands, feet, pretibia, and anogenital (any size)	≥4 cm (any location)
2	Border	Well defined	Poorly defined	N/A
3	Primary/recurrent	Primary	Recurrent	N/A
4.	Immunosuppression	Absent	Present	N/A
5.	Prior RT/chronic inflammatory process	Absent	Present	N/A
6.	Rapidly progressing tumour	Absent	Present	N/A
7.	Neurologic symptom	Absent	Present	N/A
8.	Degree of differentiation	Well- or moderately differentiated	N/A	Poor differentiation
9.	Histologic features: acantholytic (adenoid), adenosquamous (showing mucin production), or metaplastic (carcinosarcomatous) subtypes	Absent	Present	Desmoplastic SCC
10.	Depth: thickness or level of invasion	≤6 mm and no invasion beyond subcutaneous fat	N/A	>6 mm or invasion beyond subcutaneous fat
11.	Perineural involvement	Absent	Present	Tumour cells within the nerve sheath of a nerve lying deeper than the dermis or measuring ≥0.1 mm
12.	Lymphatic or vascular involvement	Absent	Absent	Present

involvement. Proximity of the tumour to the surgical margins defines the recurrence rates.

There are two surgical approaches. The tumour can be excised and the wound is primarily closed/flap covered/skin grafted, and the specimen is sent for histopathological examination. Then, based on the biopsy reports, decision on further management is taken. The other approach is, tissue is excised, then sent for frozen section examination. Re-excision can done immediately if margins are found positive, but this approach is time consuming and requires collaboration with the pathology team.

MANAGEMENT IN LOW-RISK CANDIDATES

1. Standard excision with 4–6 mm clinical margins is recommended with post-operative margin assessment
2. Cryotherapy can be used in low-risk BCC when tumour is confined to skin only and patient is not a candidate for surgical excision, excluding terminal hair-bearing areas like scalp, pubic, axillary regions and the beard area in men.

MANAGEMENT IN HIGH-RISK CANDIDATES

1. Standard excision with wide margins is recommended. Due to varied clinical characteristics of high-risk tumours, clear margins for excision cannot be defined. The excisional margin should include surrounding erythema with clinically normal-appearing skin on all sides of tumour.
2. Mohs microsurgery.

RECURRENCE

1. **Local:** patient is treated as for high-risk tumours
2. **Nodal or distant metastasis:** surgery/RT/systemic therapy/clinical trial

FOR NON-SURGICAL CANDIDATES

1. Curative radiotherapy
2. Systemic therapy if curative radiotherapy is not possible

FOLLOW-UP

Follow-up should be done 6–12 months for five years, then annually.

Treatment of SCC

Treatment of SCC is similar to BCC. Due to the aggressive nature of the tumour, wider excision of the margins, deeper tissue assessment and management of the regional nodes and strict, watchful follow-up is required. Categorisation of SCC to determine treatment, recurrence, metastasis and prognosis based on risk factors is mentioned in Table 7.3.

Ablative Treatment Used in SCC

1. **Cryotherapy:** has specific indication
2. **Radiation therapy:** low cure rate
3. Other topical therapies are not recommended as in BCC

MANAGEMENT IN LOW-RISK CANDIDATES

1. Standard excision with 4–6 mm clinical margins is recommended with post-operative margin assessment
2. Cryotherapy can be used in low-risk SCC when tumour is confined to skin only, not penetrating beyond skin (excluding terminal hair-bearing areas like scalp, pubic, axillary regions, and beard area in men)
3. Radiation therapy for non-surgical candidates

MANAGEMENT IN HIGH-RISK/ VERY-HIGH-RISK CANDIDATES

1. Standard excision with wide margins is recommended. Due to varied clinical characteristic of high-risk tumours, clear margins for excision cannot be defined. The excisional margin should include surrounding erythema with clinically normal-appearing skin on all sides of tumour.
2. Mohs microsurgery
3. For non-surgical candidates
   - curative radiotherapy
   - systemic therapy if curative radiotherapy is not possible

LYMPH NODE MANAGEMENT

For node-positive resectable cases, complete excision of primary with regional node dissection. For node-positive cases (inoperable/not fully resectable), either curative radiotherapy or, if that is not possible, then systemic therapy.

FOLLOW-UP

Follow-up should be 3–12 months for two years, then 6–12 months for the years. Annual follow-up for life is recommended.

TREATMENT OF MALIGNANT MELANOMA

Management of melanoma requires staging of the disease, depth of the invasion, histopathological characteristics and nodal assessment.

Based on these criteria, the following categories can be used in melanoma.

1. **Local melanoma:** Disease is localised. Cancerous cells confined to the lesion, not spread beyond the primary lesion.
   Includes: Stage 0 (in situ), stage I, stage II
   Stage 0, stage IA: Wide excision
   Stage IB, stage II: Wide excision with sentinel lymph node biopsy
2. **Regional melanoma:** Cancerous cell spread to regional lymph node/vessels
   Includes: Stage III
   - Stage IIIA, B, C (pathological)
     - Complete regional lymph node clearance
     - Lymph node basin surveillance (ultrasound) followed by adjuvant therapy
   - Stage III (clinical staging)
     - Wide local excision with complete lymph node dissection followed by adjuvant therapy
   - Stage III (clinical satellite/in transit) palpable or microscopic cutaneous/subcutaneous metastasis within 2 cm of primary or more than 2 cm of primary, respectively
     - **Limited resectable disease:** If margins can be completely cleared by wide local excision followed by adjuvant therapy
     - **Unresectable disease:** If margins cannot be completely cleared by wide local excision, then manage as unresectable case
3. **Distant metastatic melanoma:** Cancer spread to other parts or organs of body
   Includes: Stage IV
   - **Limited resectable disease:** If margins can be completely cleared by wide local excision followed by adjuvant therapy
   - **Unresectable disease:** Systemic therapy, local therapy, regional therapy, radiotherapy for extra-cranial palliation with palliative care

MANAGEMENT OF RECURRENCE

1. **True scar recurrence:** Re-excision with appropriate margin with lymphatic mapping/sentinal lymph node biopsy
2. **Clinical satellite/in transit recurrence**
   - **Limited resectable disease:** If margins can be completely cleared by wide local excision followed by adjuvant therapy

Table 7.4 Recommended Surgical Margin for Wide Excision of Primary Melanoma

Tumour Thickness	
In situ	0.5–1.0 cm
≤ 1.0 mm	1.0 cm
> 1.0–2.0 mm	1–2 cm
> 2.0–4.0 mm	2.0 cm
> 4.0 mm	2.0 cm

   - **Unresectable disease:** If margins cannot be completely cleared by wide local excision, then manage as unresectable case
3. **Nodal recurrence (limited to nodes)**
   - No previous node dissection:
     Complete node dissection with adjuvant therapy
   - Previous node dissection
     Resectable: Complete node dissection with adjuvant therapy
     Unresectable: Systemic therapy

SPECIAL AREAS FOR CONSIDERATION IN HEAD AND NECK REGION

Melanoma of ear: Full thickness excision with closure as skin is adherent to cartilage. Wide local excision involves removal of tumour to deep fascia, which is preserved until it is involved by tumour. Complete details about the management can be obtained from the National Comprehensive Cancer Network website, at www.nccn.org.

SYSTEMIC THERAPY FOR MALIGNANT MELANOMA

Various agents are used, including the following.

1. **Immunotherapy:** Increases immune response of the body to destroy cancer cells Programmed death receptor-1 (PD-1) inhibitor: Pembrolizumab and nivolumab
2. **Targeted therapy drugs:** Target specific genes associated with cancer cells

   BRAF inhibitors (vemurafenib or dabrafenib)
   MEK inhibitors (trametinib or cobimetinib)

LOCAL THERAPY OPTIONS IN UNRESECTABLE TUMOURS

- Intralesional injection options: Talimogene laherparepvec (T-VEC)
- Topical imiquimod
- Radiotherapy
- Palliation for symptomatic disease: Limited excision/ablation therapy

REGIONAL THERAPY OPTIONS

Isolated limb infusion/perfusion with melphalan

SURGICAL RECONSTRUCTION FOR CUTANEOUS MALIGNANCY

Ensuring a safe margin often results in a big defect not amenable for primary closure. Primary closure should be attempted side by side wherever feasible. Normal tissue is sacrificed to achieve clear margin. Hence, sometimes even if primary closure is done, it may result in aesthetic or functional deformity in the face like a distorted hairline, misaligned brow or ectropion of eyelids or lips. When primary closure is not possible, various reconstructive options from skin graft to flap can be chosen. Before the reconstruction, the resection margins of the surgical pathological specimen should be properly labelled as per the anatomical orientation.

The options are as follows:

- **Skin Graft:** The most basic amongst these is a skin graft, either split thickness or partial thickness. The advantages of split thickness grafts are readily available donor areas and possibility of resurfacing very large areas. The disadvantages are poor colour match, chances of graft contracture and subsequent deformity, especially in the visible areas of the face. By comparison, full thickness grafts are advantageous in that they have lesser contracture. Also, a full thickness graft harvested from the post-auricular or supraclavicular area gives a better colour match.
- **Local Flaps:** Local tissue rearrangement in the form of local flaps gives the best possible reconstruction in head and neck surgical defects in terms of colour and contour match. Various local flap options and their modifications are used. Some of the commonly used flaps (**see Figure 7.1**) are:

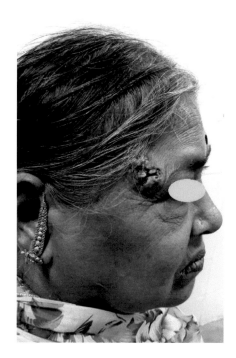

Figure 7.1a BCC right forehead.

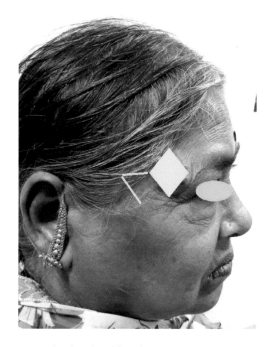

Figure 7.1b Rhomboid flap design.

- **The Rhomboid Flap** or **Limberg Flap:** it uses a geometric pattern of flap marking and employs a combination of rotation and transposition movements to resurface the

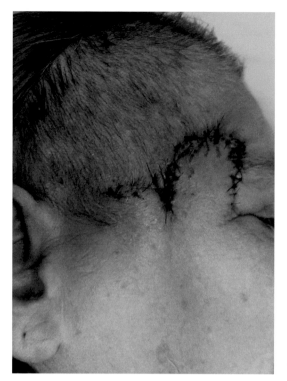

Figure 7.1c Flap transposed into defect.

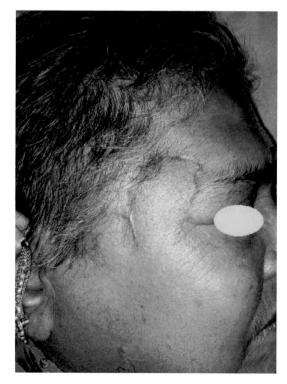

Figure 7.1d Follow-up.

defect, and also achieves primary closure of the donor.

- **Local Transposition Flap (Figure 7.2):** Can be used to cover moderate to large defects in the face and scalp. The drawbacks are the need for a skin graft for the flap donor area and distortion of hair direction if used for scalp.

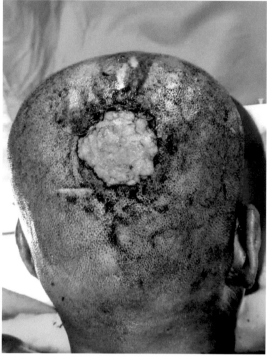

Figure 7.2a SCC occipital region.

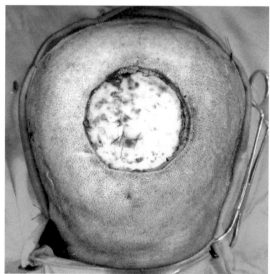

Figure 7.2b Post-excision defect.

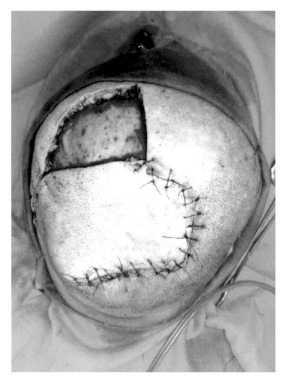

Figure 7.2c Local transposition flap inset into the defect.

- **Rotation Flap (Figure 7.3):** Moves the tissue adjacent to the defect in a wide arc to resurface defect and at the same time achieve primary closure of the donor area.
- **Modified Advancement Flaps:** The principles of advancement and Z-plasty can be used to fabricate different local flaps like "O to S plasty" or Yin-Yang flap (Figure 7.4), "A to T plasty" (Figure 7.5), V-Y advancement, etc.
- **Nasolabial Flap (Figure 7.6):** A versatile flap which can be either superiorly based or

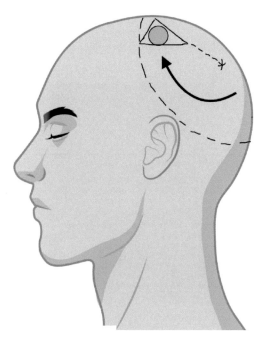

Figure 7.3 Rotation flap geometry.

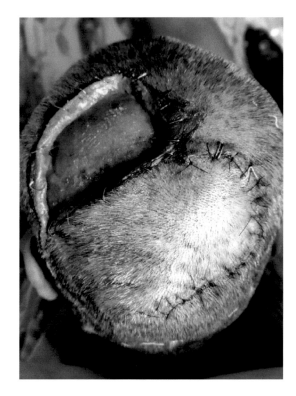

Figure 7.2d Follow-up.

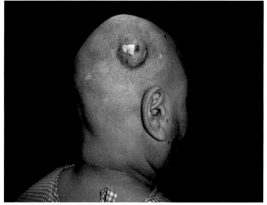

Figure 7.4a Benign hair follicle tumour of scalp.

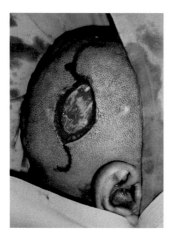

Figure 7.4b Post-excision defect with flap marking.

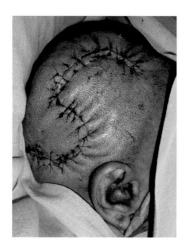

Figure 7.4c Flap inset into defect.

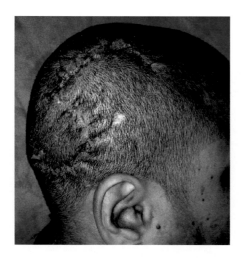

Figure 7.4d Follow-up.

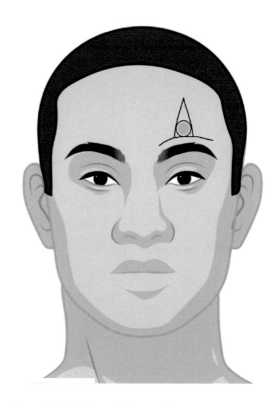

Figure 7.5a Defect with flap marking.

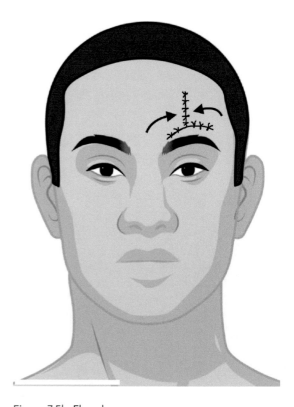

Figure 7.5b Flap closure.

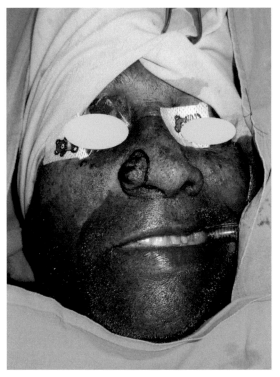

Figure 7.6a BCC right nasal ala.

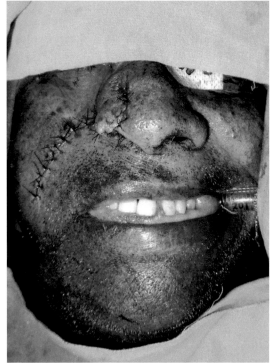

Figure 7.6c Flap inset into defect.

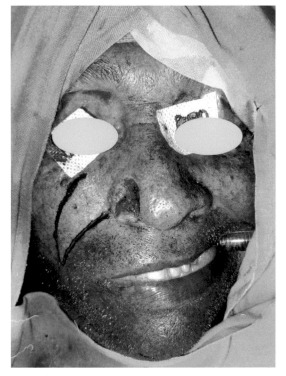

Figure 7.6b Post-excision defect with flap marking.

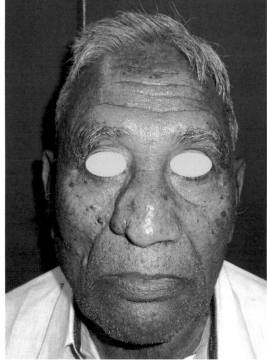

Figure 7.6d Follow-up.

inferiorly based, supplied by the communication among facial artery, terminal branch of the facial artery (i.e., angular artery) and infra-orbital artery. The scar is hidden in the nasolabial crease, which gives it distinct aesthetic advantage.

- **Bilobed Flap** (Figure 7.7): Described by Esser and modified by Zitelli, this innovative flap is mostly used for nasal tip defects. Precise geometric design ensures primary closure of the donor.

- **Tenzel Flap** (Figure 7.8): Specifically used for full thickness defect of the eyelids post cancer extirpation. It involves division of the lateral canthal tendon and semicircular musculocutaneous advancement of the lateral skin into the eyelid defect.

- **Cervico-Facial Advancement Flap:** For very large defects, the whole of the cheek skin and

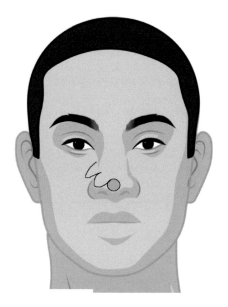

Figure 7.7a Defect with flap marking.

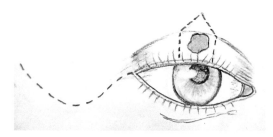

Figure 7.8a Lesion of upper lid with incision marking.

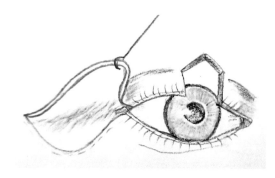

Figure 7.8b Post-excision defect with flap elevation.

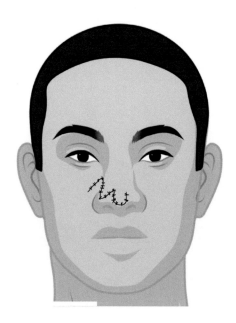

Figure 7.7b Flap after closure.

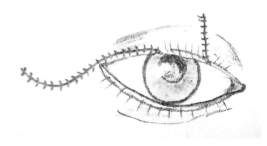

Figure 7.8c Flap inset into defect.

neck skin can be recruited into the defect to resurface it.

- **Forehead Flap:** For defects involving the nose, the time-tested forehead flap is still widely used. Both the classical midline as well as para-median forehead flaps can be used (Figure 7.9). The lateral forehead flap, based on the frontal branch of the superficial temporal artery, has limited application nowadays owing to the disfigurement of the forehead. However, it is still used in selected cases where other options are either exhausted or not feasible.

- **Regional Flaps:** For big defects not amenable for closure by local flaps, regional flaps like the deltopectoral flap (Figure 7.10), Supraclavicular flap or pectoralis major flap can be used.

- **Free Flap Reconstruction**
  Free flap reconstruction has the advantage that practically any defect can be resurfaced with tissue brought from distant parts. Radial artery forearm flap is the workhorse flap in head and neck reconstruction owing to its thin, pliable skin paddle and good colour match to the face (Figure 7.11). Other flaps with thin skin, such as the SCIP flap (superficial circumflex iliac artery perforator flap) or the MSAP flap (medial sural artery perforator flap) can give good contour.

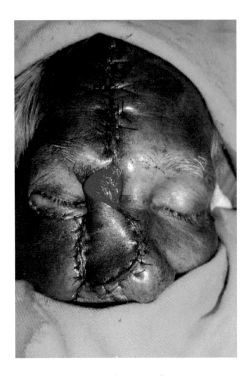

Figure 7.9b Paramedian forehead flap inset into defect.

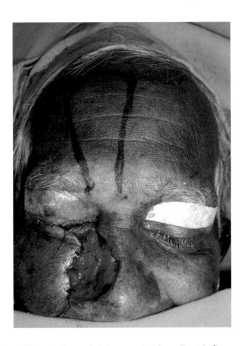

Figure 7.9a Defect of right nasal sidewall with flap marking.

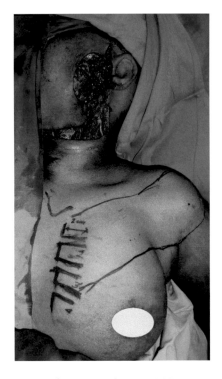

Figure 7.10a Left pre-auricular post-SCC excision defect.

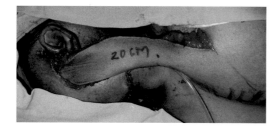

Figure 7.10b Deltopectoral flap elevated and transferred to the defect.

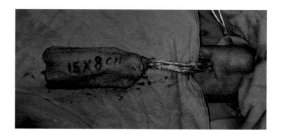

Figure 7.11b Radial forearm flap harvested.

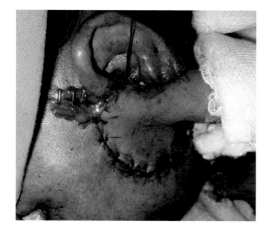

Figure 7.10c Flap inset into defect.

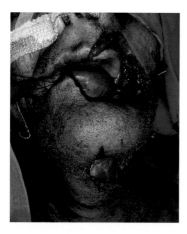

Figure 7.11a Left cheek and angle of mouth post-SCC excision defect.

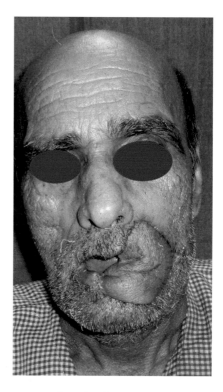

Figure 7.11c Well-settled flap.

MOHS MICROGRAPHIC SURGERY

This is presently the most recommended modality for resection of non-melanoma skin cancers of the head and neck region. This is a method of excision that ensures a clear margin of resection.

The surgeon – specially trained in this modality – after resection of lesion under magnification, using bevelled cuts, examines the histology of the lesion and does a mapping of the margins. Any margin showing residual tumour is serially excised and examined till a clear margin is achieved. This method ensures clear margin with minimum possible defect and spares normal tissues, which is very advantageous in anatomically complex areas. This modality has a cure rate of 98% in primary tumours and about 95% in recurrent tumours. The disadvantages are that it is time consuming, costly and requires special training to be certified as a Mohs micrographic surgeon.

8

Oral Cancer Surgery

ROHIT K SHARMA

INTRODUCTION

Oral cancer is a major health burden in the world. This concern is aggravated by the fact that oral cancer is more likely to occur among low socio-economic populations that are exposed to a wide array of carcinogenic factors like tobacco, alcohol and poor oro-dental hygiene. Of late, a viral etiology has been implicated, especially the human papillomavirus 16 and 18. Moreover, because of lack of awareness and limited access to good healthcare facilities, these patients tend to present late. Most oral cancers are squamous cell carcinomas, which tend to be ulcerative. Carcinomas arising from the minor salivary glands form the remainder. The management of oral cancers is based on its location, dimensions, status of neck metastasis and involvement of lower alveolus, mandible, floor of mouth and upper alveolus. Surgery in the form of resection of the primary along with neck dissection remains the mainstay of treatment of oral cancers. A large number of these patients will also require post-operative radiation therapy.

PRE-OPERATIVE MANAGEMENT

Clinical Evaluation

By definition, oral cancers include cancers arising in the lips, mucosa of the tongue, gingivae, buccal mucosa, floor of mouth and hard palate. The examiner should document the morphology, size, depth, invasion of surrounding structures and the regional metastasis to stage the tumour (Tables 8.1 and 8.2). The tumour may be exophytic, endophytic or ulcerative. The size should be measured in the maximum and minimum dimensions. The depth of the tumour should be measured from the imaginary surface of the normal mucosa, but this is clinically very difficult to correctly assess in most cases. Similarly, invasion of surrounding structures is difficult to evaluate clinically, although clinical features like trismus may indicate involvement of masticator muscles and fixity of anterior tongue may indicate involvement of floor of mouth. The presence of neck nodes should be documented as regional metastasis is one of the most important prognostic factor.

Investigations

A detailed investigative work-up is of utmost importance to confirm the diagnosis, to assess the local or distant spread and also to rule out systemic comorbidities. As the oral cancer commonly presents as an ulceroproliferative or an ulcerative lesion, punch biopsy is usually adequate to confirm the histopathological diagnosis. Rarely, an incisional biopsy may be required in lesions without an apparent mucosal breach. Fine needle aspiration cytology should be carried in the cases where palpable lymphadenopathy is present. A detailed clinical examination of the upper aerodigestive tract, preferably in the form of flexible fibre optic nasopharyngolaryngoscopy should be performed in all patients in whom oral malignancy is suspected or

DOI: 10.1201/9780367430139-8

Table 8.1 Primary Oral Cancer Classification (AJCC, 8th Edition)

Clinical	
Tx	Primary tumour cannot be assessed
Tis	Carcinoma in situ
T1	Tumour ≤2 cm in greatest dimension, ≤5 mm depth of invasion (DOI, not tumour thickness) OR tumour >2 cm but ≤ 4 cm, and ≤ 10 mm DOI
T2	Tumour ≤2 cm, DOI >5 mm and ≤10 mm OR tumour >2 cm but ≤4 cm and ≤10 mm DOI
T3	Tumour >4 cm OR any tumour >10 mm DOI
T4	Moderately advanced or very advanced local disease
T4a	Moderately advanced local disease (lip) tumour invades through cortical bone or involves the inferior alveolar nerve, floor of mouth, or skin of face, (i.e., chin or nose). (Oral cavity) tumour invades adjacent structures only (e.g., through cortical bone of the mandible or maxilla, or involves the maxillary sinus or skin of the face). Note: Superficial erosion of bone/tooth socket (alone) by a gingival primary is not sufficient to classify a tumour as T4.
T4b	Very advanced local disease tumour invades masticator space, pterygoid plates or skull base and/or encases internal carotid artery.

Table 8.2 Regional Lymph Node Staging (AJCC, 8th Edition)

Nx	Regional lymph nodes cannot be assessed
N0	No regional lymph node metastasis
N1	Metastasis in a single ipsilateral lymph node, ≤3 cm in greatest dimension and ENE (—)
N2	Metastasis in a single ipsilateral lymph node, >3 cm but ≤6 cm in greatest dimension and ENE (—); OR mets in multiple ipsilateral lymph nodes, ≤6 cm in greatest dimension and ENE (—); OR mets in bilateral or contralateral lymph nodes, ≤6 cm in greatest dimension and ENE (—)
N2a	Metastasis in single ipsilateral lymph node >3 cm but ≤6 cm in greatest dimension and ENE (—)
N2b	Metastasis in multiple ipsilateral lymph nodes, ≤6 cm in greatest dimension and ENE (—)
N2c	Metastasis in bilateral or contralateral lymph nodes, ≤6 cm in greatest dimension and ENE (—)
N3	Metastasis in a lymph node >6 cm in greatest dimension and ENE (—); OR metastasis in any lymph node(s) with clinically overt ENE (+)
N3a	Metastasis in a lymph node > 6 cm in greatest dimension and ENE (—)
N3b	Metastasis in any lymph node(s) with clinically overt ENE (+)

confirmed. This helps in ruling out an occasional second primary malignancy. Blood tests should include haemoglobin, blood counts, serum urea and electrolytes, liver and kidney function tests, blood grouping and cross matching. The author's center has a policy of photographing all the lesions before any form of treatment to supplement the documentation.

Radiology

In a large number of patients with oral cancer, an experienced surgeon may be able to plan a treatment that may hold good even after a radiological examination. An MRI alone would suffice in lesions limited to the tongue, which is always better for soft tissue lesions. Deeper invasion of the tongue musculature and involvement of the base of the tongue can be clearly demonstrated by an MRI with contrast that may be missed on clinical evaluation. Invasion of the mandible is one of the most important parameters during the management of oral carcinomas. A CT scan would be able to indicate bony involvement in lesions which abut the upper or lower alveolus. A plain X-ray of the mandible is not sufficient to demonstrate bony invasion. An orthopantogram is better, but nowadays an easy accessibility of CT scans precludes its necessity. Generally, a tumour clinically abutting the mandible and not showing a bony invasion on a CT scan is suitable for a marginal mandibulectomy. Patients with a definitive bone invasion by an oral cancer are a candidate for segmental mandibulectomy. Lesions growing over the alveolus from either side also indicate segmental mandibulectomy. A plain chest X-ray is helpful in ruling out lung metastasis, but an HRCT thorax is preferable. (See Figure 8.1)

The Multidisciplinary Team or the Tumour Board

The multidisciplinary team, also commonly called the Tumour Board, usually comprises the surgeon, radiation and medical oncologist, radiologist and pathologist. Their work is central to evaluate and plan the management of head and neck cancers. This is of greater importance in the context of oral cancers because of the complexities in their management and outcomes. The responsibility of the Tumour Board is to ensure a thorough evaluation and planning prior to the commencement of the treatment. The diagnosis and staging must be confirmed in its meetings. The members of the board should be aware of the contemporary guidelines based on clinical evidence. Any changes in the clinical scenario should be put forward during the review meetings.

Pre-Operative Nutrition

Patients with oral cancers are more prone to malnutrition because of difficulty in swallowing, reduced mouth opening, cancer-induced cachexia and adverse effects of radiotherapy. Malnutrition is directly correlated to poor wound healing and increased risk of complications. Services of a dietitian should be obtained both before and after the surgery for better management of nutrition. Where oral intake is inadequate, parenteral nutrition should be given.

Dental Work-Up

A number of functions of the oral cavity like speech and swallowing might be affected by the oral cancer or the various treatment modalities applied. A dental evaluation is pertinent prior to any modality of treatment applied to oral cancer. These patients in due course of treatment may develop mucositis, xerostomia, abnormal taste, trismus, dental caries and necrosis of the jaw bone. Dental prophylaxis should address teeth with caries, sharp and jagged edges and plaques. Loose teeth should be extracted. Preferably no dental treatment is to be performed in the teeth expected to come in the surgical margin as this can pose a risk of micro-metastasis into the mandible. Postoperative dental rehabilitation should be discussed and a plan chalked out. A compromise in the orodental prophylaxis may lead to reduction in quality of life, leading in turn to adverse outcomes.

Counselling and Psychosocial Issues

A thorough discussion with the patient and relatives regarding the status of the disease and the management plan is essential. This should include the goals of the treatment and commonly expected complications. Patients with head and neck cancer and especially oral cancers are prone to psychosocial issues. These may be anxiety, depression, suicidal tendencies and issues of poor quality of life and medical outcome. A simple psychiatric assessment and management of these will go a long way to achieve good results.

PRE-ANAESTHESIA CONSIDERATIONS

Oral cancer patients have considerable comorbidities, including COPD, cardiovascular, malnutrition, difficult airway, poor oro-dental hygiene and loose teeth. They are often chronic smokers, oral tobacco users and alcohol abusers. Some of these patients might have received radiotherapy, which makes the airway access difficult to anesthetist. If possible, these conditions should be managed pre-operatively by the appropriate specialist, otherwise significant post-operative morbidities may result, like complications of anaesthesia, sepsis, poor wound healing and flap failure. In cases where a difficult airway is anticipated, especially

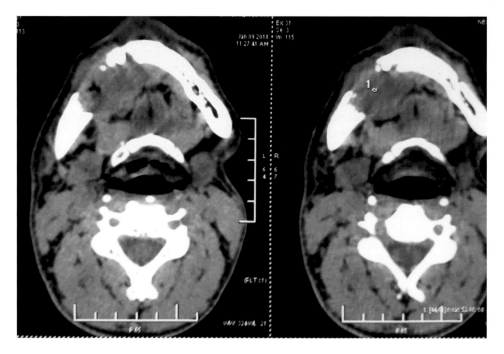

Figure 8.1a Carcinoma, oral cavity, eroding the mandible.

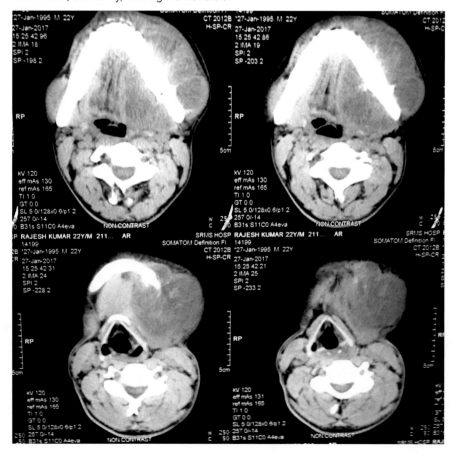

Figure 8.1b Chondrogenic osteosarcoma arising from the mandible.

in the patients with reduced mouth opening, there should not be any hesitation in performing a planned tracheostomy.

Anaesthesia, Cleaning and Draping in Operating Theatre

General anaesthesia is preferred in most patients undergoing surgery for oral cancers. Standard antiseptic procedure should be meticulously followed for cleaning and draping on operation table. If the method of reconstruction is decided pre-operatively, then the site for harvesting the flap should also be prepared along with the surgical field.

LIPS

The treatment of choice for management of lip cancer is surgery. Radiotherapy is indicated post-operatively in advanced disease, in patients where general conditions do not permit surgery or if the patient does not consent to it. Though the primary objective of the surgical excision of the lip carcinoma remains satisfactory excision of the lesion, the maintenance of lip function (speech and competence of oral commissure) and appropriate cosmesis are also equally important. The margin of resection of the lip is 5 mm, as compared to 10 mm in the other areas of the oral cavity.

Carcinoma of Lip, Less Than 30%

- Carcinoma of lip involving less than 30% of its length is usually amenable to a V resection. This can be applicable to both the lower and upper lip.
- The surgery for smaller lesions can usually be performed under local anaesthesia, usually in a concentration of 2% xylocaine with 1:2,00,000 of adrenaline, up to a maximum concentration of 1:1,00,000. Occasionally, if general anaesthesia is required, then the endotracheal tube should be fixed in so as not to distort the lips, or preferably a nasal intubation should be done.
- The incisions are marked externally with a minimum of 5 mm normal margin and the lower lip is held by the assistant between the thumb and the index finger during the procedure on both sides.

- A No. 15 blade is used to complete the skin incision. From here an electrocautery can be employed to complete the subcutaneous dissection so as to get a better control on homeostasis.
- Bleeding from inferior labial arteries is usually controlled by a bipolar electrocautery or suture ligation.
- The closure begins after confirming the negative margins on the frozen section where, as a first step, a nylon stay suture is applied at the vermilion border to achieve a good cosmesis.
- If there is tension while closing, a curvilinear incision can be made at the junction of the upper lip and the chin over which the two cut ends can be advanced.
- Some sutures are applied at the muscular layer, then the closure is carried out in the internal mucosal lining and then the skin externally. For muscular layer and mucosal lining, catgut or Vicryl 3–0 is used, whereas nylon is used for the skin.

Carcinoma of Lip, More Than 30%

- Primary closure of the carcinoma of upper or lower lip is difficult and should be avoided, as it results in very poor functional and cosmetic results. If done, there will be drooling of saliva as the oral commissure on both sides is pulled medially on the excised lip. Advancement flaps are useful in cases where more than a third defect is expected after excision.
- For resection of median lesions on the upper lip with involvement of more than 30%, advancement can be carried out by excising the skin and soft tissue lateral to the nasal ala on both sides (Burow's triangles) resulting in better symmetry (see Figure 8.2a through 8.2e).
- Lip switch flaps (Abbe or Estlander) are used in defects of more than 50% of the lower lip. The Abbe flap is used for the defects in the central parts of the lower lip, wherever the oral commissure is preserved. The Estlander flap is used especially on the lateral aspect where the oral commissure needs to be excised (see Figures 8.3a through 8.3i).
- For example, for a growth on the lower lip, a full thickness resection is performed in a triangular fashion. A flap from the upper lip is planned from the same side. It has to be the same in vertical dimension as that of

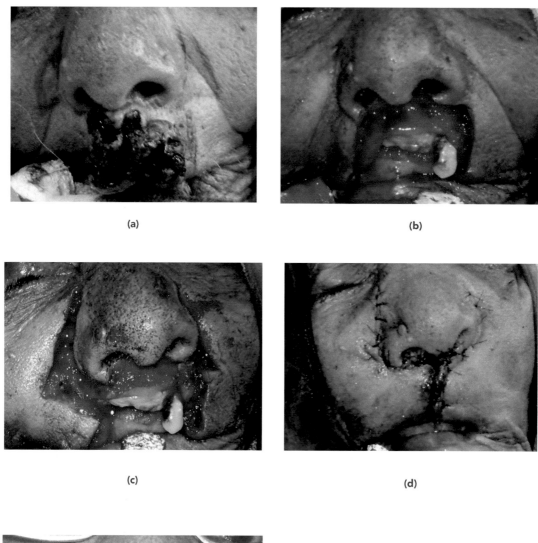

(a)

(b)

(c)

(d)

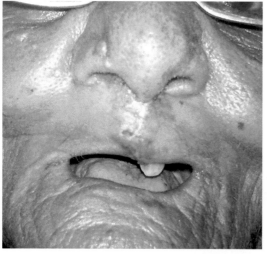

(e)

Figure 8.2 (a) Burow's triangles medial to the nasolabial folds with margins of resection marked. (b) Defect after excision of growth on upper lip. (c) Skin and soft tissue from Burow's triangle is excised (d) Skin is sutured after advancement (e) Satisfactory cosmetic and function result after four weeks.

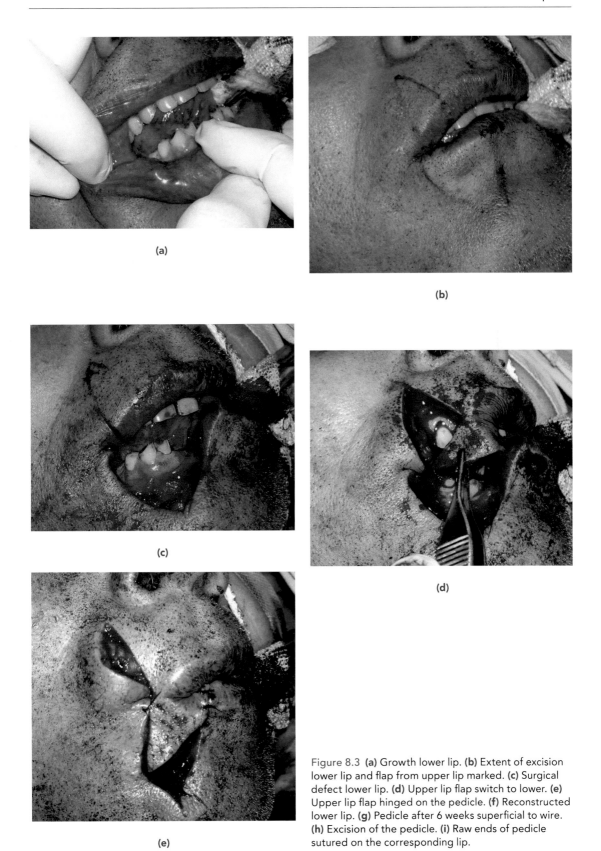

Figure 8.3 (a) Growth lower lip. (b) Extent of excision lower lip and flap from upper lip marked. (c) Surgical defect lower lip. (d) Upper lip flap switch to lower. (e) Upper lip flap hinged on the pedicle. (f) Reconstructed lower lip. (g) Pedicle after 6 weeks superficial to wire. (h) Excision of the pedicle. (i) Raw ends of pedicle sutured on the corresponding lip.

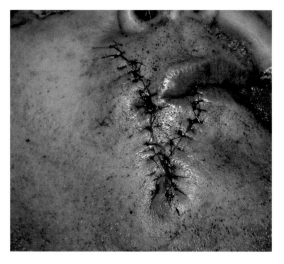

(f)

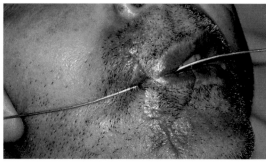

(g)

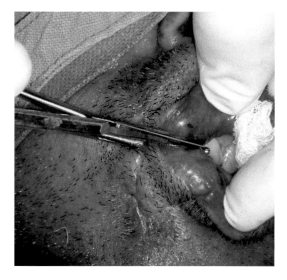

(h)

(i)

Figure 8.3 (Continued)

the defect, and the width of the flap has to be around half of that of the defect. This equalises the final dimensions of both the lips.

- Muscular layer of the flap and the resected margin is now sutured with 3–0 Vicryl. The defect of the donor site is also closed, beginning with the muscular layer. Mucosa on both sites is sutured with 3–0 Vicryl and the skin with 4–0 nylon. All the suturing in the lip is made in interrupted fashion.
- As the pedicle of the donor site still remains attached to the resected site, the mouth opening is minimal and the patient must take special precautions not to stretch and traumatise

it. Until the pedicle is not transected, the patient must be on a liquid/semi-solid diet.

- The pedicle is transected at about four weeks. A mosquito artery forceps is inserted behind the pedicle and then it is cut with a no. 15 blade.
- A larger lesion of the central component of the lower lip can also be reconstructed by a Karapandzic flap. Curvilinear incisions are made on both sides from the inferior margin of the defect towards the oral commissure, keeping it superficial to the orbicularis oris muscle. These bilateral incisions can be extended into the nasolabial folds. The

skin and subcutaneous tissue are mobilised. The muscle is preserved along with its vascularity and nerve supply. By this medial mobilisation on both sides, adequate closure and satisfactory cosmesis can be achieved with the local tissue itself, but the resultant oral cavity may be smaller (see Figures 8.4a through 8.4e).

Carcinoma Tongue: Partial Glossectomy—Peroral Approach with Primary Closure

- For the early lesions of anterior two-thirds of tongue with normal tongue mobility, a partial glossectomy is usually feasible via a peroral approach.

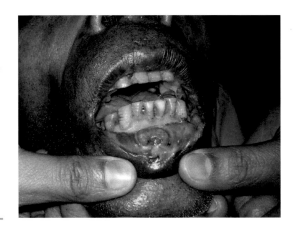

(a)

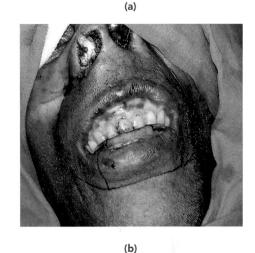

(b)

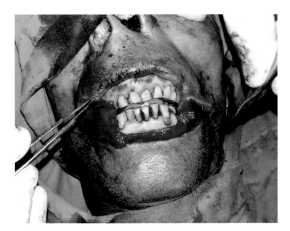

(c)

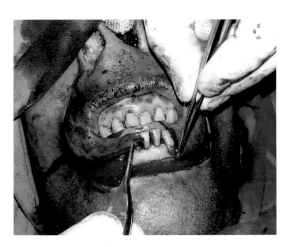

(d)

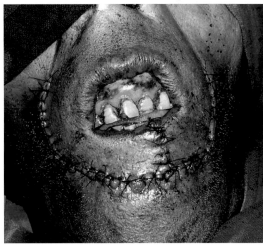

(e)

Figure 8.4 (a) Carcinoma, lower lip, with involvement of more than 30%. (b) Resection margins and Karapandzic flaps marked. (c) After excision of primary Karapandzic flaps are raised. (d) Flaps advanced medially. (e) Karapandzic flaps after final closure.

- The surgery is carried out under general anaesthesia. A self-retaining mouth gag (Doyen or Fergusson Ackland) is applied.
- A stay suture with silk (1–0 on needle) is passed through the tip and/or the edges of the lesion.
- A beginner can mark the surgical margins with a marking pen or a needle cautery tip not less than 1.0 cm from the most peripheral induration.
- For the lesions on the lateral border and the tip, wedge excision gives a better cosmetic and functional result. A vertical wedge excision is preferred over the horizontal. Midline lesions may require an elliptical excision.
- For better homeostasis, the author prefers electrosurgery for dissection in the oral cavity. It is used in the cutting mode during mucosal incisions and in coagulating mode in the deeper muscular dissection.
- During the course of surgery, the lingual artery may be found traversing within the surgical margins and will require ligation with silk sutures (1–0 or 2–0).
- Clinical surgical margins of 1 to 1.5 cm should be obtained. If the dissection is done with help of a cautery, the margins are expected to contract, hence a pathological margin of 5 mm may be considered appropriate.
- Frozen sections, if contemplated, should be obtained from the surgical bed to assess the adequacy of resection.
- The operative team should change gloves and gowns and re-drape the patient before beginning the neck dissection.
- It is the author's policy to perform a supra omohyoid neck dissection (SOHND) or an extended SOHND in patients with N0 necks. In patients with N1 cervical metastasis, an SOHND, extended SOHND or a modified neck dissection may be performed. Beyond N1, a modified or a radical neck dissection may be more appropriate. Refer to chapter 16, "Neck Dissection," for details.
- The wound should be irrigated with diluted povidone iodine and then closed after confirming the negativity of the margins. The deeper muscular layer should be closed first, followed by the mucosal margins, using a monofilament suture like Vicryl 3–0 or 2–0, or a chromic catgut (see Figures 8.5a through 8.5f).

Partial Glossectomy with Reconstruction

- The technique of excision remains the same in larger lesions, as described earlier in partial glossectomy with primary closure. The use of a flap can be considered in these cases.
- Microvascular free flap is the preferred method to reconstruct the tongue, but regional flaps like pectoralis major myocutaneous flap and skin grafting may also be used in select settings.
- In our experience, even a significantly smaller tongue occurring out of primary closure functions satisfactorily and most patients do not complain about problems in speech and deglutition. This could be because these patients had severer symptoms due to a larger growth, compared to reduced functional problems resulting from a smaller post-operative tongue occurring due to primary closure.
- See chapter 22 for details of each flap.

Resection of Premalignant and Malignant Buccal Superficial Lesions, Peroral Approach

- Premalignant lesions can be resected superficially, including the mucosa and some part of the buccinator muscle.
- For malignant superficial mucosal lesions, resection of the mucosal membrane, buccinator and some part of masseter, along with the fat pad, is resected. As compared to premalignant lesions, a wider surgical margin of minimum 1 cm should be obtained.
- In most malignant lesions, especially T2, where a deeper resection has been done, a microvascular free flap has to be considered.
- A very small lesion could be left for healing with primary intention; however, a full thickness skin graft should be considered in other superficial lesions (see Figures 8.6a through 8.6c).

Resection of Oral Cavity Tumours, Lip Split and Paramedian Mandibulotomy

- Indication—for access to oral cavity, pharyngeal and parapharyngeal tumours.

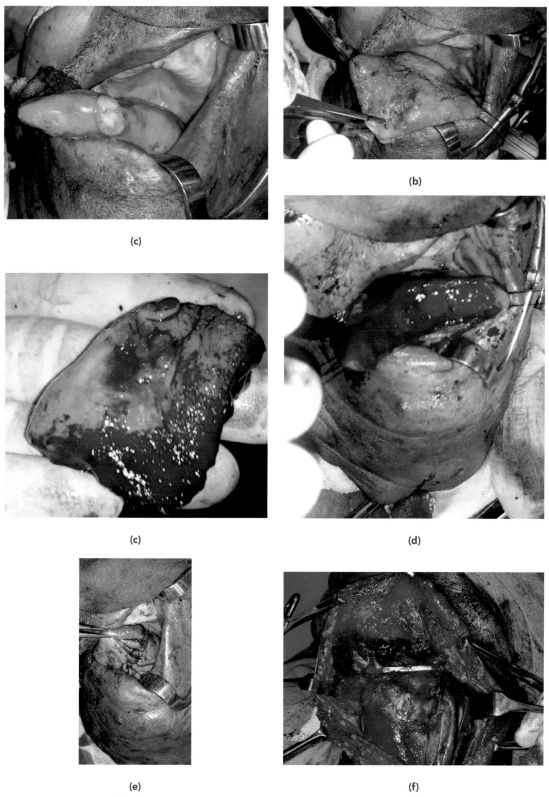

Figure 8.5 **(a)** Growth of about 2 cm on left lateral border of tongue. **(b)** Resection margins of at least 1.0 cm are marked in a wedge shape. **(c)** Resected tongue specimen. **(d)** Surgical defect on the tongue. **(e)** Resected surfaces of the wedge defect are closed after approximating the margins. **(f)** Extended supraomohoid dissection is completed.

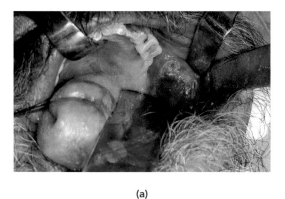

(a)

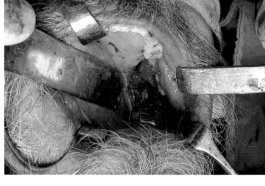

(b)

(c)

Figure 8.6 **(a)** T1 lesion of left buccal mucosa. **(b)** Surgical defect on buccal mucosa seen after resection by coagulation electrosurgery. **(c)** Skin graft harvested from the inner aspect of thigh is applied to the defect.

- In the author's series, the commonest indication of paramedian mandibulotomy is carcinoma tongue with deep muscle infiltration or oropharyngeal involvement.
- A dental consultation is obtained to rule out septic tooth in the vicinity of the bony cut, to perform any extraction if needed and to plan for the prosthetic management of the extracted tooth.
- Once the patient is placed under general anaesthesia, a thorough oral cavity examination should be done to confirm the surgical plan.
- If planned, an appropriate neck dissection is performed prior to the mandibulotomy.
- A lip split incision can be circum-mental, with a midline Z or a straight split.
- Some surgeons describe a midline Z for good alignment; however, in our experience, if the labial margins are approximated properly, the midline straight lip split also gives an optimum result.
- Now the lip is completely split and the spurt from the labial arteries is usually controlled by electrosurgery.

- The incision is then extended to the ipsilateral gingivobuccal sulcus, leaving a margin of mucosa on the mandible to enable a proper closure after the resection.
- The cheek flap is not elevated beyond the mental nerve, to prevent anaesthesia of the chin.
- The mandibular cuts are now marked. The midline straight osteotomy described by Trotter is not preferred as it may lead to loss of central incisor, which gives a poor cosmetic result. Moreover, after securing it with miniplates, there may be hinge-like action on the joint, leading to poor healing.
- The paramedian cuts are marked on the mandible. It can be done in two ways, as commonly described in the literature. One method is to make a vertical bone cut between the roots of the lateral incisor and the canine and then fashion the inferior half of the cut obliquely. The other way is to make the bony cuts in a step-ladder fashion.
- Irrespective of type of mandibular cut, the miniplates are screwed and then removed

before making the bony cut so as to obtain an exact alignment during closure.
- The oncologic clearance is then carried out with adequate margin of 1–1.5 cm.
- Primary mucosal closure or, if planned, a reconstructive procedure is undertaken.
- The pre-contoured miniplates are now fixed (Figures 8.7a through 8.7i).

Resection of Primary Carcinoma of Oral Cavity with Segmental Mandibulectomy

- Primary resection of oral cavity carcinoma is combined with segmental mandibulectomy where there is a clinical or radiological evidence of mandibular invasion, post-radiotherapy recurrence and thin atrophied (pipe stem) mandible.
- During examination the relation of the tumour with the mandible must be noted.
- A contrast CT scan is a prerequisite, which can indicate whether the growth is invading the mandible or just abutting.
- Planning for flap reconstruction is done accordingly.
- A number of patients may require a tracheostomy, but for some, peroral endotracheal intubation may suffice.
- An appropriate ipsilateral neck dissection is done and the specimen left attached to the oral primary or removed.
- The neck dissection incision is extended superiorly onto chin and lower lip in the midline to perform a lip split.
- The midline lip split incision as described in paramedian mandibulotomy is adequate.
- The cheek flap would have to be elevated beyond the mental nerve in this situation so as to gain exposure of the outer surface of the mandible.
- Wide local mucosal and mucoperiosteal cuts of at least 1 cm margin are made around the oral primary.
- In cases where segmental resection is planned, the mandibular cuts are marked, again at least 1 cm away from the involved bone.
- The bone is cut with a powered saw or a drill from outside to in, first anteriorly and then posteriorly.

- A flat instrument like a tongue depressor is inserted intraorally so as to protect the soft tissue from injury once the saw comes out medially.
- The oral primary along with the mandible and the neck dissection specimen are removed in toto.
- The frozen section specimen is now sent from the surgical defect just as the reconstruction begins.
- Free fibular microvascular flap (Figures 8.8a through 8.8g) or a pedicled flap (pectoralis major myocutaneous; see Figures 8.9a through 8.9h) is then carried out, as described in the chapter 22, "Reconstruction in head and neck tumours".

Resection of Primary Carcinoma of Oral Cavity with Marginal Mandibulectomy

- Marginal or rim resection of the mandible is performed where the oral primary is in close contact with the mandible and there is no clinical or radiological evidence of involvement of the mandible.
- If the lesion is small and anterior, excision with marginal mandibulectomy can be done by a peroral approach and a skin graft to repair the defect along with a neck dissection.
- In the rest of the patients, the surgery begins with an appropriate neck dissection on the ipsilateral side.
- For most of these patients, the incision and exposure for marginal mandibulectomy remains same as segmental resection with the lower cheek flap commonly raised.
- The mucosal and periosteal cuts are made around the oral primary with at least 1 cm margin followed by the bony cuts.
- A powered saw is used to make the bony cut in a curvilinear fashion and not as straight cuts with angles. A curved marginal mandibulectomy helps to dissipate the pressure on the residual bone evenly. The straight bony cuts have a tendency to get fractured at the angles.
- If the residual defect is small, then buccal mucosa can be primary closed with the floor of mouth or with a part of the tongue; however, a pedicled or a free flap would be required in other cases (see Figures 8.10a through 8.10f).

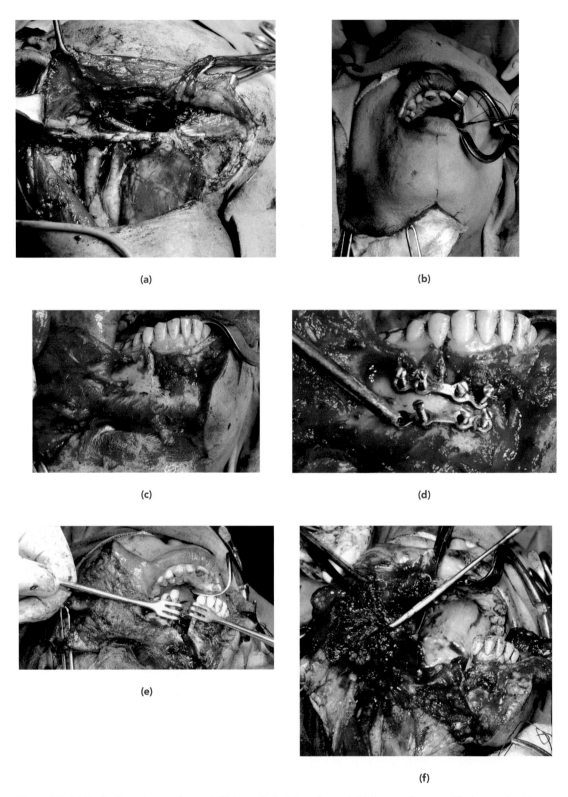

Figure 8.7 **(a)** Neck dissection performed. **(b)** Lip split incision planned. **(c)** Paramedian mandibulotomy incision marked on the right side. **(d)** Temporary miniplate fixation done to achieve perfect post-operative alignment. **(e)** Paramedian mandibulotomy performed. **(f)** Growth tongue and floor of mouth resected. **(g)** Pectoralis major myocutaneous (PMMC) flap planned. **(h)** PMMC flap elevated and brought into oral cavity. **(i)** Tongue and floor of mouth reconstructed with the flap.

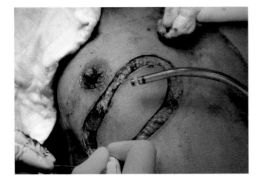

(g)

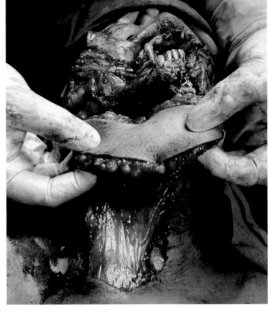

(h)

Figure 8.7 (Continued)

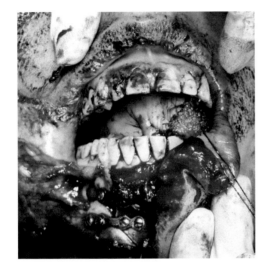

(i)

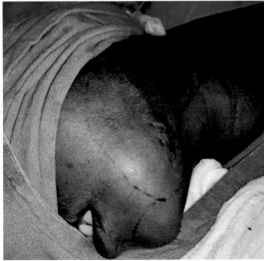

(a)

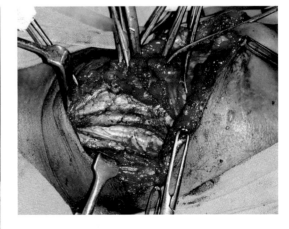

(b)

Figure 8.8 (a) Growth of buccal mucosa involving the alveolus and skin. (b) Modified radical neck dissection performed. (c) Soft tissue dissection during excision. (d) Segmental mandibulectomy performed. (e) Harvesting the free fibula flap. (f) Free fibular flap ready for placement. (g) Soft tissue and bony defect is reconstructed.

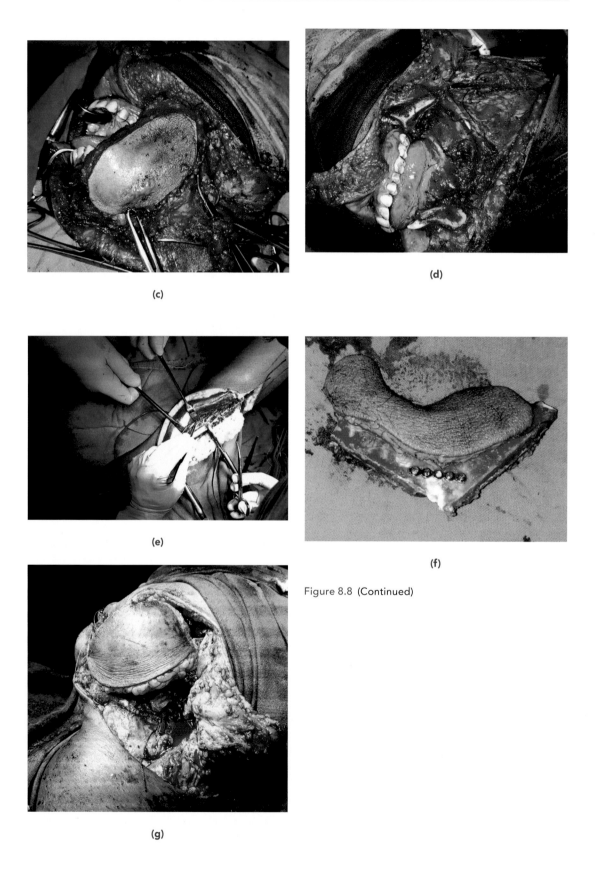

(c)

(d)

(e)

(f)

Figure 8.8 (Continued)

(g)

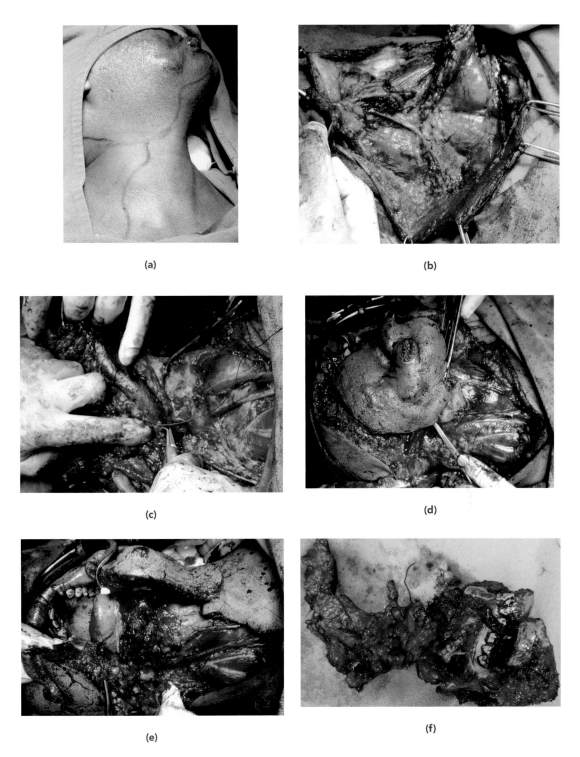

Figure 8.9 (a) Incision planned for lip split and neck dissection. (b) Level V dissection is performed. (c) Levels II, III, IV are dissected along with the internal jugular vein. (d) Carcinoma cheek involving the facial skin, lower alveolus and floor of mouth in the oral cavity. (e) Surgical defect after composite resection. (f) Surgical specimen after composite resection (segmental mandibulectomy with modified radical neck dissection). (g) Pectoralis major myocutaneous and deltopectoral flaps raised to reconstruct. (h) Flaps sutured to reconstruct the inner and outer surface of cheek and skin graft applied to the donor site.

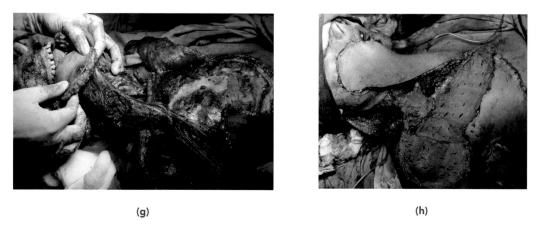

(g)   (h)

Figure 8.9 (Continued)

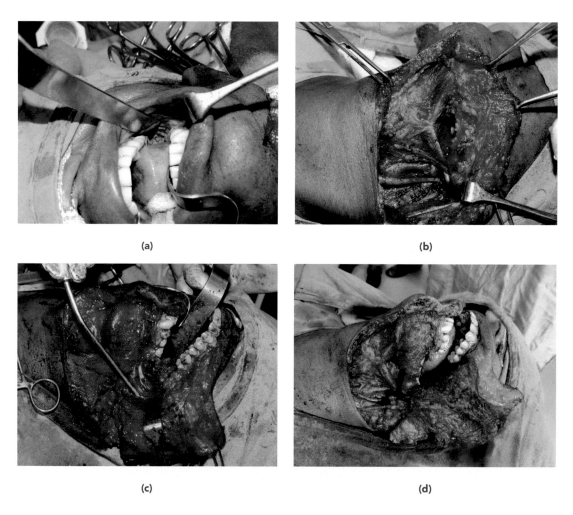

(a)   (b)

(c)   (d)

Figure 8.10 (a) Carcinoma buccal mucosa abutting the left lower mandible. (b) Supra-omohyoid neck dissection is performed with an N0 neck. (c) Left buccal mucosa primary resected with curvilinear cut is made on the mandible to perform a marginal mandibulectomy. (d) Marginal mandibulectomy is completed. (e) Reconstruction performed with PMMC. (f) Final closure after reconstruction.

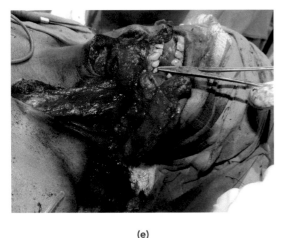

(e)

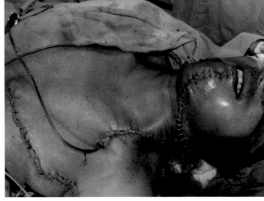

(f)

Figure 8.10 (Continued)

Resection of Primary Carcinoma Oral Cavity Involving Upper Alveolus

- Lesions limited to upper alveolus clinically and radiologically can be excised via the peroral approach.
- A CT scan will delineate the disease as well as accurately indicate any bony erosion.
- Consultation for a dental prosthesis, if planned, has to be taken prior to the surgery.
- Electrosurgery is preferred to make the incision around the growth with at least 1 cm margin of normal mucosa.
- Periosteal elevators are used to elevate the soft tissue. A powered saw is used to make the bone cuts accurately. Alternatively, a drill, osteotomes and a Kerrison rongeur may be used for the same purpose.
- Bony cuts on the hard palate lateral maxillary wall are completed before the posterior separation behind the maxillary tubercle. Posterior separation may require a heavy scissors to separate the muscular attachments. At this juncture, maxillary antrum may be seen because of defect on the floor.
- The maxillary sinus mucosa should be curetted and skin graft should be applied. This mucosa, if left, may hypertrophy and cause the patient the odd taste of maxillary sinus secretions. Cavity is packed with medicated ribbon gauze or Jelonet Paraffin gauze dressing so as to keep the skin graft in contact with the tissues in the surgical defect.
- The dental prosthesis (prepared beforehand) is now applied.

Resection of Carcinoma Buccal Mucosa Abutting/Involving Both Upper and Lower Alveoli

- Extensive lesions involving the buccal mucosa as well as both the alveoli are not amenable for peroral resection. Moreover, invasion of skin is more likely to occur in such lesions.
- The incision is planned carefully and involvement of the skin of the cheek is taken into account. Incision is deepened to leave the growth attached to the bones of upper and lower alveolus.
- Marginal or segmental mandibulectomy is performed as described earlier. Cuts on the mandible are extended to include the retromolar trigone if it is involved.
- Upper alveolar resection is performed as described previously.
- The specimen is resected in toto.
- An appropriate neck dissection is performed before or after the resection of oral carcinoma.
- This resultant defect, which is likely to be quite large, is closed using regional or microvascular free flap (see Figures 8.11a through Figure 8.11g).

FROZEN SECTION AND HISTOPATHOLOGICAL ANALYSIS

Intraoperative frozen section should be obtained wherever available. However, surgery may be done even if it is not available. The frozen section

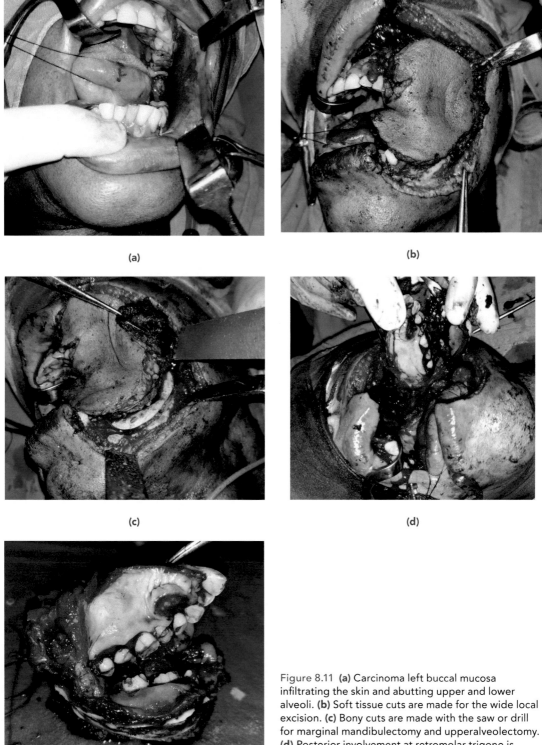

(a)

(b)

(c)

(d)

(e)

Figure 8.11 (a) Carcinoma left buccal mucosa infiltrating the skin and abutting upper and lower alveoli. (b) Soft tissue cuts are made for the wide local excision. (c) Bony cuts are made with the saw or drill for marginal mandibulectomy and upperalveolectomy. (d) Posterior involvement at retromolar trigone is dissected. (e) Specimen after complete excision. (f) The resulting large defect. (g) Reconstruction done by using PMMC flap on inside and DP flap on outside.

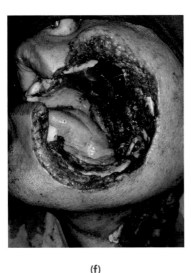

(f)

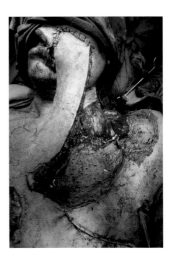

(g)

Figure 8.11 (Continued)

analysis may help in typifying the malignancy, but in oral carcinomas it is more commonly used to determine the adequacy of surgical margins. The specimen for the frozen section analysis is preferably obtained from the surgical defect with a surgical knife, though it can be taken from the resected specimen. Apart from determining the adequacy of surgical margins, no other histopathological parameter can be obtained by this technique. Yet, the histopathological analysis still must be meticulously performed so as to determine the depth of invasion, lymphovascular and perineural spread. The frozen section specimen is sent dry, whereas the specimen for histopathology is sent in formalin.

POST-OPERATIVE CARE AND COMMON COMPLICATIONS

- Peri-operative antibiotic coverage is very helpful in controlling infection. For clean surgery, a third-generation cephalosporin like ceftriaxone is used. However, an aminoglycoside like amikacin must be added in clean contaminated surgeries.
- In the immediate post-operative period, for patients undergoing extensive oral cavity resections, adequate precautions are taken to prevent airway compromise.
- Some patients who undergo resection of the oral cancer may also undergo a peri-operative

tracheostomy, whenever post-operative oedema is anticipated. The ward staff should be very thorough in performing tracheostomy care. Decannulation should be performed once the oedema subsides.
- Maintenance of oral hygiene is pertinent to obtain good results. This may be difficult to achieve, as the mouth opening is very poor in a large number of patients. Apart from antiseptic gargles, a gauze or cotton swab dipped in antiseptic solution like chlorhexidine is used to frequently clear the retained secretions, blood and food.
- Oral intake in the immediate post-operative period is expected to be inadequate. Intake/output charts should be maintained. Any deficiency in oral intake should be compensated by IV fluids. If the condition of the patient does not permit oral nutrition, then a feeding tube must be inserted.
- Suction drains should be frequently checked in the post-operative period for patency and maintenance of negative pressure. The fluid chamber should be emptied every 24 hours and the volume of drainage documented. The drains are removed once the volume obtained is less than around 20 ml in 24 hours.
- Good peri-operative care goes a long way in optimising the healing process, preventing infection and forming oro-cutaneous fistulae.

9

Salivary Glands Tumour Surgery

NITIN M NAGARKAR AND RIPU DAMAN ARORA

INTRODUCTION

There are major and minor salivary glands in the head and neck region.

1. Major salivary glands: parotid, submandibular and sublingual.
2. Minor salivary glands: 600–1000 small glands distributed throughout the upper aerodigestive tract.

Salivary gland neoplasms are relatively rare and contribute to approximately 6% of head and neck tumours. Pleomorphic adenoma is the commonest tumour of major salivary glands. Parotid gland tumour contributes about 80% of these tumours and consists mainly of pleomorphic adenoma while mucoepidermoid carcinoma, warthin tumour and carcinoma ex pleomorphic adenoma contribute less than 20%.

The submandibular gland contributes about 10–15% of salivary gland tumours with pleomorphic adenoma predominance. Rest are contributed by minor salivary glands where malignant tumour dominate instead of pleomorphic adenoma.

The salivary gland tumours have following specific characteristics features as compared to other head and neck tumours:

- Variable and diverse histological appearance, making it difficult to distinguish on FNAC between benign and malignant tumours.
- Most common tumour is pleomorphic adenoma, which has premalignant potential

- Tumours have indolent growth pattern but high frequency to recur.
- Can reoccur after several years of disease-free survival.

PAROTID SURGERY

Indications

- Parotid neoplasm – parotidectomy done for both treatment and diagnosis.
- Chronic parotitis – refractory to medical management and unsuccessful sialoendoscopy.
- Resection of lymph nodes at risk of malignancy ex-skin melanoma, SSC of pre-auricular area, etc.

Contraindications

- Comorbidities for general anaesthesia.
- Nonresectable or extensive tumour of parotid gland.

Pre-Operative Evaluation

- Imaging (US/CT scan and MRI)
  - To confirm the location.
  - Relationship between lump and retromandibular nerve.
  - Location in superficial or deep lobe.
  - Better evaluation of third dimension of tumour.
  - Features suggestive of malignancy – central necrosis, infiltration of adjacent structures and cervical lymphadenopathy.

DOI: 10.1201/9780367430139-9

- MRI gives better definition between tumour and surrounding tissue.
- FNAC – best done with ultrasound guidance for the great majority of cases.
- Biopsy – avoided due to risk of tumour implantation except in lymphoma.
  - Diffuse salivary enlargement – Sjogren's, sarcoidosis and other granulomatous disorders.

Classification of Parotid Gland Surgery

- **Superficial parotidectomy:** Removal of parotid gland superficial to the facial nerve; it is the most common type of parotid surgery.
- **Total conservative parotidectomy:** Removal of the entire gland (i.e., superficial and deep lobes) while preserving the facial nerve branches.
- **Total or radical parotidectomy:** Removal of the entire gland along with the involved facial nerve.
- **Extended radical parotidectomy:** Removal of other surrounding structures like skin, mandible and external auditory canal.
- **Partial or adequate parotidectomy:** Excision of the tumour with a cuff of normal parotid tissue. It is generally performed for small, benign lesions in the tail of the parotid.

Operative Steps

- **Anaesthesia**
  - General anaesthesia
  - Muscle relaxants should be avoided to allow optimal nerve monitoring, if need be
- **Antibiotic Prophylaxis**
  - Case is usually clean, but the interruption and retention of salivary tissue may create an environment for bacterial sialadenitis to develop.
  - In chronic sialadenitis, antibiotics should be considered for 5–7 days.
  - Amoxicillin-clavulanic acid or first-generation cephalosporin is usually administered.
- **Positioning**
  - Patient is positioned on his or her back and the face is turned 180° to the side opposite the lesion.
  - The head and neck are placed in hyperextension by putting a folded drape on the side of the shoulder and a neck roll.

- **Operative Preparation and Draping**
  - Infiltrate with vasoconstrictor along planned skin incision to reduce thermal injury to skin from electrocautery to skin vessels.
  - Prepare skin using 10% povidone iodine.
  - Head drape: Place towels so the ear, mastoid tip and sternocleidomastoid muscle are well exposed.
  - Keep corner of eye and mouth exposed to see facial movement when facial nerve mechanically or electrically stimulated.
- **Incision**
  - **Modified Blair's incision** – most adopted incision. It begins from root of helix in front of the tragus in the preauricular crease extending along the lobule and curving anteriorly to join a neck crease approximately two fingerbreadths below the mandible at the level of the hyoid (see Figure 9.1a through Figure 9.1c).
  - **Rhytidectomy or facelift incision** – this incision allows better cosmesis. It extends along the hairline, allowing the entire superficial musculoaponeurotic system (SMAS) flap to be raised anteriorly.
  - In case of overlying skin involvement, both the incisions are modified so as to remove the infiltrated skin with tumour.
- **Elevation of Skin Flap**
  - After incision the skin is carefully elevated off the tragal cartilage using fine skin hooks and a no. 15 scalpel blade.
  - Alternatively, a fine needle tip electrocautery can be used for the skin incision.
  - An anteriorly placed superficial cervicofacial flap is raised up to the anterior border of the parotid gland in the plane between the SMAS and the parotid fascia.
  - In the neck, subplatysmal flap is raised.
- **Identification of Great Auricular Nerve**
  - Identify the great auricular nerve (GAN) and the external jugular vein (EJV) at the anterior border of sternocleidomastoid muscle (Figure 9.2).
  - The posterior branch of the GAN is dissected toward the earlobe and must be preserved, as it could potentially be used as a cable graft in case of resection of the facial nerve.

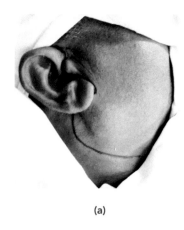

(a)

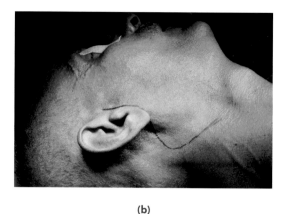

(b)

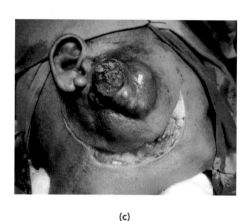

(c)

Figure 9.1 **(a)** Modified Blair's incision. **(b-c)** Modifications of lower limb according to the extent of lesion.

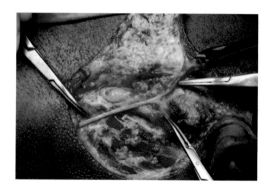

Figure 9.2 Greater auricular nerve with anterior and posterior branch.

- The greater auricular nerve occasionally needs to be sectioned in order to mobilise the parotid gland off the sternocleidomastoid muscle.
- The anterior branch of the GAN is divided.
- **Separate Parotid Gland from Sternocleidomastoid**
  - o The anterior border of SCM is skeletonised and separated from the parotid gland.
  - o The posterior belly of the digastric muscle is identified by retracting the parotid gland superiorly.
- **Mobilisation of Parotid in Preparation for Facial Trunk Identification and Dissection**
  - o Place 2–0 silk "stay sutures" into earlobe for posterior retraction and into the cheek flap for anterior retraction.
  - o Identify and skeletonise the posterior belly of the digastric muscle. Do not dissect cephalad of the muscle injury of the facial nerve can result.

- o The parotid gland tissue is then elevated off the cartilage of the external auditory canal up to the tragal pointer.
- o The mastoid tip should be skeletonised up to the depth of the tragal pointer.
- **Identification of Landmarks for Facial Nerve**
  - Tragal pointer: The facial nerve is 1 cm deep and inferior. This relationship may be altered by the presence of tumour, previous surgery or infection.
    - o It points to the facial nerve in only 20% of cases.
  - Tympanic ring.
  - Tympanomastoid suture line-facial nerve is 6–8 mm deep to the tympanomastoid suture that is situated at the apex of vagino-mastoid angle.

- Posterior belly of digastric muscle is the most used landmark (Figures 9.3a and 9.3b).
  - Facial nerve is identified at the same depth, just superior to muscle as the nerve exits the stylomastoid foramen.
  - In this location, the facial venous plexus lies just above the nerve. In case of inadvertent injury and bleeding, application of local pressure may suffice to control the bleeding.
- Styloid process: The facial nerve lies in the angle between the styloid and digastric, and crosses the styloid.
- Two deep right-angled retractors are used to gently retract the parotid gland in an anterior direction so that the parotid tissue overlying the main trunk of the facial nerve is stretched.

- A long and curved dissection heamostat forceps is used to gently spread the parotid tissue in this region along the direction of the nerve. This part of the dissection should be carried out in small increments, ensuring haemostasis before the next tissue plane is dissected.
- **Dissect Facial Nerve from Parotid Gland (Figures 9.3b, 9.4a and 9.4b)**
  - Identify the pes anserinus, then trace the upper and lower divisions of the facial nerve anteriorly.
  - Use fine curved blunt-tipped scissors for the remainder of the nerve dissection. Tunnel and spread the tissues overlying the facial nerve and its branches and divide the parotid tissue overlying the nerve.

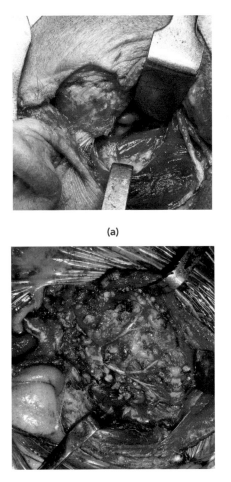

(a)

(b)

Figure 9.3a and 9.3b Landmarks for facial nerve.

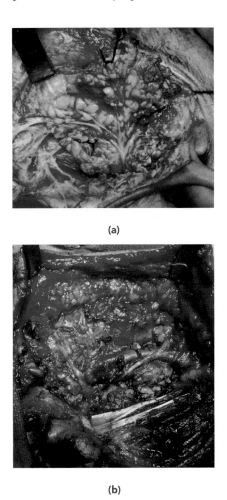

(a)

(b)

Figure 9.4a and 9.4b Identification of branches of facial nerve.

- It is important to dissect directly on the nerve so as not to lose sight of it. Never divide parotid tissue beyond exposed facial nerve.
- Divide the parotid fascia and parotid tissue superiorly and inferiorly to release the parotid posteriorly and to permit anterior mobilisation of the gland/tumour.
- Dissect carefully along each branch and strip the superficial lobe off the branches of the facial nerve.
- Identify the retromandibular vein as it crosses medial to the facial nerve.
- Tumour with a cuff of the superficial parotid lobe is removed.
- Completed superficial parotidectomy. The nerve is seen related superficially to the retromandibular vein (Figure 9.4b).
- Retrograde approach.
  - o A retrograde approach involves identification of the branches of the facial nerve and then following them to identify the main trunk.
  - o This approach is not recommended routinely. However, it can be used in large tumours which are impinging on the stylomastoid foramen.

Total Parotidectomy for Deep Lobe Tumour

- Taking care to avoid unnecessary traction on the nerve, identify, dissect and circumferentially free up the facial nerve from the underlying deep lobe or tumour to provide access to the deep lobe.
- A superficial parotidectomy can be done, or the superficial lobe can simply be reflected anteriorly, keeping the parotid duct intact and replacing it at the end of the surgery (Figure 9.5).
- The retromandibular vein and the external carotid artery may need ligation just above the lower border of the mandible (Figure 9.6).
- If the deep lobe tumour extends to the parapharyngeal space, it can be freed using blunt dissection. If necessary, the stylomandibular ligament can be divided to improve access to the tumour.

Management of the Facial Nerve

- If the facial nerve is encased within the malignant tumour and there is pre-existing facial paresis or palsy, it should be resected with negative margins, both proximally and distally, followed by appropriate reconstruction.
- If the facial nerve function is intact pre-operatively, an attempt must be made to structurally preserve the nerve, if oncological margins permit.

Facial Nerve Reconstruction (Figures 9.7a and 9.7b)

- If structurally intact, observe.
- If transected, do end-to-end anastomosis.
- If primary anastomosis is not possible, interposition or cable graft (greater auricular nerve, sural nerve and ansa hypoglossi) must be considered.

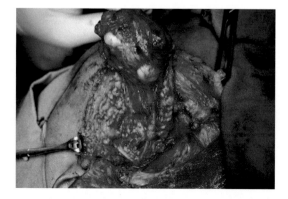

Figure 9.5 Retracted superficial lobe of parotid.

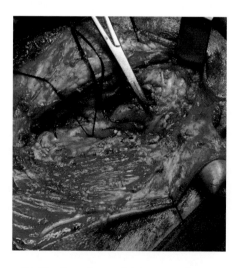

Figure 9.6 Ligation of superficial temporal artery.

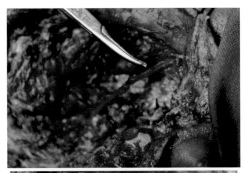
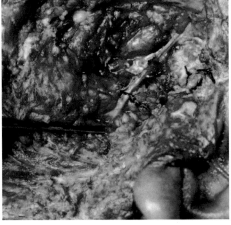

Figure 9.7a and 9.7b End-to-end of facial nerve branch.

- If the proximal stump is inadequate, hypoglossal facial anastomosis or a cross facial nerve graft must be considered.
- Muscle transfer is considered, if no proximal stump of facial nerve is available.

Reconstruction

- It may be required if there is loss of skin or resection of the mandible. A cervical rotation flap may be attempted for skin defects. Other options include submental flap, a pectoralis major, myocutaneous flap or a free flap (Figure 9.8).

Lymphadenectomy

- Neck dissection may be considered for T3 and T4 tumours.
- Size greater than 4 cm.
- High-grade tumours.
- Extraparenchymal spread.

Wound Closure

- Obtain meticulous haemostasis: Use ties and bipolar electrosurgery.
- Employ a sealed suction drain until drainage <25 ml/24 hours.
- For skin closure, use subcutaneous and subcuticular absorbable sutures.

Post-Operative Care
Suction Drain Management

- The suction drain is left in for 36 hours minimum.
- General rule: Remove drain only after three consecutive eight-hour shifts demonstrate less than 25 cc total output.
- Suture removal is usually done after sixth-seventh day depending on the wound healing

Complications
Cosmetic problems (Figure 9.9)

- Surgical depression caused by removal of the parotid gland. This depression also decreases with time, but does not disappear entirely.
- A superiorly or inferiorly based sternomastoid flap has been proposed to reconstruct the hollow cavity after parotidectomy.
- Skin-flap necrosis is rare and is usually located in the distal tip of the post-auricular skin flap.

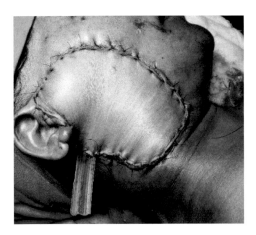

Figure 9.8 Reconstruction of surgical defect with flap after radical parotid surgery.

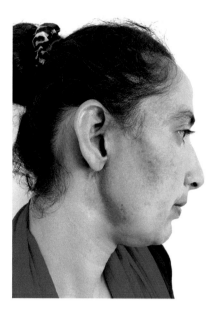

Figure 9.9 Cosmetically well-healed modified Blair incision used in Figure 9.1a.

- Care must be taken in designing the parotid flap to avoid curving too far posteriorly, to avoid this complication.
- Hypoesthesia of greater auricular nerve
  - The area of numbness will improve within one year of the operation, but a small area of skin may remain anaesthetised.
- Facial palsy
  - Temporary facial nerve palsy may be seen in 10–50% of cases, while permanent palsy may occur in up to 5% of the cases.
  - Nerve paresis most commonly affects the marginal mandibular branch.
  - Recovery is generally seen within 6–12 months.
- Gustatory sweating (Frey's syndrome)
  - Aberrant innervation of cutaneous sweat glands overlying the parotid by postganglionic parasympathetic salivary nerves results in localised sweating during eating or salivation.
  - It can develop within weeks to months after parotidectomy.
  - It can be prevented by raising a thick skin flap, rotating a superficial temporal artery-based temporoparietal flap, rotation of the sternocleidomastoid muscle or rotating a portion of the SMAS.
  - Various interventions may be employed, like topical application of antiperspirants;

injection of botulinum toxin and surgical implantation of materials like silicon sheet or acellular dermis may rarely be required.
- Salivary leakage
  - The raw gland surface can result in a collection of saliva below the skin or leakage of saliva from the wound.
  - Conservative measures include drainage of sialocele with pressure dressings. Glycopyrrolate can be used to decrease salivary secretions. Botulinum toxin has also been used in this setting.
  - Extensive salivary leakage may require surgical reexploration.
- Infection
  - Infection is rare following parotidectomy and is avoided by using an aseptic technique and antibiotic prophylaxis. Treatment of infection consists of drainage and wide-spectrum antibiotics.

SUBMANDIBULAR GLAND SURGERY

Clinical Examination

- Bimanual examination for calculi in duct and confirmation of submandibular gland tumour.
- Rule out fixity to mandible.
- Examine tongue for any paralysis due to hypoglossal nerve invasion and loss of taste or general sensation due to lingual nerve invasion.
- Trismus favour invasion of mandibular depressor muscles.
- Check for any node.

Pre-Operative Evaluation

Imaging (US/CT Scan and MRI)

Ultrasound is the investigation of choice for submandibular gland diseases. However, malignant tumours require CT scan for better characterisation for the following reasons.

- To confirm the location and probable diagnosis.
- Better evaluation of dimensions of tumour.
- To show features suggestive of malignancy – central necrosis, infiltration of adjacent structures and cervical lymphadenopathy.

- MRI gives better definition between tumour and surrounding tissue.

Fine needle aspiration (FNAC) is done in the majority of cases and best done with ultrasound guidance for the great majority of cases.

Indications

- Submandibular gland tumour.
- Sublingual/minor gland tumour.
- Chronic sialoadenitis.
- As a part of neck dissection.
- Large plunging ranula.
- Large calculi of submandibular duct or gland.

Anaesthetic Considerations

- Trismus requires fibre-optic intubation.
- Wide surgical resection, like composite resection, requires reinforced endotracheal tubes.
- Elective tracheostomy is planned in major resections for better post-operative outcome.

Surgical Technique

- About 4–5 cm horizontal incision is marked about two fingerbreadths (5–6 cm) below the lower border of mandible.
- Lignocaine (1% or 2%) or saline with adrenaline (1:1,00,000 or 1:2,00,000) is infiltrated in surgical field.
- Skin incision is made with knife while platysma is cut with low-intensity monopolar electrocautery.
- Sub-platysmal flap is raised with sharp dissection or electrocautery up to lower border of mandible. Electrocautery should be used carefully in low-power mode and when looking for marginal mandibular nerve.
- This nerve runs in the fascial plane and can be saved by ligating the facial vein and performing the dissection below it in the subfacial planes. However, this step should be avoided in malignant diseases or when performing the excision as a part of neck dissection.
- The marginal mandibular nerve should be identified. It lies over the submandibular gland in the fascia, and is dissected and saved by putting in loose suture to hang it from

the platysma (see Chapter 16, Figure 16.11). Sometimes identification is difficult, and this is where a nerve monitoring system is useful. Rarely, in large metastatic facial lymph node dissection, one may proceed without its identification.

- The lower pole of the submandibular is grasped, dissected and retracted cephalic, exposing anterior and posterior bellies of digastric.
- The facial artery is identified as it enters the gland postero-superiorly just below the posterior belly of digastric at the level of angle of mandible. This artery is secured, ligated and divided, unless it is to be saved if any local flap (nasolabial, mucosal-muscular buccal flap) is planned (see Chapter 16, Figure 16.12).
- The specimen is retracted antero-inferiorly and dissected from the lower margin of ramus, ligating and dividing retromandibular vein with its tributaries as they exit parotid gland inferiorly.
- As dissection proceeds anteriorly, facial vessels are encountered again and must be ligated and divided.
- Dissection proceeds further anteriorly below ramus with bipolar tongs and fascia along with associated tissue over mylohyoid muscle is dissected exposing posterior border of mylohyoid. The mylohyoid artery and its branches must be coagulated satisfactorily, otherwise haemorrhage ensues, which delays further dissection.
- Now the mylohyoid muscle is retracted antero-superiorly while the submandibular specimen is retracted inferiorly, thereby bringing into view the lingual nerve with submandibular ganglion (see Chapter 16, Figure 16.13). The submandibular gland specimen is retracted superiorly to dissect it over the hyoglossus, which also exposes the hypoglossus, nerve as it lies over this muscle (see Chapter 16, Figure 16.14).
- Once the hypoglossal nerve is identified, specimen and mylohyoid are again retracted inferiorly and antero-superiorly, respectively, to expose the lingual nerve. Wharton's duct is identified and dissected to the floor of mouth and cut with bipolar tongs at 10–12W. A vein runs with the duct and needs to be coagulated carefully, otherwise troublesome haemorrhage

occur later. Now the lingual nerve and ganglion is divided with bipolar tongs while avoiding injury to lingual nerve.

- Specimen is delivered and marked.
- Complete haemostasis is achieved.
- Mini drain or glove drain is kept and incision closed in layers.

Post-Operative Care

- Antibiotic and pain are managed as per protocol.
- Oral feeding is started once intestinal movements return.
- Drain is removed after 1–2 days when drain becomes negligible.
- Sutures/staples are removed after 5–7 days.

Operative Complications

- Haemorrhage: Facial vessels causing haemorrhage – a loose knot or clip can be dangerous in the post-operative period as any collection in the submandibular fossa will cause respiratory obstruction. These vessels should be ligated carefully.
- Marginal mandibular nerve injury usually occurs due to failure to identify the nerve. Patients with paresis usually recover after few months and this doesn't require any specific intervention.
- Hypoglossal nerve injury is rare but not unusual, especially with inexperienced surgeons who use electrocautery in high-power mode during dissection. Anatomical injury can be managed by primary repair or nerve graft.

10

Oropharyngeal Tumour Surgery

SMRITI PANDA AND HITESH VERMA

INTRODUCTION

The oropharynx is part of the upper aero-digestive tract juxtaposed between the nasopharynx and the hypopharynx. In the craniocaudal axis it extends from the hard palate superiorly to the tip of the epiglottis inferiorly. Its anterior limit is the faucial pillar formed by the palatoglossus muscles. Posteriorly it is bound by the buccopharyngeal fascia anterior to the alar space. Neoplasms arising from the oropharynx can be divided into those arising from its epithelial lining and those with a mesenchymal origin. The former can originate either from the squamous epithelium, typically a squamous cell carcinoma, or from the minor salivary glands. Tumours derived from mesenchymal tissues range from benign lesions like lipoma, schwannoma or leiomyoma to tumours of malignant potential like teratoma, rhabdomyosarcoma or mucosal melanoma. While upfront surgery forms the mainstay of treatment for benign mesenchymal tumours, minor salivary gland tumours and a few sarcomas, management strategies for squamous cell carcinoma by radiation or chemoradiation are often part of the contemporary standard of care. The oropharynx is one of the few subsites in the head and neck where surgical techniques have been heavily influenced by technological advancements. Advancements in the field of laser and robotics, along with the discovery of the association with human papillomavirus, has created a resurgence in the field of surgical management of oropharyngeal cancers. Even though the focus of the current literature is on minimally invasive techniques, it is essential to understand the conventional open approaches to the oropharynx as well.

CLASSIFICATION OF APPROACHES TO THE OROPHARYNX

1. **Conventional Approach**
   a. Transoral
   b. Paramedian mandibulotomy or mandibular swing
   c. Midline labiomandibular glossotomy
   d. Lateral pharyngotomy
   e. Suprahyoid pharyngotomy
   f. Lower cheek flap with segmental mandibulectomy
   g. Lingual release and pull-through
2. **Minimally Invasive Approach**
   a. Transoral laser microsurgery (TOLM)
   b. Transoral robotic surgery (TORS)
   c. Transoral endoscopic ultrasonic surgery (TOUSS)

INVESTIGATIONS FOR OROPHARYNGEAL TUMOUR

Preliminary work-up for a patient presenting with an oropharyngeal mass can be divided into detailed head and neck examination and radiological, pathological and metastatic screening.

Clinical Examination

Important information can be garnered right at this step, even before radiology. Presence of

DOI: 10.1201/9780367430139-10

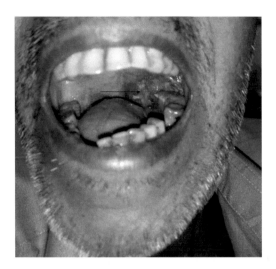

Figure 10.1 Clinical examination showing ulcero-infiltrative growth arising from the oropharynx, involving tonsil, soft palate and retromolar trigone with restricted mouth opening.

surface ulceration and induration points towards a malignant etiology (Figure 10.1). A smooth, mucosa-covered mass is oftentimes benign or originating in the submucosal minor salivary glands. Pulsatility of the mass hints towards a vascular

origin, mandating appropriate radiology before embarking on histopathological sampling. Clinical examination in white light can be supplemented with flexible in-office endoscopy equipped with narrow-band imaging (NBI) for detailed mapping of the tumour and identifying surrounding pre-malignant lesions (Figure 10.2). Certain factors at this stage can assist in decision making regarding the appropriate surgical approach. Presence of trismus (inter-incisor distance less than 2.5 cm), protuberant central incisors, mandibular tori, bulky tongue, limited neck extension and deeply infiltrative tumour (Figure 10.1) are adverse features for a transoral approach.

Radiology

Cross-sectional imaging aims to determine the exact anatomical extent, presence of neck metastasis and relationship with critical neurovascular structures. Both contrast-enhanced computed tomography (CECT) and contrast-enhanced magnetic resonance imaging (CEMRI) offer complementary information (Figure 10.3). In this section, we will discuss the role of radiology in selecting

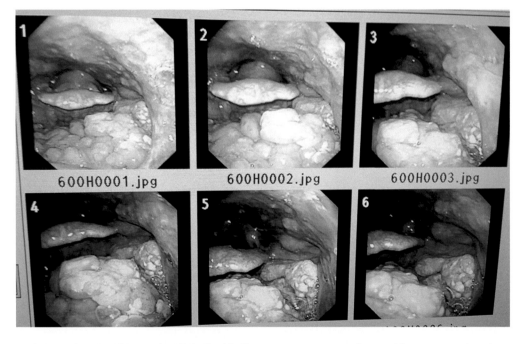

Figure 10.2 Panels 1, 2 and 3 are white-light flexible fibre-optic images revealing proliferative growth in the left side oropharynx involving tonsil, base of tongue, lateral pharyngeal wall and vallecula. Panels 4, 5 and 6 are NBI images showing unhealthy mucosa crossing the midline which was clearly underestimated by white-light examination.

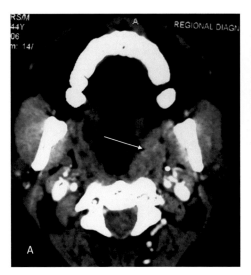 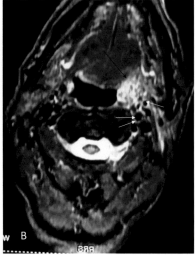

Figure 10.3 (a) CECT showing enhancing soft tissue density in left oropharynx with fat plane between medial pterygoid muscle and great vessels. (b) CEMRI of the same patient shows better soft tissue delineation from terminal branches of ECA (single white arrow) and ICA (double arrows).

the appropriate surgical approach. The following conditions preclude transoral approaches: Tumour infiltrating mandible, invasion of parapharyngeal fat, invasion lateral to the styloid apparatus, involvement of the masticator space, encasement of the carotid system (defined by >270-degree contact with carotids and loss of fat plane) by either tumour or primary, confluence of the primary oropharyngeal tumour and neck node, invasion of extrinsic tongue musculature and tumour involving larynx or requiring sacrifice of both lingual arteries. Additionally, radiology helps to identify anatomical aberrations like retropharyngeal internal carotid artery which if ignored can again jeopardise a minimally invasive approach. Lastly, radiology helps to differentiate a parapharyngeal space mass (paraganglioma, schwannoma) causing oropharyngeal bulge from a true oropharyngeal tumour.

Metastatic Work-Up

Imaging directed to identify distant metastasis is of prime importance whenever a malignant etiology is suspected. For low-grade tumours, small primaries without bulky neck nodes (solitary, <3 cm) and in resource-constrained settings, usually a chest X-ray will suffice. A high-resolution CT of the chest or a non-contrast CT of the chest with lung window also provides acceptable information. The

role of ^{18}F-FDG PET-CT is limited for metastasis screening. Absolute indications would be screening for an unknown primary, high-grade tumours with a propensity for non-pulmonary metastasis (mucosal melanoma) and disease surveillance following radical treatment.

PATHOLOGY

Cross-sectional imaging should always precede biopsy. Biopsy should be from the edge of the tumour with the tumour-host interface adequately sampled. Reporting should be based on the features seen on haematoxylin and eosin (H&E) and supplemented by immunohistochemistry (IHC) whenever required. Current staging system requires IHC information pertaining to p-16, a surrogate marker for human papilloma virus (HPV) in oropharyngeal squamous cell carcinoma.

PRE-OPERATIVE PREPARATION

Pre-operative preparation will be discussed as follows.

1. **Transoral access:** Pre-operative dental evaluation is indicated in case of soft palate tumours where the intent is to rehabilitate with a palatal obturator. The prosthodontics team is provided with exact resection margins to

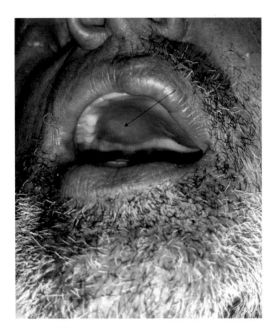

Figure 10.4 Definitive obturator with dental restoration in a patient with palatal defect following maxillectomy and orbital exenteration.

fabricate the impression of the palate followed by designing of the surgical obturator (Figure 10.4). The obturator is also required in cases where reconstruction is performed with a palatal mucoperiosteal rotation flap. This helps in maintaining apposition between the defect and the flap and prevents the formation of a dead space. Prosthodontics consultation is also optional in transoral approaches for other subsites to fabricate a cast for the lower dentition which can be fitted before the application of the mouth gag. This prevents trauma to the tongue and floor of mouth mucosa from prolonged use of a mouth gag.

2. **Mandibulotomy:** An orthopantomogram should be obtained before a mandibulotomy. This provides a reference with respect to the mandibular height. Also, the osteotomy site can be pre-planned based on the divergence of the tooth roots.

3. **Assessing risk of aspiration:** Surgeries of the oropharynx can be associated with a significant risk of post-operative swallowing disability. Micro-aspiration needs to be documented pre-operatively with FEES (Functional Endoscopic Evaluation of Swallowing+/-Sensory Testing) or with MBS (Modified Barium Swallow). Pre-existing COPD and other pulmonary pathology can compromise post-operative recovery should aspiration develop following surgery. Pulmonary function tests (FEV1/FVC) and assessing the ability of a patient to climb two flights of stairs should be a part of the routine assessment.

4. **Pre-Anaesthetic:** To facilitate nasotracheal intubation, pre-operative nasal decongestion and topical anaesthesia should be administered in the patient hold-up area.

ANAESTHESIA CONCERNS

Due to the inherent problem of airway sharing, surgery for oropharyngeal tumours requires dedicated efforts from the anaesthesia team. All oropharyngeal procedures are to be performed under nasotracheal intubation. Awake fibre-optic intubation is now considered state of the art for the same. Tracheostomy is generally reserved as the last resort for failed nasotracheal intubation or highly vascular tumours and those completely obscuring the view of the endolarynx.

SPECIAL CONSIDERATIONS FOR TOLM

Intubation is performed with a laser-safe endotracheal tube. Commercially available laser-compatible tubes consist of two cuffs: The superior one inflated with methylene blue and the inferior one inflated with saline. Non-flammable gases are generally preferred. Whenever the expertise is available, total intravenous anaesthesia (TIVA) should be considered. Fi02 (percentage of inhalational oxygen) should be kept at 30%. In case of an airway fire, all inhalational circuits are to be disconnected, the burnt endotracheal tube should be removed, the upper airway should be thoroughly irrigated, the patient re-intubated with a new tube, and the endoscopy assessed for damage.

SPECIAL CONSIDERATION FOR TORS/TOUSS

Since the head end of the patient is occupied by the robotic arms or the flexible endo-eye of the TOUSS, the endotracheal tube as well as the anaesthetic circuit must be shifted to the foot end of the patient. To fulfil the above requirements, specialised endotracheal tubes like north-facing RAE (Ring Adair Elwin) are utilised. The other alternative is nasal intubation with an armoured flexometallic tube.

SURGICAL APPROACHES TO THE OROPHARYNX: TECHNICAL CONSIDERATION

Conventional transoral access

Transoral approach for the oropharynx without the utilisation of specialised equipment like TORS/TOLM/TOUSS has very limited scope.

Indications

1. Tumours arising from the soft palate, tonsil, posterior pharyngeal wall, the base of tongue.
2. The entire circumference of the tumour should be visualised after applying the mouth gag.
3. The tumour should be freely mobile on palpation.
4. Exophytic tumours.

Contraindications

1. Deeply infiltrative tumours.
2. Invasion of the underlying bone, extrinsic muscles of the tongue, the floor of mouth, superior constrictor, buccopharyngeal fascia.

Technique

Exposure of the tumour can be optimised by positioning the patient with a sand-bag under the shoulders causing extension at the cervico-thoracic joint and flexion at the atlanto-axial joint. Mouth gags used for transoral access are Boyle Davis, Crowe Davis, Jennings and Dingman. Boyle Davis, Crowe Davis and Dingman have an in-built tongue depressor which the Jennings mouth gag lacks (Figure 10.5). The Dingman mouth gag has additional attachments for cheek retraction. Principles of transoral excision of a tonsillar tumour are similar to a routine tonsillectomy. Radical tonsillectomy preferably should not be performed with this route. For the base of tongue resection, additional retraction can be achieved by passing 1–0 or 2–0 silk sutures through the base of the tongue.

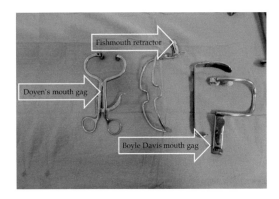

Figure 10.5 Widely used retractors for conventional transoral approach.

Paramedian Mandibulotomy with Mandibular Swing

Indications

1. Tumours of anterior 2/3 tongue extending to the base of tongue.
2. Tonsillar tumours not suitable for TORS/TOUSS/TOLM due to poor exposure (trismus or limited neck extension).
3. Tonsillar tumours with lateral extension into parapharyngeal fat.

Contraindications

1. Tumours requiring either marginal mandibulectomy or segmental mandibulectomy.
2. Edentulous patients with atrophic mandible which will not sustain the stress of mandibular fracture and plating.
3. Tumours following radiation to the mandible may develop osteoradionecrosis after paramedian mandibulotomy.

Technique

The initial steps begin with the elevation of a lower cheek flap using a skin crease incision with lip split. If neck dissection is indicated, the same can be accomplished before the paramedian mandibulotomy. After the lip split, the osteotomy site over the mandible is exposed. The periosteum is scored with monopolar cautery. The site for osteotomy is conventionally between the ipsilateral lateral incisor and canine as the tooth roots generally diverge. The orthopantomogram can also provide guidance to choose the region between the two diverging tooth roots. Paramedian location is chosen as it does not compromise the neuro-vascular structures emerging from the mental foramen. The osteotomy is either performed in step-ladder fashion or following pre-plating. This helps in accurate apposition of the two bone fragments in the end. The mucosal incision is made next in the gingiva-lingual sulcus, preserving at least 5 mm of mucosa over the mandible. The incision is extended till tonsillo-lingual sulcus. The only floor of mouth muscle which requires division is the mylohyoid. The attachments of genioglossus and geniohyoid remain undisturbed. Once the mucosal incision has been completed, the mandible can be swung laterally. To prevent malunion or non-union, it is important to fix the mandible by applying two six-hole mini-plates over the osteotomy site and the under-surface of the mandible.

Median Labio-Mandibular Glossotomy

This approach was first described by Roux and Trotter. Contrary to the previously described paramedian mandibulotomy, this approach utilises the relatively avascular plane in the midline raphe of the tongue. Therefore, a midline mandibulotomy is performed.

Indications

1. Tumours originating from the soft palate, the base of tongue and posterior pharyngeal wall.
2. Midline tumours of the oropharynx not suitable for transoral excision.
3. Extended applications include procedures for clivus, upper cervical vertebra and the cervicomedullary junction.

Contraindications

1. Previous radiation to the mandible.
2. Edentulous mandible.

Technique

In the original description of this procedure, a pre-operative tracheostomy was mandatory. It also involved the extraction of the mandibular incisor to facilitate osteotomy. The tongue is split in the midline through avascular midline raphe. The tumour is exposed by retracting the two ends of the mandible

as well as the two halves of the tongue. Since the attachments of genial tubercle are disturbed, during closure geniohyoid and genioglossus muscles need to be reapproximated at the midline by drilling holes and passing non-absorbable sutures.

Lateral Pharyngotomy

Indications

1. Tumours of the base of tongue, vallecula and lateral pharyngeal wall.
2. Favourable for inferiorly located tumours.
3. Unlike mandibulotomy, this approach is suitable for post-radiation salvage.

Contraindications

1. Involvement of apex of pyriform sinus.
2. Difficult to approach tumours located high up in the base of tongue, tonsil and soft palate.
3. Extensive contralateral spread.

Technique

Incision chosen for this approach can be a horizontal skin crease at the level of thyroid cartilage or a vertical incision parallel to the anterior border of the sternocleidomastoid. Skin flaps are elevated in the subplatysmal plane, superiorly till the hyoid and inferiorly till the upper border of cricoid. The plane between the carotids and the laryngotracheal complex is dissected. It is essential to carefully preserve the superior laryngeal nerve and artery. Similar to the steps in a total laryngectomy, the inferior constrictor is divided from its attachment on the oblique line. Using a blunt elevator, pyriform sinus mucosa is freed from the thyroid perichondrium. For the inferior access, the pyriform sinus is opened using a vertical incision. The tumour is visualised inferiorly. For the superior access, the incision can be extended to the thyrohyoid membrane.

Suprahyoid Pharyngotomy

See Figure 10.6.

Indications

1. Tumours of the tonsil, lateral pharyngeal wall, the base of tongue and vallecula not amenable to transoral excision.

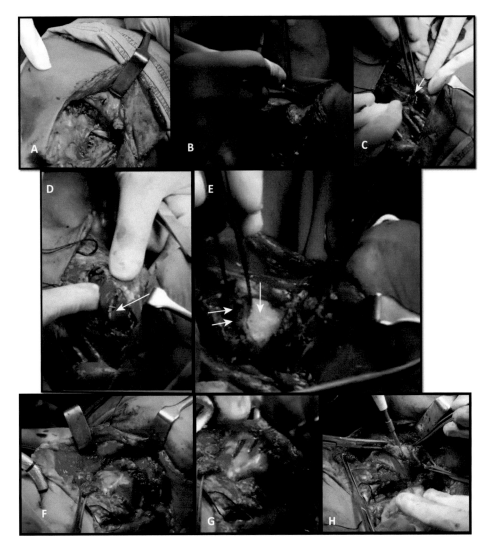

Figure 10.6 Steps involved in suprahyoid pharyngotomy and lateral pharyngotomy in a case of carcinoma at base of tongue. (A) Horizontal skin crease incision used for completion of level 2, 3 and 4 clearance. (B) The same incision is extended, followed by elevation of subplatysmal flap. (C) Mobilisation of the larynx is begun by dissection in the groove between the carotid artery and the larynx is partially devascularised by ligating or applying a clip over the superior laryngeal pedicle (arrow). (D) Superior laryngeal nerve is seen coursing over the thyrohyoid membrane (arrow). (E) Strap muscles (double arrows) are detached from their attachment from the hyoid (Allis forceps). (F) Thyroid cartilage with perichondrium reflected inferiorly. (G and I) Greater cornu of hyoid is divided. (H) Suprahyoid release.

2. There is an overlap of indications with the lateral pharyngotomy approach.
3. Since mandibular resection is not required, post-radiotherapy salvage can be undertaken.

Contraindications

1. Tumours with involvement of the pyriform sinus apex.
2. Pre-epiglottic space involvement.
3. Tumours where excision would require a total

laryngectomy due to either oncological or functional reasons.

Technique

A horizontal skin crease incision is made at the level of the thyrohyoid membrane. Superior exposure is till the base of tongue musculature. The hyoid bone is scored with monopolar cautery. Attachments of suprahyoid muscles are divided from the hyoid,

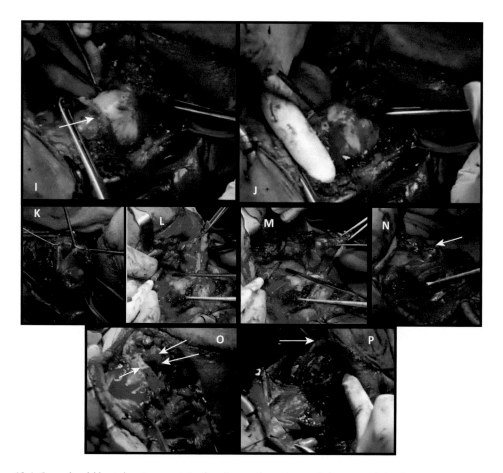

Figure 10.6 Care should be taken to ascertain the disease-free status of the pre-epiglottic space pre-operatively. Hypoglossal nerve and lingual artery (looped in vascular slings) are to be carefully preserved. (J) Thyroid cartilage is incised above the level of the anterior commissure and the vocal cords. (K) Laryngeal entry visualised in a cranio-caudal direction. (L and M) Oropharynx visualised with epiglottis being retracted inferolaterally. (N) Arytenoids are secured to the remnant of thyroid cartilage. (O) Three 1–0 PDS sutures are passed, encompassing thyroid cartilage (single arrow) and base of tongue (double arrow). (P) Final step involves laryngeal suspension to the mandible. Drill holes for this purpose are shown being fashioned in this picture.

taking care not to manipulate beyond the greater cornu. This will prevent traumatising the lingual artery and hypoglossal nerve. The pre-epiglottic space is entered. Once the epiglottis and base of tongue are visualised, the inferior aspect of the base of tongue is grasped with a Babcock forceps. At this stage, the tumour should be well visualised and subsequent excision can be carried out with appropriate margins.

Lingual Release and Pull-Through

This approach is an alternative to mandibulotomy. Indications are similar to mandibulotomy mentioned earlier. The advantage lies in the absence of a facial scar, lip splitting and mandibular osteotomy or plating. As this is a soft tissue approach, prior head and neck irradiation is not a contraindication.

Technique

The incision for this approach is a horizontal skin crease incision from one mastoid tip to another at the level of the hyoid bone. The flap is elevated subplatysmally to the lower border of the mandible, taking care to identify and preserve the marginal mandibular nerve. To completely release the mandible from the overlying soft tissue, the mucosal incision is made over the gingiva-buccal sulcus from one retromolar trigone to another. By connecting the outer skin and inner mucosal incision, one can elevate the skin and soft tissue from over

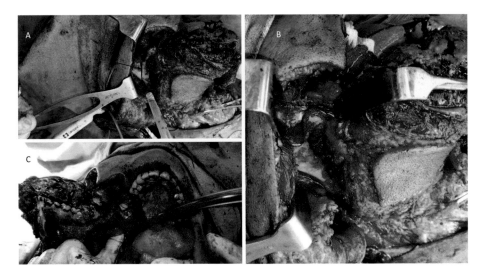

Figure 10.7 Mandibular Resection. A. Osteotomy made in the subcondylar region. B. Arrow points towards the insertion fibres of temporalis muscle which should be resected to prevent post-operative trismus. C. Midline osteotomy completed. Finger placed lateral to the medial pterygoid muscle in an avascular plane.

the mandible. While making the mucosal incision over the gingivobuccal sulcus, it is important to leave a 5 mm cuff of mucosa over the bone to facilitate closure. The approach to this point is known as the visor approach. For the "pull-through", the incision is made over the floor of mouth to deliver the tongue and base of tongue into the neck. Once in the neck, the tumour is visualised and appropriate resection is undertaken.

Mandibular Resection

See Figure 10.7.

Indications

1. Oropharyngeal tumour with frank mandibular invasion: Through and through cortical erosion or medullary invasion.
2. Post-radiation salvage cases where oncological principles mandate a marginal mandibulectomy.

Contraindication

Resection of the mandible for the sake of access in upfront cases.

Technique

A lower cheek flap is the favoured soft tissue approach for a mandibular resection accompanying

oropharyngectomy. A skin crease incision is made together with a lip split. Cheek flap is reflected laterally over the mandible to be resection by incising the mucosa over the gingivobuccal sulcus. If the masticator space is uninvolved, the masseter is preserved and only its attachment with mandible is divided. Coronoidectomy should be included in mandibular resection. This is accomplished by dividing the fibres of temporalis attaching to the coronoid process and the ascending ramus of the mandible. This has profound significance towards achieving adequate mouth opening in the post-operative period. An important structure of concern while working in the masticator space is the internal maxillary artery. The first part is just medial to the neck of the mandible. The second part if medial to the lateral pterygoid muscle. One should carefully identify and ligate this branch. Staying anterior to the styloid process, one can avoid injury to the internal carotid artery.

MINIMALLY INVASIVE APPROACHES

The various approaches that have so far been described have very limited application in the contemporary management of oropharyngeal tumours. Though both surgery and radiation or concurrent chemoradiation are equally advocated for early-stage oropharyngeal tumours, there has been a paradigm shift towards minimally invasive approaches. Minimally invasive techniques

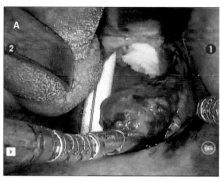
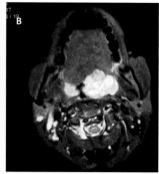
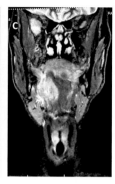

Figure 10.8 A. Pedunculated proliferative tonsillar lesion ideally suited for a minimally invasive transoral approach. B. CEMRI of the same patient showing absence of infiltration of extrinsic tongue musculature. C. CEMRI showing a deeply infiltrative tongue lesion reaching midline, requiring sacrifice of both lingual pedicles. This patient should not be offered a minimally invasive approach. If surgery is planned, reconstruction with a bulky sensate flap is required.

promise to significantly reduce the requirement of nasogastric tube placement, peri-operative tracheostomy, shorter length of hospital stay and in carefully selected cases, offer histopathology stratified treatment intensification or deintensification. However, one should bear in mind that patient selection can make or break the prospect for a minimally invasive approach. The indications can be divided into anatomical/access related, tumour related and patient factors.

Indications and Contraindications

Anatomical

Rich et al. identified eight anatomical factors known as the 8 Ts for TOLM, which can be extended to TORS or TOUSS.

1. Teeth: Protruding central incisors.
2. Trismus: Mouth opening less than 2.5 cm of interincisor distance.
3. Tori: Mandibular or palatal tori significantly hamper transoral access.
4. Tilt: The range of movement at the spine should be adequately assessed, pre-operatively. Presence of cervical spondylolisthesis or kyphoscoliosis is a contraindication.
5. Transverse diameter of the mandible: Reduced transverse diameter of the mandible prevents successful application of mouth gags and retractors.
6. Tongue: A bulky base of tongue can be assessed with a Mallampatti score or from a reduced retroglossal space on fibre-optic

endoscopic evaluation.
7. Treatment: Previous radiation to the head and neck, especially with 2-D planning, can cause significant subdermal and submucosal fibrosis, which can hamper a transoral route.
8. Tumour: This will be covered in the following section.

Tumour-Related

1. A pedunculated proliferative tumour is favoured over an infiltrative tumour (Figure 10.8). The third dimension of a tumour needs to be assessed with MRI. This is important to prevent a positive deep margin.
2. All T4b disease: including the ones where prevertebral fascia is involved.
3. Mobility of the tumour needs to be ascertained during examination under anaesthesia (EUA).
4. Invasion of mandible or infiltration into the parapharyngeal fat.
5. Unresectable nodal disease or retropharyngeal lymphadenopathy with extranodal spread.
6. Distant metastasis: The only possible exception would be an oropharyngeal adenoid cystic carcinoma with pulmonary metastasis.

Vascular

1. Presence of a retropharyngeal internal carotid artery.
2. Tumour adjacent to carotid bulb resulting in its sacrifice of exposure.
3. Any tumour where resection would entail the

sacrifice of both lingual arteries or the hypo-glossal nerve should be avoided.

Functional—rule of 50%, meaning any tumour requiring resection of >50% of the following:

1. Extrinsic tongue musculature or
2. Posterior pharyngeal wall or
3. Tongue base and entire epiglottis.

Patient Factors

1. Poor general condition or multiple comor-bidities: Overall assessment of an individual's general condition can be performed using instruments like ECOG performance status (ECOG PS) or Karnofsky Performance Score (KPS). Generally, radical treatment is under-taken if ECOG PS is greater than 2 or KPS is greater than 70. Assessment for comorbidity can be done using the Charlson Comorbidity Index or the Modified Frailty Score.
2. Risk of bleeding: Patients who have uncon-trolled peri-operative blood pressure or in whom discontinuation of anti-coagulants is deemed unsafe should not be considered for this treatment modality due to high risk of secondary haemorrhage.

TRANSORAL LASER MICROSURGERY

TOLM was introduced in 1990 for laryngeal lesions. Soon centres in Germany extended its utility to oropharyngeal tumours as well. The advantages offered by CO_2 laser (10600 nm) over monopolar cautery are reduced thermal damage, reduced blood loss, better wound healing, preven-tion of collateral damage to uninvolved tissues, and preserving the integrity of the hyo-mandibular complex.

Overview

Using the CO_2 laser in the oropharynx requires greater expertise than using it in the larynx. The straight line of sight offered by the CO_2 laser makes it difficult to manoeuvre in the curved cross-section of the oropharynx, especially the base of tongue. It is ideally suited for soft palate, tonsil and posterior pharyngeal wall tumours. The CO_2 laser can be directed to the area of interest

using a microscope-micromanipulator system (400 mm focal length) or a hand-held system, or in more recent use, a flexible fibre-optic system (OmniGuide) or incorporated into a robotic arm during TORS (Flexible CO_2 laser or Thulium YAG laser). Our preference is to use the CO_2 laser in the ultra-pulse mode with a Surgi-Touch blade. To the best of our knowledge it strikes the right bal-ance for efficient tissue ablation, reduced charring and minimum collateral damage. Apart from the anaesthetic requirements outlined previously, it is important for every person present in the operat-ing room to follow laser safety precautions. Laser safety glasses should be worn by all, except for the surgeon using the microscope. The patient's eyes and exposed skin should be covered with soaking wet gauze. Flammable ointments and adhesives should not be used. A reserve of ice-cold water should be available with the scrub nurse. The oper-ating room should have a laser warning board out-side to prevent unwanted persons from entering the premises.

The principle of TOLM differs in that "tumour transection in situ" is often employed. Small tumours can be resected in toto by taking 3–5 mm mucosal margin in the oropharynx. In the case of larger tumours, sequential small sections are resected in all three dimensions. Few centres rou-tinely employ frozen section confirmation of mar-gin. It is essential to maintain three-dimensional orientation of the resected sections. One technique to do so is to mount the specimen on dehydrated cucumber or corkboard and paint the margin. The wound can be left to heal by secondary intention. Indications for reconstruction will be considered in a separate section.

TRANSORAL ROBOTIC SURGERY

The limitations of TOLM paved the way for TORS. TORS provides three-dimensional binoc-ular visualisation, tremor filtration, 540 degrees of wristed movements and ability to manoeuvre along the contour of difficult-to-access areas like the base of tongue and vallecula. Development of the FK (Feyh Kastenbauer) retractor and the LARS (laryngeal advanced retraction sys-tem) allowed exposure from the oropharynx to the larynx (Figure 10.8). This provided enough room for three robotic arms including a three-dimensional 0-degree or 30-degree endoscopic camera. One of the robotic arms carries a 5 mm

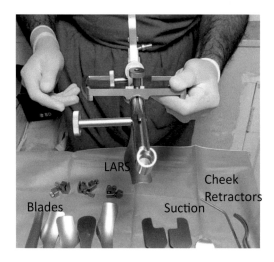

Figure 10.9 Components of a laryngeal advanced retraction system (LARS).

or 8 mm monopolar cautery Bovie for resection. A Maryland dissector is used for grasping or tissue retraction. The latest Xi system also offers Prograsp and Maryland bipolar scissors. Being 8 mm in diameter, these two instruments are challenging to manoeuvre in the limited space present in the oropharynx (Figures 10.9 through 10.11). The surgeon at the remotely located surgeon's console controls the movement of the robotic arms. The surgeon seated at the head end aids with tissue retraction, suctioning and haemostasis of larger vessels with hemoclips (Figure 10.11). The robotic patient side-cart is positioned at 30 degrees relative to the patient. The latest Xi system contains a centring green laser light with cross-hairs to assist in positioning. Due to the advantages of TORS listed above in comparison with TOLM, in toto resection is often possible. The majority of the defects can be left to heal by secondary intention; indications for reconstruction are dealt with later.

TRANSORAL ENDOSCOPIC ULTRASONIC SURGERY

TOUSS works according to the same principles as TORS. It utilises the same retractor system. The difference lies in the energy source, which is ultrasonic energy in TOUSS and visualisation by a flexible endoscopic camera, the ENDOEYE FLEX. ENDOEYE Flex is available in 5 mm 2-D and 10 mm 3-D endoscopes with 100-degree rotation at the tip.

The ultrasonic scalpel known as Thunderbeat is used for cutting and coagulation. Because the cutting occurs over a distance of 100 microns, collateral injury is minimised. The Thunderbeat is also available with a bipolar sealing device which can coagulate vessels to a maximum diameter of 7 mm. Principles of resection are the same as TORS. While using the Thunderbeat, caution should be exercised in placing the active blade away from critical structures. The surgeon operates from the head-end of the patient, using the Thunderbeat and laparoscopic forceps or scissors in either hand. The role of the assistant is to aid in suctioning and focussing and positioning the ENDOEYE FLEX.

SUBSITE-SPECIFIC CONSIDERATION

In this section, we will address the practical subsite-specific concerns.

Tonsil

In the order of contemporary relevance, we will discuss the suitable approaches for tonsillar tumours.

1. **TORS/ TOUSS**
Tumour is exposed with either the Boyle Davis mouth gag or the FK retractor. In our experience we prefer the former in case of purely tonsillar tumours. Lateral oropharyngectomy is the appropriate terminology for a radical tonsillectomy. Using the monopolar Bovie which is held by the robotic arm ipsilateral to the tumour, mucosal incisions are made, taking 5 mm margin. The anterior margin is taken over the buccal mucosa and retromolar trigone, superior margin over the soft palate, inferior margin over the tonsillolingual sulcus and the base of tongue, and posterior margin over the lateral pharyngeal wall and posterior pharyngeal wall. Deep margin is tailored to the radiologic extent. For exophytic tumours, the superior constrictor muscle can be preserved. In rare cases, the superior constrictor muscle must be sacrificed. The vascular feeders from the facial artery, ascending pharyngeal artery and descending palatine artery need to be carefully clipped when dissecting lateral to the stylopharyngeus muscle. Lack of tactile feedback is an important limitation. This is compensated for by the excellent depth perception of the

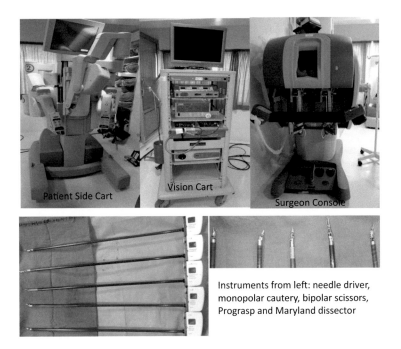

Instruments from left: needle driver, monopolar cautery, bipolar scissors, Prograsp and Maryland dissector

Figure 10.10 Da Vinci S Surgical System.

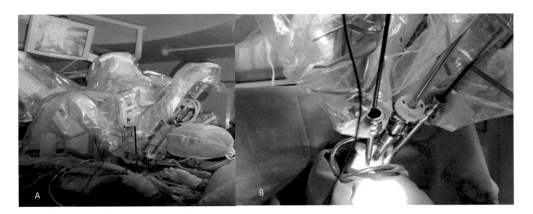

Figure 10.11 Robotic set-up for transoral robotic surgery. A. Robot docked at the head end with surgeon assisting with suction and haemostasis. B. Zoomed-in view showing instruments loaded onto right and left robotic arms and binocular endoscopic 3-D camera in the central arm.

instrument. One should be vigilant of visible pulsations in the tonsillar resection bed which points towards the proximity of the internal carotid artery.

2. TOLM

In the oropharynx, TOLM is an excellent cost-effective alternative to TORS/TOUSS. With the tumour exposed, as in TORS, resection can be accomplished with either a microscope-micromanipulator or hand-held device. We prefer the former because of magnification and better depth perception and absence of a cumbersome instrument in a physically constrained space. We now describe tumour transection in situ. The tumour is transected in the mid-portion into a superior and inferior half. After each half is resected separately, marginal biopsies are taken and oriented to the main specimen: superior pole, inferior pole, anterior and posterosuperior margin, anterior and posteroinferior

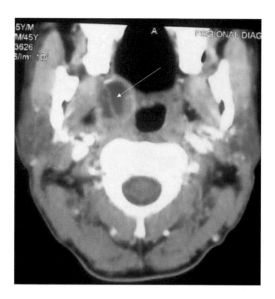

Figure 10.12 Benign tonsillar cyst.

margins and finally a deep margin from the superior constrictor.

3. Transoral Resection

There is a very limited role for this approach. It should be restricted to tonsillar cysts (Figure 10.12), benign papillomas and lastly for radical tonsillectomy as a part of unknown primary work-up (Figures 10.13 and 10.14).

4. Paramedian Mandibulotomy

Due to morbidity associated with this procedure and excellent cure rates documented with chemoradiation, paramedian mandibulotomy is hardly ever considered for oropharyngeal tumours. The only indication for this approach in our practice is for radioresistant tumours of the tonsil that are not suitable for minimally invasive techniques, the best example being minor salivary gland tumours. Paramedian mandibulotomy is performed as described before. Tumour must be released from both the parapharyngeal aspect as well as from the mucosal aspect. Once level I, II and III are cleared, posterior belly of digastric and muscles belonging to styloid apparatus are divided. Vascular control is taken around common carotid artery, external carotid artery and internal carotid artery. On retracting these vessels anterolaterally, the parapharyngeal and retropharyngeal space are exposed. The fibrofatty tissue is cleared followed by developing a well-demarcated plane between buccopharyngeal fascia and the great vessel. We usually keep a slice of gelfoam to allow identification from the mucosal aspect. Mucosal incisions for a radical tonsillectomy are tailored to the tumour

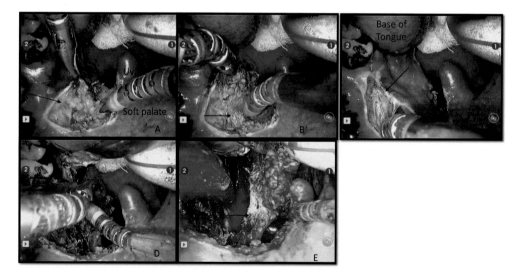

Figure 10.13 Steps involved in transoral robotic radical tonsillectomy. A. Superior mucosal incision over the soft palate. B. Superior constrictor divided. C. Mucosal incision over the anterior tonsillar pillar. D. Additional retraction applied over base of tongue to expose the tonsillo-lingual sulcus. Margin at the level of the tonsillo-lingual sulcus and the base of tongue is tailored to the inferior extent of the tumour. E. Final resection is undertaken at the level of posterior pharyngeal wall.

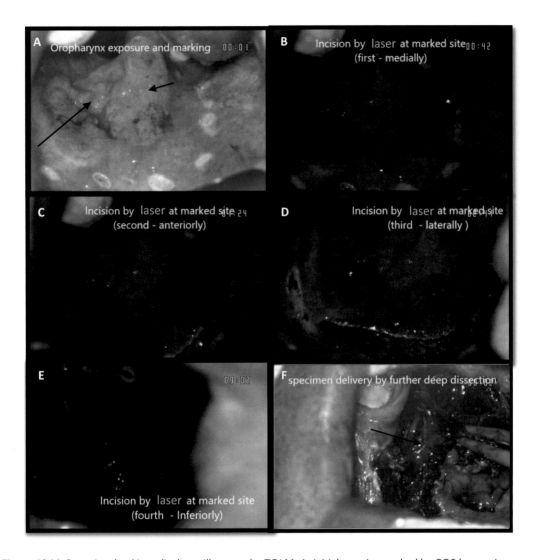

Figure 10.14 Steps involved in radical tonsillectomy by TOLM. A. Initial margins marked by CO2 laser using a micromanipulator taking 5 mm mucosal margin. Tumour is seen involving the left tonsillar fossa (long arrow) and the uvula (short arrow). B. Initial mucosal cuts are made starting medially. Preferred setting is ultrapulse mode. Visualisation is maintained by continuous suctioning of smoke. Avoiding charring, maintaining traction and counter-traction and anterior haemostasis are key to optimising surgical outcomes intraoperatively. C. Dissection is extended onto the soft palate and anterior tonsillar pillar (panel D) following the principles enumerated above. E. Margin at the level of tonsillo-lingual sulcus and base of tongue. F. Tumour dissected away from the medial pterygoid (arrow).

taking 5 mm margins over the buccal mucosa, the retromolar trigone, the tonsillo-lingual sulcus, the base of tongue, posterior pharyngeal wall and lateral pharyngeal wall. Attention is focussed on vascular pedicles of facial, lingual and ascending pharyngeal artery lateral to stylopharyngeus. In the case of extensive tumours, the internal maxillary artery should also be controlled.

5. **Mandibular Resection**
In our practice, mandibular resection with lateral oropharyngectomy is undertaken in the post-chemoradiation salvage setting. The technique has been covered previously.

Reconstruction Options for Tonsil
1. Defects following transoral resection.

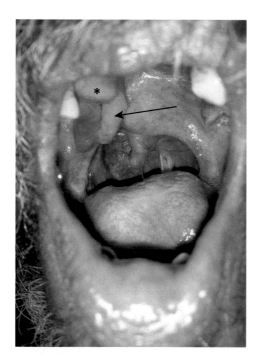

Figure 10.15 Soft palate defect on the right reconstructed with right-sided palatal mucoperiosteal flap (indicated by arrow). It is pedicled on the right greater palatine artery (indicated by asterisk).

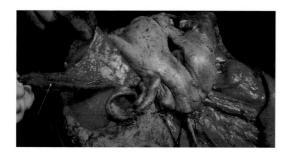

Figure 10.16 Temporoparietal facial flap (TPPF) can be harvested conventionally using a pre-auricular C-shaped incision as shown. Skin is elevated in the subcutaneous tissue layer only as deep as the hair follicles. TPPF comprises fascia between subcutaneous layer and temporalis fascia, supplied by superficial temporal artery.

De Almeida et al. have classified oropharyngeal defects following TORS. In the case of Class 1 and Class 2 defects involving one or two oropharyngeal subsites with no high-risk features, defects can be left to granulate by secondary intention. For Class 3 defects, where there is at least one high-risk feature (oro-cervical communication, great vessels exposed in the pharynx, >50% soft palate resection), reconstruction can be achieved with local flaps. Options available include the following:

a. Submental flap (SMF)
b. Infrahyoid flap (IF)
c. Palatal mucoperiosteal flap (Figure 10.15)
d. Temporoparietal flap (TPPF) (Figure 10.16)
e. Facial artery myo-mucosal flap (FAMM)

For Class 4 defects, with more than one adverse feature, regional flaps like pectoralis major myo-cutaneous flap (PMMF) or free flaps like radial forearm free flaps (RAFF) and anterolateral thigh (ALT) flaps should be considered.

The sternomastoid flap (SM) (Figure 10.17) is a modification of superiorly based (occipital artery) muscle-only sternal flap for transoral oropharyngeal defects. The indications are for Classes 1–3 defects. Besides patients with no mucosal defect, the flap is used for buttressing possible microscopic leaks as well.

The superior constrictor advancement rotation flap (SCARF) is suitable for tonsillar defects extending to the soft palate and the lateral pharyngeal wall. A stab incision is made at the contralateral tonsillo-lingual sulcus and superior constrictor with the overlying palatal muscles are advanced to the palatal defect.

2. Reconstruction indications for conventional approaches
a. Local flaps listed above can be considered when there is through-and-through oro-cervical communication.
b. Regional flaps are suitable for post-chemo-radiation salvage.
c. Osseocutaneous flaps – osseocutaneous radial forearm free flap or free fibular flap (FFF) – can be considered with concomitant mandibular defects. PMMF is an alternative in patients with poor general condition and vessel-depleted neck.

Soft Palate

1. **TORS/TOUSS/TOLM**
The soft palate is a favourable subsite for all three transoral techniques. The principles of mucosal resection are like a tonsillar resection. One line of difference is the preference for Dingman retractor over Boyle Davis or FK retractor.

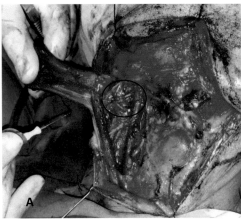
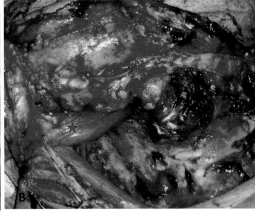

Figure 10.17 Harvesting (A) and insetting (B) of a modified sternomastoid muscle-only flap for an oropharyngeal defect. The flap is based on the occipital artery and includes only the sternal head (indicated by star). To preserve the flap pedicle, dissection of level IIb (circle) should be done carefully.

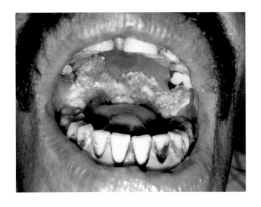

Figure 10.18 Verrucous lesion over the soft palate with extension to hard palate and retromolar trigone. The extensive nature of the lesion along with trismus makes this patient a suitable candidate for open approaches.

2. **Conventional Transoral Resection**
Can be employed for limited benign tumours, premalignant lesions and verrucous lesions.

3. **Paramedian Mandibulotomy**
Reserved for soft palate tumours with trismus (Figure 10.18). The technique has been described previously.

RECONSTRUCTION FOLLOWING SOFT PALATE EXCISION

Soft palate reconstruction is challenging due to the functional deficits brought forth by its resection: Velopharyngeal insufficiency.

Urken et al. have classified soft palate defects as follows.

1. SP0 – no soft palate defect
2. SP1 – defect <1/4 of the soft palate
3. SP2 – defect involving <1/2 of the soft palate, not involving the uvula
4. SP3 – defect involving >1/2 of the soft palate, including the uvula

Class 1 defects and those following transoral resection with an intact muscular framework can be left to heal by secondary intention. Class 2 defects can be reconstructed with local flaps like the palatal mucoperiosteal flap (see Figure 10.15), FAMM or posterior pharyngeal wall flap. Palatopharyngoplasty is performed as an adjunct class 2 defect onwards. By creating a raw surface between the posterior end of the soft palate and the posterior pharyngeal wall or by incorporating a posterior pharyngeal wall flap with other local flaps, the nasopharyngeal isthmus can be narrowed. Class 3 defects are preferably reconstructed with RAFF, ALT or rectus abdominis flap. The various techniques for flap insetting are patch, jump and Gehanno.

BASE OF TONGUE RESECTION

1. **TORS/TOUSS (Figures 10.19 and 10.20)**

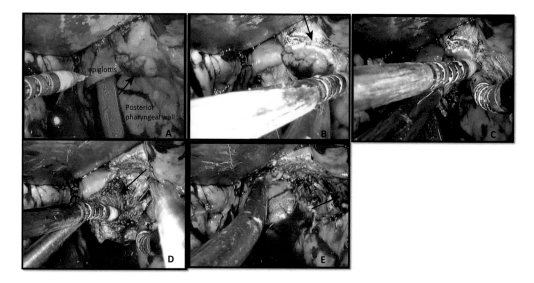

Figure 10.19 Operative steps involved in transoral robotic base of tongue resection. A. Exophytic tumour arising from the base of tongue. B, C. First mucosal incision made over the lateral aspect of the tumour, taking 5 mm margin. D. Arrow pointing towards intrinsic muscles of the tongue. E. Post-operative defect revealing intact superior constrictor.

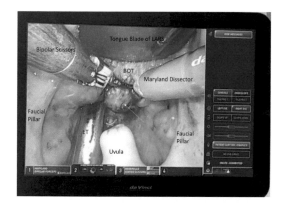

Figure 10.20 View through the vision cart of Da Vinci Xi System. Intraoperative image of base of tongue haemangioma. TORS/TOUSS procedures require in-depth knowledge of inside-out anatomy.

Tumour is exposed with the FK retractor or with the LARS. A 30-degree downward facing endoscope is preferred in case of TORS. The inside-out anatomy of the lingual artery is important to avoid any vascular catastrophe (see Figure 10.17). The lingual artery lies lateral to the geniohyoid. One will not encounter the lingual artery while dissecting in the substance of the intrinsic muscles. Cadaveric studies have shown that the lingual artery lies 1.6 cm lateral to foramen cecum and 2.7 cm inferior. To further minimise blood loss, the lingual artery can be ligated in the neck. The lingual artery can be located in the neck inferior to the hypoglossal nerve, superior to the greater cornu of hyoid bone and deep to the fibres of hyoglossus muscle. For mucosal incision, the inferior margin is the most challenging. For deeply infiltrative tumours, counter-pressure is applied over the hyoid and the deep margin is taken up to the pre-epiglottic space.

2. TOLM

Unlike tonsil and soft palate, TOLM is not suitable for extensive malignant lesions arising from the base of tongue.

3. Paramedian Mandibulotomy

This is ideally suited for anterior two-thirds tongue malignancy extending to the base of tongue with poor mouth opening.

4. Visor Approach and Lingual Approach

It is an alternative to mandibular swing with similar indications. Can also be combined with marginal mandibular resection which is considered a relative contraindication with paramedian mandibulotomy. It is also suitable for post-chemoradiotherapy salvage situations.

5. **Lateral Pharyngotomy with Suprahyoid Pharyngotomy**
The base of tongue lesions extending to vallecula and pre-epiglottic space can be approached by combining these two methods. In case of involvement of the pre-epiglottic space, suprahyoid pharyngotomy may result in tumour tissue violation. Supraglottic laryngectomy is the ideal operation in such cases.

Special Considerations to Optimise Speech and Swallowing Outcomes Following Base of Tongue Resection

1. **Hyomandibular complex**
   a. Every attempt should be made to preserve the attachments of the genioglossus and the geniohyoid muscles. In case of the floor of mouth resection in that region, these muscle attachments need to be suspended to the mandible by drilling holes and using non-absorbable sutures

   b. **Hyoid suspension**
   With an extensive base of tongue resection, the laryngeal elevation is hampered. To mechanically elevate the larynx and reduce post-operative aspiration, hyoid can be suspended to the mandible by passing non-absorbable sutures fixed to holes drilled over the lower border of the mandible (Figure 10.21).

2. **Epiglottosplasty**
   Another strategy to reduce aspiration is to reduce the size of the laryngeal inlet. The mucosal incision is made over the free edge of the epiglottis. Excess cartilage is trimmed, then the free edges of the mucosa are sutured, resulting in a tubular and narrowed laryngeal opening.

3. **Hypoglossal nerve and lingual artery** Neurovascular pedicle to at least one side should be preserved at any cost. If not, the patient becomes an oral cripple, dependent on PEG feeding and tracheostomy for the rest of his/her life.

4. **Reconstruction**
   a. Following TORS/TOUSS, de Almeida classification and algorithm are followed as enumerated for tonsil tumours.

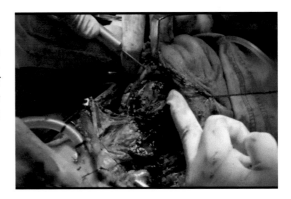
Figure 10.21 Drill holes in mandible for hyoid suspension.

   b. Following an open approach to the base of tongue, the aim of reconstruction differs from anterior 2/3 tongue reconstruction. Here bulk and sensate features of a flap take precedence over pliable and mobile flaps. Regional flaps satisfying these criteria include PMMF and latissimus dorsi flap. If free flaps are being used, RAFF and ALT are the preferred options.

COMPLICATIONS AND MANAGEMENT

Post-operative complications can be divided into major or minor or classified using instruments like the Clavien-Dindo scale. In this section, we will focus on the pertinent complications expected following oropharyngeal tumour surgery.

1. **Secondary haemorrhage**
Bleeding from the surgical site occurring beyond 24 hours can be due to labile blood pressure in the peri-operative period, coagulation abnormalities, major vessel exposure into the pharynx, orocervical communication and secondary infection. Investigation and treatment should be instituted hand in hand. Bleed into the airway should not be taken casually. Tachycardia, wide pulse pressure, pallor, prolonged capillary refill are indications of an ongoing blood loss. Nasogastric tube, if not already inserted, should be connected to continuous drainage and output and character of drain monitored closely. With torrential bleed, the airway is secured by tracheostomy followed by locating the bleeder and ligating it. If expertise is not available for intraoral haemostasis,

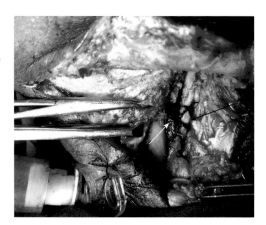

Figure 10.22 A case of carotid blow-out following radical concurrent chemoradiation in a case of carcinoma base of tongue T4N3bM0. Airway was secured with tracheostomy followed by ligation of common carotid artery (black arrow). Tumour with extracapsular spread (white arrow) is seen abutting common carotid artery.

transcervical ligation of the lingual artery or facial artery should be performed. If facilities for endovascular embolisation are available and the patient's haemodynamic condition permits, CT angiography followed by endovascular treatment can be considered. One should refrain from external carotid artery ligation or common carotid artery (Figure 10.22) ligation as the initial management of the latter is associated with significant morbidity and mortality and major vessel ligation precludes future endovascular procedures altogether. Bleed from a major vessel in the neck not associated with a fistula can be repaired. However, caution must be exercised in the presence of a fistula. Vascular adventitia in these cases is weakened and ligation is the only safe option. Haemostatic agents like Fibrin Glue, Tissue-Seal and oxidised cellulose have only an adjunctive role and should never be used as stand-alone management for secondary haemorrhage.

2. **Orocervical communication and fistula formation**

Conservative management with pressure dressing, anticholinergics and antibiotics can be considered in case of small fistulas where there is no history of prior radiation and without exposure of great vessels. In the presence of any of these high-risk features, conservative management can avert a major vessel blow-out. This kind of patient needs to be re-explored in the operating theatre with expertise available for fistula repair with vascularised tissue.

3. **Flap necrosis and dehiscence**

Risk factors include prior radiation, prior surgery to the neck depleting neck vessels, positive margin, improper technique, hypoalbuminemia, poor nutrition, atherosclerosis, diabetic vasculopathy and hypothyroidism. Partial flap loss without the presence of a fistula can be managed conservatively. Complete flap loss with orocervical communication cannot be expected to heal by secondary intention. One should resort to a second flap if a flap was required for reconstruction in the very first surgery.

4. **Intractable aspiration and PEG dependence**

We have already discussed surgical manoeuvres to facilitate swallowing and will discuss the rehabilitation aspects later. The last resort for intractable aspiration is total laryngectomy or lifelong PEG feeding and tracheostomy dependence.

5. **Osteoradionecrosis, malunion, non-union, hardware exposure** (Figure 10.23)

These are some of the potential complications that plague paramedian mandibulotomy. Osteoradionecrosis can be minimised by vigorous oro-dental treatment before radiotherapy and minimising radiation dose to the mandible (<60 Gy) by conformal techniques. Management options include hyperbaric oxygen therapy, prolonged antibiotics, sequestrectomy and introduction of non-irradiated vascular tissue.

Malunion and non-union can be minimised by double plating and using titanium reconstruction plates. If this complication develops, a redo of internal fixation should be considered, with or without inter-dental wiring.

REHABILITATION

1. **Velopharyngeal insufficiency**

A soft palate prosthesis can be used for rehabilitation in patients with intact dentition. Techniques for palatopharyngoplasty have been enumerated previously. Various injection techniques are described to augment the posterior pharyngeal wall, including fat, fascia, autologous cartilage and injectable collagen.

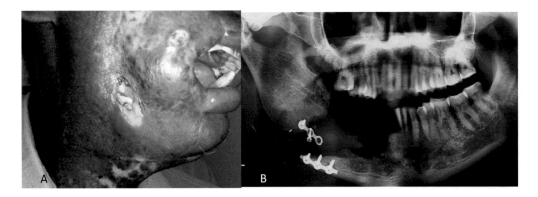

Figure 10.23 Osteoradionecrosis. A. Sequestrum with skin defect and plate exposure. B. Orthopantomogram showing pathological fracture, plate fracture and multiple lytic areas in the body of the mandible.

2. Swallowing rehabilitation

The oropharyngeal phase of swallowing is severely compromised following resection of any part of the oropharynx. This manifests as increased oropharyngeal transit time, increase in oropharyngeal residue and diminished laryngeal elevation, all amounting to aspiration. Manoeuvres to strengthen the base tongue and assist in hyo-mandibular elevation include chin tuck, Mendelson manoeuvre, Masako manoeuvre and Shaker technique. Patients who have also undergone resection of the epiglottis or a supraglottic laryngectomy will benefit from a supraglottic or a super supraglottic swallow.

FURTHER READING SUGGESTIONS

1. Osborne RF, Brown JJ. Carcinoma of the oral pharynx: An analysis of subsite treatment heterogeneity. Surg Oncol Clin N Am. 2004 Jan;13(1):71–80.
2. Blanchard P, Baujat B, Holostenco V, Bourredjem A, Baey C, Bourhis J, et al. Meta-analysis of chemotherapy in head and neck cancer (MACH-NC): A comprehensive analysis by tumour site. Radiother Oncol J. 2011 Jul;100(1):33–40.
3. Golusiński W, Golusińska-Kardach E. Current role of surgery in the management of oropharyngeal cancer. Front Oncol. 2019 May 24 [cited 2020 Feb 14];9.
4. Hohenstein NA, Chan JW, Wu SY, Tahir P, Yom SS. Diagnosis, staging, radiation treatment response assessment, and outcome prognostication of head and neck cancers using PET imaging: A systematic review. PET Clin. 2020 Jan;15(1):65–75.
5. Lewis JS, Thorstad WL, Chernock RD, Haughey BH, Yip JH, Zhang Q, et al. p16 Positive oropharyngeal squamous cell carcinoma: An entity with a favorable prognosis regardless of tumor HPV status. Am J Surg Pathol. 2010 Aug [cited 2020 Feb 14];34(8).
6. Jaffer NM, Edmund D, Au FW-F, Steele CM. Fluoroscopic evaluation of oropharyngeal dysphagia: Anatomy, technique and common etiologies. AJR Am J Roentgenol. 2015 Jan;204(1):49–58.
7. Matyja G. Objective evaluation of respiratory function of the larynx after partial laryngectomy of various range. Ann Acad Med Stetin. 2001;47:145–61.
8. Rubinstein M, Armstrong WB. Transoral laser microsurgery for laryngeal cancer: A primer and review of laser dosimetry. Lasers Med Sci. 2011 Jan;26(1):113–24.
9. Wessberg GA, Hill SC, McBride KL. Median labiomandibular glossotomy. Int J Oral Surg. 1981 Oct;10(5):333–7.
10. Rich JT, Milov S, Lewis JS, Thorstad WL, Adkins DR, Haughey BH. Transoral laser microsurgery (TLM) +/- adjuvant therapy for advanced stage oropharyngeal cancer: Outcomes and prognostic factors. The Laryngoscope. 2009 Sep;119(9):1709–19.
11. Weinstein GS, O'Malley BW, Rinaldo A, Silver CE, Werner JA, Ferlito A. Understanding contraindications for transoral robotic surgery (TORS) for oropharyngeal cancer. Eur Arch Oto-Rhino-Laryngol. 2015 Jul;272(7):1551–2.
12. Asher SA, White HN, Kejner AE, Rosenthal EL, Carroll WR, Magnuson JS. Hemorrhage after transoral robotic-assisted surgery. Otolaryngol-Head Neck Surg. 2013 Jul;149(1):112–7.
13. Williams CE, Kinshuck AJ, Derbyshire SG, Upile N, Tandon S, Roland NJ, et al. Transoral laser resection versus lip-split mandibulotomy in the management of oropharyngeal squamous cell carcinoma (OPSCC): A case match study. Eur Arch Oto-Rhino-Laryngol. 2014 Feb;271(2):367–72.

14. Qureshi HA, Abouyared M, Barber B, Houlton JJ. Surgical options for locally advanced oropharyngeal cancer. *Curr Treat Options Oncol.* 2019 Apr 1;20(5):36.

15. Hinni ML, Nagel T, Howard B. Oropharyngeal cancer treatment: The role of transoral surgery. *Curr Opin Otolaryngol Head Neck Surg.* 2015 Apr;23(2):132–8.

16. Fernández-Fernández MM, Montes-Jovellar L, Parente Arias PL, Ortega Del Alamo P. TransOral endoscopic UltraSonic Surgery (TOUSS): A preliminary report of a novel robotless alternative to TORS. *Eur Arch Oto-Rhino-Laryngol.* 2015 Dec;272(12):3785–91.

17. de Almeida JR, Park RCW, Villanueva NL, Miles BA, Teng MS, Genden EM. Reconstructive algorithm and classification system for transoral oropharyngeal defects. *Head Neck.* 2014 Jul;36(7):934–41.

18. Panda S, Thakar A, Sikka K, Sharma SC. Role of sternomastoid muscle interposition in concomitant transoral oncologic resection and neck dissection. *Head Neck.* 2019;41(8):2724–31.

19. Jackson I. Mark L. Urken (Ed), Multidisciplinary head and neck reconstruction: A defect-oriented approach. *Eur J Plast Surg.* 2010 Apr 1;33(2):115.

20. Chung E-J, Lee D-J, Kang H-D, Park M-I, Chung C-H, Rho Y-S. Prospective speech outcome study in patients with soft palate reconstruction in tonsillar cancer. *Oral Oncol.* 2011 Oct;47(10):988–92.

21. Yin LX, Moore EJ, Van Abel KM. Transoral robotic surgery (TORS)—inside out anatomy and exposure of the operating field. *Curr Otorhinolaryngol Rep.* 2019 Dec 1;7(4):260–7.

22. Vallur S, Dutta A, Arjun AP. Use of Clavien—Dindo classification system in assessing head and neck surgery complications. *Indian J Otolaryngol Head Neck Surg.* 2019 Jul 25 [cited 2020 Feb 14].

23. Remacle M, Bertrand B, Eloy P, Marbaix E. The use of injectable collagen to correct velopharyngeal insufficiency. *The Laryngoscope.* 1990 Mar;100(3):269–74.

11

Hypopharyngeal Tumour

AVINASH CHAITANYA S AND RAJEEV GUPTA

INTRODUCTION

Hypopharynx, also known as laryngopharynx, is the lowermost part of the pharynx after the naso- and oro-pharynx. It lies posteriorly and laterally to the larynx and it acts as the passage for the entry of food into the oesophagus. Hypopharynx is divided into three subsites anatomically. They are the pyriform sinus, posterior pharyngeal wall and the post-cricoid region. Anatomically it extends from the hyoid to the inferior border of the hyoid. It is bounded anteriorly by the larynx, with the epiglottis, aryepiglottic folds and arytenoids forming the marginal zones. It is lined by stratified squamous epithelium.

Pathology

Because the hypopharynx is lined by squamous epithelium, squamous cell carcinomas outnumber all other histologies combined. Other types include adenocarcinomas, neuroendocrine and salivary gland origin tumours.

Etiology

As in other cancers of the head and neck region, tobacco and alcohol have an important role in the etiopathogenesis of hypopharyngeal cancers. They have a potent role individually and a synergistic role in combination. Apart from these, chronic gastro-esophageal reflux and conditions like post-cricoid webs are also considered as the etiological factors associated with carcinomas of the hypopharynx, especially the post-cricoid region.

CLINICAL FEATURES

Hypopharyngeal tumours have the following common presenting features:

1. Progressive dysphagia is one of the most common presentations. It starts with a pricking sensation in the throat while swallowing and progresses to dysphagia to solids and then to liquids.
2. Cervical lymphadenopathy is the presenting complaint in the majority of patients. It is common for pyriform sinus tumours to be asymptomatic for dysphagia and present with nodes in the neck.
3. Change in the quality of voice and breathing difficulty are suggestive of local spread of the tumour to the larynx. They occur at a later stage.
4. Referred pain to ear while swallowing is usually due to glossopharyngeal nerve.
5. As the patient has long-standing dysphagia to solids in most cases, the patients tend to present in a malnourished state, managing only liquids orally.

The subsites of hypopharynx not only differ in their anatomy but have distinct clinical features and prognosis when it comes to malignancy. Each of the subsites should be dealt with as a different entity.

DOI: 10.1201/9780367430139-11

The **pyriform sinus** is the most common sub-site of hypopharynx to be involved by malignancy. It has a preponderance in the elderly, with males over the age of 60 years being the most common group. Smoking and alcohol consumption are commonly associated with the occurrence in this region. These are marginal zone cancers and have the highest propensity to spread anteriorly to the larynx.

Due to the relatively large space in the pyriform sinus, the malignancies tend to present at a later stage. Nearly 25% of the patients have nodal metastasis as their presenting symptoms and dysphagia occurs at a relatively later stage.

Despite this, they are the subset with the best prognosis among the hypopharyngeal cancers.

Carcinoma of the **post-cricoid region** of the hypopharynx is associated with the worst prognosis. In contrast to pyriform sinus malignancies, it occurs at a younger age and has a preponderance in females. It presents with early onset, rapidly progressive dysphagia. Most of these patients are typically lean with low BMI. History of addictions is generally absent. Oesophageal webs and Plummer-Vinson syndrome are usually associated with the post-cricoid carcinomas. Despite aggressive treatment with extensive surgery and radiation, these cancers tend to recur early with local or distant failures.

Posterior pharyngeal wall cancers present with odynophagia and referred pain. They are less common than the pyriform sinus tumours but have similar etiological factors. Their location makes them less amenable to surgical resection due to limited reconstruction options. Radiation fields are limited due to their proximity to the spine.

CLINICAL ASSESSMENT

A high index of clinical suspicion is essential in differentiating the hypopharyngeal malignancies from other causes of dysphagia. A history of persistent and progressive dysphagia with referred pain to ear should point the clinician to the differential diagnosis. Cervical lymphadenopathy should always be considered for further evaluation. Laryngeal crepitus is almost always absent in cancer in the hypopharynx; although it may be present in early stages. An indirect laryngoscopy or video-assisted laryngoscopy helps to visualise

the lesion and also take a biopsy in the outpatient clinic.

Cancer of the post-cricoid region and apex of pyriform sinus may sometimes be missed on routine laryngoscopy. Upper GI endoscopy might be required at times to visualise and diagnose the post-cricoid lesions. Stenotic lesions like webs in the cricopharynx also hinder the vision of the endoscope and dilatation of the strictures may be required prior to biopsy.

INVESTIGATIONS

The diagnosis of hypopharyngeal cancer is driven by the presenting symptoms. A patient presenting with dysphagia is investigated with endoscopy as a screening tool. Being an office procedure, it is cost effective and fast. In the same sitting, upper GI endoscopy can be used to obtain tissue for biopsy to confirm the diagnosis. As with any other subsite, biopsy is the mainstay for confirming the diagnosis of a hypopharyngeal malignancy. In a selective few cases, direct laryngoscopy or hypopharyngoscopy under general anaesthesia may be required for assessing the disease and procuring the tissue for biopsy.

In an ideal setting, imaging should precede the biopsy to avoid biopsy-related artefacts like tumour oedema, bleeding or necrosis, which may lead to overestimation of the tumour size. All patients should undergo direct laryngoscopy for complete assessment of the extent of the tumour and structures involved. Fixity of the vocal cord, subglottic involvement and apex of pyriform sinus also can be assessed on direct laryngoscopy. Direct laryngoscopy helps to better assess the areas like apex of pyriform sinus, post-cricoid region, subglottis, ventricle, anterior commissure and laryngeal surface of epiglottis which are hidden on indirect laryngoscopy.

A patient presenting with cervical lymphadenopathy as the presenting complaint is initially assessed with an FNAC from the node to ascertain it to be metastatic cancer. Simultaneously, the site of the primary can be evaluated. A history of dysphagia or hoarseness leads us to the primary, which can be confirmed with endoscopy.

With the diagnosis established by the biopsy, it is then essential to ascertain the extent of the disease with a cross-sectional imaging of the neck. A contrast-enhanced CT of the neck is an excellent choice of imaging. It provides adequate information of the site and size of the primary with involvement of the adjacent structures. Following are the important features to be looked for in the pre-operative scans.

1. **Laterality:** Whether the tumour is confined to the pyriform sinus on one side or it is crossing to the other side. This helps in pre-operative counselling and planning for reconstruction.
2. **Involvement of laryngeal structures:** It is common for the tumour to extend anteriorly to involve the arytenoid, cricoid and adjacent laryngeal structures. Involvement of the laryngeal cartilages becomes one of the absolute indications for surgery.
3. **Extent:** Involvement of the base of tongue or pharyngeal wall of the oropharynx superiorly and oesophageal extension inferiorly is an important factor for determining the type of pharyngeal reconstruction required.
   Superior extent is significant in post-cricoid malignancy where gastric pull-up is planned as the reconstruction method. The gastric conduit, like any flap, has precarious blood supply in the distal-most part and is generally associated with dehiscence and leaks in anastomosis above the base tongue level. Inferior extent is to be seen to rule out large segment upper oesophageal disease.
4. **Nodal involvement:** It is common for hypopharyngeal malignancies to present with unilateral or bilateral nodal metastasis. Involvement of the carotid or prevertebral fascia by the extra-capsular spread from the node is to be assessed for staging the disease more accurately, to decide operability and to decide on the adjuvant treatment.
5. **Thyroid gland involvement:** Rather than for the thyroid gland function, one lobe of thyroid is generally preserved to preserve the parathyroids. If, on pre-operative imaging, it is established that disease is infiltrating the thyroid gland, then the patient can be counselled for total thyroidectomy and prolonged hypocalcaemia.
6. **Great vessels assessment:** Encasement of the carotid vessels is a contraindication for surgical treatment. They may be involved either by the disease extension for the primary or by the nodes.
7. **Involvement of the prevertebral fascia:** The spread of the tumour from the primary or cervical node is to be assessed for determining the operability.

Historically, barium swallow used to be the investigation performed in case of dysphagia. Its use has slowly diminished in clinical practice as it yields less information and has a potential for aspiration and related complications. Even after replacing barium with other water-soluble compounds for oral contrast, they have not gained acceptance over cross-sectional imaging like computed tomography.

Role of metastatic work-up with PET CT is ideally limited to recurrent or residual cases. It has also been used in cases with multiple large metastatic nodes as the chances of having distant metastasis at presentation is high in such patients. Post-cricoid carcinomas are also evaluated with an initial PET-CT in most centres. Because it is an aggressive malignancy with a high rate of distant failures, it is pertinent to rule out distant metastasis prior to embarking on such a morbid surgical treatment. PET-CT is now preferred over many tests, like CT chest, bone scan, etc.

TREATMENT OPTIONS

Surgical treatment has always been the gold standard of treatment for laryngeal and hypopharyngeal cancers. Total laryngectomy with partial or total pharyngectomy has had a very successful role in the treatment of malignancies of this region. With the advent of newer radiation techniques, there is an increasing trend for organ preservation. Laryngeal preservation is attempted in all subsites of the hypopharynx with comparable results.

Pyriform sinus tumours tend to be limited to one side with extension to the larynx in advanced cases. After removal of the tumour with adequate margins, generally there is ample mucosa remaining to close the pharynx primarily. As in laryngectomy, the neopharynx can be closed in I-shape or Y-shape. Adequate-sized lumen should be present for better functional outcomes. In case of inadequate remnant pharyngeal wall, various flaps can be used to reconstruct the pharyngeal wall. PMMC, radial forearm and DP flaps are used routinely for these reconstructions.

Posterior pharyngeal wall tumours are generally not taken up for surgery due to the limited reconstruction options. Radiation is the preferred modality in such cases. If surgery is planned, total laryngectomy with tubed flaps/gastric pull-ups/free jejunal transfer are used for pharyngeal wall reconstruction.

Post-cricoid region tumours are notorious in having early and excessive dysphagia. In early stage non-circumferential non-stenotic lesions, the patient is generally able to tolerate oral feeds. In such cases radiation is the preferred mode of treatment. Patients with absolute dysphagia tend to have cicatrising lesions extending into the upper oesophagus. These patients must undergo total laryngo-pharyngo-oesophagectomy.

SURGICAL MANAGEMENT

The aim of surgery is to remove all the gross tumour burden in the neck with preservation of oral feeding. Due to the location of the hypopharyngeal tumours, it is imperative to sacrifice the larynx for compete clearance. Total laryngectomy with partial or total pharyngectomy with pharyngeal reconstruction is the surgical procedure. The steps of the procedure are as follows.

1. **Anaesthesia:** Procedure is done under general anaesthesia with oro-tracheal intubation or upfront tracheostomy with a flexometallic tube. Nasogastric (NG) tube is placed if feasible. If the NG tube is not negotiable, it is left in the nasopharynx so that it can be inserted after resection of the tumour.
2. **Direct laryngoscopy:** Even if prior laryngoscopy had been performed for the purpose of biopsy, it should be performed prior to the definitive surgery to assess any change in the disease status in the time gap. This is done to assess the extent of tumour and amount of mucosa that can be preserved. The amount of pharyngeal mucosa that can be preserved determines the requirement of any reconstruction and its type. Superior and inferior extent of the growth also needs to be ascertained for the same purpose.
3. **Incision:** The midline lower neck skin crease incision extends from the posterior border of sternomastoid muscle of one side to the other. In case of previously tracheostomised patients,

the skin around the tracheostoma should be included to avoid stomal recurrence and for better wound healing. Classical apron incision can be planned for a better approach to the level 2 region.
4. **Raising the flaps:** After incising the skin, subplatysmal flaps should be raised superiorly up to the submandibular gland and inferiorly up to the clavicle for maximum exposure of the area to be dissected.
5. **Neck dissection:** Elective neck dissection of bilateral levels 2–5 is done, preserving the IJV, SCM and SAN. All nodes and fascia are dissected out and sent separately for HPE. Bilateral paratracheal clearance is done before resecting the primary. Care should be taken to avoid devascularisation of the parathyroid blood supply.
6. **Resection of the primary:** Omohyoid and sternohyoid and sternothyroid are divided at the lower border. Superior and inferior thyroid vessels are identified, ligated and divided on the diseased side. On the opposite side, inferior and superior thyroid vessels are preserved in continuity along with the ipsilateral thyroid gland. Superior laryngeal vessels are ligated. The thyroid lamina is denuded and the pharyngeal mucosa is separated from the cartilage. Hyoid bone is skeletonised, preserving the hypoglossal nerve and lingual vessels. Vallecula is entered from the side opposite the tumour. Pharyngeal mucosal cuts are taken with adequate margins in case of partial pharyngectomy. The tracheal cut is made and the endotracheal tube is replaced with a sterile tube placed into the distal tracheal lumen. The lower pharyngeal cut is made at the cricopharynx, and the specimen is delivered. The distal tracheal lumen is sutured to the skin with 1–0 Prolene to prevent it from retracting into the chest.
7. **Pharyngeal reconstruction:** Pharyngeal mucosa can be closed primarily if there is adequate mucosa to cover the nasogastric tube without tension. The pharyngeal mucosa is sutured submucosally in layers with 3–0 and 4–0 PDS sutures. Care should be taken that the mucosa is not projected outside the suture line. The base of tongue is closed in a straight line (I-shaped closure) or with a tripoint (Y-shaped closure) with a reinforcement.

8. If sufficient mucosa is not available, the pharyngeal reconstruction is done with myocutaneous or fasciocutaneous flaps. Pedicled flaps like PMMC are used as a patch to reconstruct the pharynx. Microvascular free tissue flaps like radial forearm free flaps can be used in the same fashion.

9. In case of circumferential disease, the pharynx is divided superiorly and the pharyngeal wall is separated from the prevertebral fascia. The pharyngeal tissue along with the larynx, and sometime oesophagus in case tumour involves cricopharynx, is resected. The reconstruction is done with tube PMMC for defects above the cricopharynx or with free jejunal transfer or gastric conduit pull-up for longer segment defects.

POST-OPERATIVE CARE

1. Patient is shifted to the ICU for further monitoring. Essential parameters like haemoglobin and electrolytes are stabilised and the patient is observed for signs of reactionary haemorrhage and haematoma under the skin flaps.

2. Patient is kept on IV fluid overnight and Ryle's tube feeding is started the next morning. In patients having gastric pull-up, feeding jejunostomy is preferred over nasogastric tube. High-protein diet is recommended.

3. Prophylactic antibiotics are used as per the hospital protocol and are generally sufficient for a period of five days.

4. Use of prokinetics and anti-emetics is warranted as regurgitation of feeds from the stomach into the oesophagus and pharynx can lead to anastomotic leaks.

5. Care of the tracheostoma: The new tracheostoma has the tendency to get obstructed in the immediate post-operative period with the dried blood or dried tracheal secretions. Care should be taken to clean the stoma with a swab stick dipped in liquid paraffin or glycerine. Keeping the stoma moist with a wet sterile gauze can also help in avoiding the drying of the secretions.

6. Calcium management: As in case of total thyroidectomy, post-operative serum calcium of parathormone assessment should be done from the second post-operative day to prevent hypocalcaemia-related symptoms.

OTHER SURGICAL OPTIONS

For lesions limited to a small region, total laryngectomy with pharyngectomy is overkill. Thus, various organ-conservative surgeries have been tried and introduced. Lateral pharyngotomy can be used as an approach to the pharynx as done for the oropharyngeal tumours. It involves extensive soft tissue dissection for resection of the tumour. Thus, the complication rates are usually high, with pharyngocutaneous fistula being the most common.

Transoral resection under magnification with a microscope can be attempted for small lesions. With the advancements in technology and the introduction of laser (TOLS) and robotic surgery (TORS), small tumours can now be excised with minimal morbidity as a day-care procedure. T1 lesions limited to one subsite can be resected with tumour-free margins transorally without the morbidity and complications of open pharyngotomy.

Since the primary aim of these procedures is to avoid radiation, the selection criteria for them is very strict. Clinically node negative, small lesions without any adverse features are preferred for TOLS and TORS.

ADJUVANT TREATMENT

Achieving negative surgical margins and removal of the gross disease in the neck is the aim of the surgical management. Adjuvant radiation is mandated in case of large tumour volume with extra laryngeal spread (T3, T4 disease), node positivity (N+ status) and adverse pathological features like LVI and PNI. Intensification of the adjuvant with chemotherapy is done for margin positivity and extranodal spread of the tumour.

As a standard, 60–66 Gy radiation is given to the primary and node positive region in 30–33 #. Node negative necks are treated with reduced doses of up to 54 Gy. Spinal cord sparing is done after 40 Gy. IMRT is preferred over conventional RT techniques to reduce radiation-associated toxicities.

Cisplatin is used as the drug of choice for concurrent chemoradiotherapy due to its additional radiosensitising effects. It is given as either a weekly 40 mg/m^2 or three-weekly dose of 50–100 mg/m^2. The maximum cumulative dose, and thus the toxicity, is more in the three-weekly regimen.

Figure 11.1 summarises the algorithm for management of hypopharyngeal malignancies.

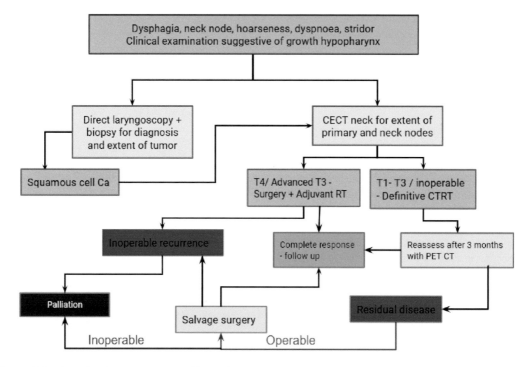

Figure 11.1 Algorithm for management of hypopharyngeal malignancies.

REHABILITATION

Patients treated surgically end up with a permanent speech handicap. They can be rehabilitated with electrolarynx or oesophageal speech to enable them to communicate effectively. Patients with primary pharyngeal closure have the option of using tracheo-esophageal prosthesis for speech production, as in cases of laryngectomy.

COMPLICATIONS

1. Pharyngo-cutaneous fistula: It is the most common complication. Early feeding, tongue mobilisation, malnourishment and haematoma formation under the flaps are the common causes of this complication. Post-radiation reduced tissue vascularity and healing are the predisposing factors in salvage cases.

2. Aspiration: One of the common causes of morbidity and mortality.
3. Pneumothorax: Commonly seen after gastric pull-up.
4. Paralytic ileus: As in all other abdominal cases, paralytic ileus is a common side effect.
5. Hypocalcaemia: Can occur if the parathyroids or their blood supply are not preserved.

CONCLUSION

Cancers of the hypopharynx are common malignancies, with smoking and alcohol acting as etiological agents. Surgery with adjuvant radiation remains the standard of care. Organ preservation with concurrent chemoradiation is now being practiced for early cancers with excellent results. Post-cricoid cancers still remain one of the most dreaded cancers in terms of surgical morbidity and prognosis.

12

Laryngeal Cancer Surgery

VIPIN ARORA,RAVI MEHER, DIVYA VAID AND SUVERCHA ARYA

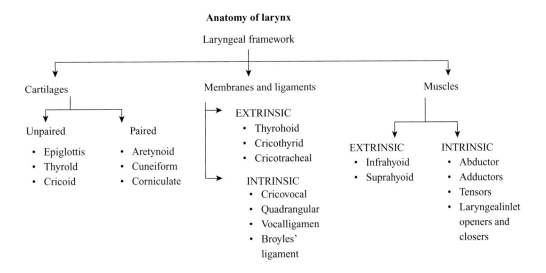

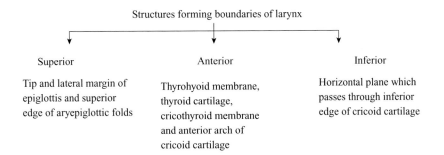

Flow Diagram 1

DOI: 10.1201/9780367430139-12

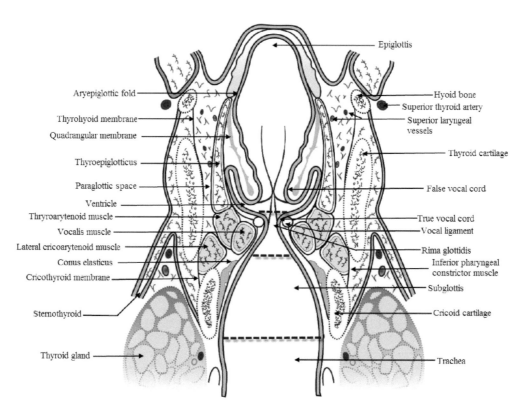

Figure 12.1 Coronal section through the larynx.

Anatomy of the Larynx

See Flow Diagram 1 and 2 Figures 12.1 and 12.2.

Natural barriers to tumour spread

- Laryngeal cartilages
- Hyoepiglottic ligament
- Thyrohyoid membrane
- Quadrangular membrane
- Conus elasticus
- Anterior commissure: Part of glottis where true vocal cords meet anteriorly. Extent: From vocal ligaments to midline of inner surface of thyroid cartilage.
- Cricothyroid membrane

LYMPHATIC DRAINAGE

This is based on the development of supraglottis from second and fourth (buccopharyngeal) arches and that of glottis and subglottis from the sixth (respiratory) arch. As a result, the vocal folds anteriorly and laterally act as the "watershed" for lymphatic drainage of the larynx although they themselves have minimal drainage. Regional drainage is demarcated as follows.

- Supraglottis: Level II and level III via superior laryngeal vessels; bilateral drainage
- Anterior glottis and subglottis: Anteriorly through cricothyroid membrane to level VI and to level IV laterally
- Posterior glottis and subglottis: Paratracheal nodes in level VI through cricotracheal membrane and laterally to level IV

PATHWAYS OF TUMOUR SPREAD

1. **Pre-epiglottic space (Boyer's space)**
   - Boundaries:
     - Anteriorly: Thyroid cartilage and thyrohyoid membrane.
     - Superiorly: Hyoid bone, hyoepiglottic ligament and valleculae.
     - Posteriorly: Anterior surface of epiglottis and thyroepiglottic ligament.
     - Laterally communicates with paraglottic space.

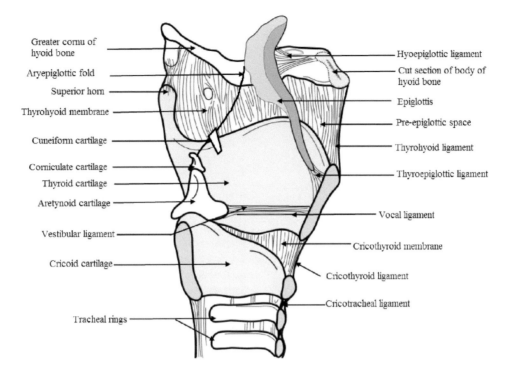

Figure 12.2 Sagittal section through the larynx.

- Contents:
  - Fat and areolar tissue.
  - Lymphatic drainage: Level II and Level III.
  - Pre-epiglottic space is frequently invaded by tumours because epiglottis has multiple small fenestrations.
  - Supraglottic tumours involving this space are staged as T3.
2. **Para-glottic space**
   - Boundaries:
     - **Medially:** Quadrangular membrane, laryngeal ventricle and conus elasticus.
     - **Laterally:** Thyroid cartilage anteriorly and mucosa of medial wall of PFS posteriorly.
     - **Inferolaterally:** Cricothyroid membrane.
     - **Anteriorly:** Continuous with pre-epiglottic space.
     - Supraglottic and glottic tumours involving this space are staged as T3.
3. **Anterior subglottic wedge**

MALIGNANT LESIONS OF THE LARYNX

See Tables 12.1 and 12.2.

TNM Classification for Laryngeal Cancer [AJCC 8th Edition] (See Table 12.3 through 12.7)

Management of Laryngeal Cancer

Work-up (according to the NCCN guidelines) is as follows:

- History and head and neck examination
- Fibre optic examination
- Direct laryngoscopy and biopsy of primary site +/- FNA of the neck nodes
- CT with contrast of primary and neck and thin angled cuts through larynx and/ or MRI with contrast of primary and neck
- Chest CT (with or without contrast) in cases of advanced nodal disease
- Audiogram, videostrobe for selected patients
- FDG-PET/CT in advanced stage disease
- Nutritional status, dental, speech and swallowing evaluation
- Pulmonary function test if conservation surgery is planned

Table 12.1 Primary Laryngeal Malignancies

Epithelial	Squamous cell carcinoma
	• Verrucous SCC
	• Spindle SCC
	• Adenoid SCC
	• Basaloid SCC
	• Clear cell carcinoma
	• Adenosquamous carcinoma
	• Giant cell carcinoma
	• Lymphoepithelial carcinoma
Malignant salivary gland tumours	Adenocarcinoma
	Acinic cell tumour
	Mucoepidermoid carcinoma
	Adenoid cystic carcinoma
	Carcinoma ex pleomorphic adenoma
	Epithelial—myoepithelial cell carcinoma
	Salivary duct carcinoma
Neuroendocrine tumours	Carcinoid tumour
	Small cell carcinoma
	Malignant paraganglioma
Malignant soft tissue tumours	Fibrosarcoma
	Malignant fibrous histiocytoma
	Leiomyosarcoma
	Rhabdomyosarcoma
	Angiosarcoma
	Kaposi sarcoma
	Malignant haemangiopericytoma
	Malignant nerve sheath tumour
	Alveolar soft part sarcoma
	Synovial sarcoma
	Ewing sarcoma
Malignant tumours of bone and cartilage	Chondrosarcoma
	Osteosarcoma
Haematolymphoid tumours	Lymphoma
	Extramedullary plasmacytoma

Table 12.2 Secondary Laryngeal Malignancies

Contiguous primary site	Hypopharynx
	Oropharynx
	Thyroid
Distant primary site	Kidney
	Skin (melanoma)
	Breast
	Lung
	Prostate
	Gastro-intestinal tract

Table 12.3 Supraglottis Cancer

Primary tumour (T)	
TX	Primary tumour cannot be assessed
T0	No evidence of primary tumour
Tis	Carcinoma in situ
T1	Tumour limited to one subsite of supraglottis with normal vocal cord mobility
T2	Tumour invades mucosa of more than one adjacent subsite of supraglottis or glottis or region outside supraglottis (e.g., mucosa of base of tongue, vallecula, medial wall of pyriform sinus) without fixation of larynx
T3	Tumour limited to larynx with vocal cord fixation and/or invades any of the following: post-cricoid area, pre-epiglottic space, paraglottic space and/or inner cortex of thyroid cartilage
T4a	Tumour invades through outer cortex of thyroid cartilage, and/or invades tissues beyond the larynx, e.g., trachea, soft tissues of neck including deep/extrinsic muscle of tongue (genioglossus, hyoglossus, palatoglossus and styloglossus), strap muscles, thyroid, oesophagus
T4b	Tumour invades prevertebral space, encases carotid artery or mediastinal structures

Table 12.4 Glottis Cancer

Primary Tumour (T)	
TX	Primary tumour cannot be assessed
T0	No evidence of primary tumour
Tis	Carcinoma in situ
T1	Tumour limited to vocal cord(s) (may involve anterior or posterior commissure) with normal mobility T1a Tumour limited to one vocal cord T1b Tumour involves both vocal cords
T2	Tumour extends to supraglottis and/or subglottis; impaired vocal cord mobility
T3	Tumour limited to larynx with vocal cord fixation and/or invades paraglottic space and/or inner cortex of thyroid cartilage
T4a	Tumour invades through outer cortex of thyroid cartilage, and/or invades tissues beyond the larynx, e.g., trachea, soft tissues of neck including deep/extrinsic muscle of tongue (genioglossus, hyoglossus, palatoglossus and styloglossus), strap muscles, thyroid, oesophagus
T4b	Tumour invades prevertebral space, encases carotid artery or mediastinal structures

Table 12.5 Subglottis Cancer

Primary tumour (T)	
TX	Primary tumour cannot be assessed
T0	No evidence of primary tumour
Tis	Carcinoma in situ
T1	Tumour limited to subglottis
T2	Tumour extends to vocal cord(s) with normal or impaired mobility
T3	Tumour limited to larynx with vocal cord fixation
T4a	Tumour invades cricoid or thyroid cartilage, and/or invades tissues beyond the larynx, e.g., trachea, soft tissues of neck including deep/extrinsic muscle of tongue (genioglossus, hyoglossus, palatoglossus, and styloglossus), strap muscles, thyroid, oesophagus
T4b	Tumour invades prevertebral space, encases carotid artery or mediastinal structures

Table 12.6 : N-Regional Lymph Nodes Metastasis

NX	Regional nodes cannot be assessed
N0	No regional lymph node metastasis
N1	Metastasis in a single ipsilateral lymph node ≤ 3 cm in greatest dimension, without clinical extranodal extension
N2a	Metastasis in a single ipsilateral lymph node > 3 cm but not more than 6 cm in greatest dimension, without clinical extranodal extension
N2b	Metastasis in multiple ipsilateral lymph nodes, none > 6 cm in greatest dimension, without clinical extranodal extension
N2c	Metastasis in bilateral or contralateral lymph nodes, none > 6 cm in greatest dimension, without clinical extranodal extension
N3a	Metastasis in a lymph node > 6 cm in greatest dimension, without clinical extranodal extension
N3b	Metastasis in single or multiple lymph nodes, with overt extranodal extension irrespective of size

Table 12.7: M-Distant Metastasis

M0	No distant metastasis
M1	Distant metastasis

TREATMENT OPTIONS FOR LARYNGEAL CANCER

SUPRAGLOTTIC LARYNX

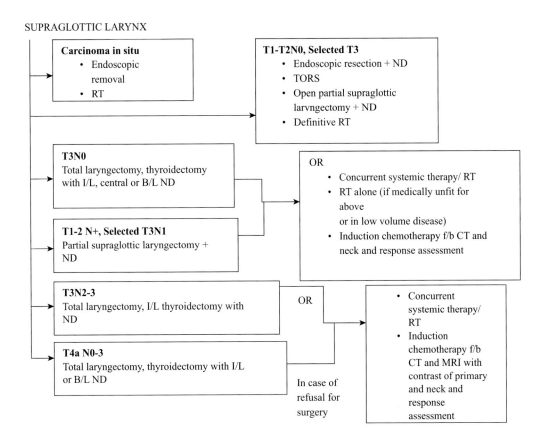

(RT- Radiotherapy, I/L- Ipsilateral, B/L- Bilateral, ND- Neck Dissection)

Flow Diagram 2

Treatment of Advanced Laryngeal Cancer

Concurrent systemic therapy/RT or induction systemic therapy followed by RT or systemic therapy/RT or palliative RT/clinical trial are the various options for advanced laryngeal cancers.

SURGERY FOR LARYNGEAL CANCER

Organ Preservation Laryngeal Surgery (See Table 12.9)

The principles of organ preservation surgery are as follows.

1. Local control.
2. Accurate prediction of three-dimensional extent of tumour.
3. Preservation of at least one functional cricoarytenoid unit: The cricoarytenoid unit is the basic functional unit of the larynx (one arytenoid, cricoid, associated musculature and nerve supply). It is the cricoarytenoid unit, not the vocal folds, that allows for physiologic speech and swallowing without the need for a tracheostomy.

Transoral Laser Microsurgery

Transoral laser microsurgery (TLM) has similar oncologic outcomes as open partial laryngectomy with less functional morbidity.

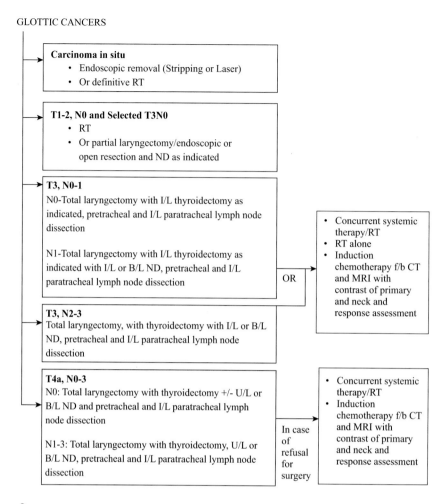

GLOTTIC CANCERS

Flow Diagram 3

Its advantages are as follows:

- Decreased tracheotomy requirement.
- No pharyngocutaneous fistulae.
- Less disfigurement.
- Less pain.
- Better voice quality.
- Earlier swallowing.
- Lower risk of overtreatment.
- Shorter hospital stay.
- Can be repeated many times for local recurrences as well as second primary tumours.

Contraindications are as follows:

- Unresectable cancer.
- Advanced cancer that requires reconstruction.
- Patients with functional disorders after extensive partial resection such as severe, persistent aspiration or secondary stenosis.

Transoral laser surgery has comparable results with open partial surgeries and radiotherapy if tumour-free margins are obtained.

TLM could be recommended as a curative treatment for the following:

- **Early glottis cancers:** T1 or T2 without nodal or distant metastases, selected T1a, T1b or T2a with anterior commissure involvement.
- **Moderately advanced glottis cancers:** Possible for selected T3 and T2b with anterior commissure involvement.
- **Supraglottic cancers:** Possible for all T-stage tumours especially T1, T2 and selected T3 with minimal infiltration of pre-epiglottic space, paraglottic space, or T4 with only circumscribed involvement of thyroid cartilage, provided it has been fully visualised during preceding diagnostic microlaryngoscopy surveys.

For supraglottic cancers, glottic-preserving partial laryngectomy using TLM contradicts the classic rules of oncologic surgery as there is sectioned and piecemeal removal of tumour in many cases.

- A laser-safe double-cuff endotracheal tube is used or anaesthesia is delivered through intravenous infusion with muscle relaxant and maintained through venture entrainment system.
- Optimal exposure is necessary for safe tumour resection. Spreadable blades of bivalve laryngoscopes may be used for adequate exposure of laryngeal structures. For maximal view, pressure may be applied to cricoid by tapes.
- After the laser system has been pre-tested, an optimal setting with dot size of 1 mm, exposure time of 0.1 second and a power of 5–10 watts, in a repeated mode, is done.
- Surgery is performed with CO2 laser coupled to operating microscope and laser beam manipulated with micromanipulator, taking all laser safety precautions. Zero degree, 30 degree and 70 degree Hopkins rod telescopes may be helpful.
- Operating microscopes and haemostatic effect of CO2 are helpful in detecting boundary between tumour and healthy tissue.
- Small tumours along the free margins of the epiglottis and aryepiglottic fold can be excised en bloc while larger ones require systematic stepwise excision.
- In cases of infrahyoid tumour extension, pre-epiglottic space must be completely removed

and may be extended to false vocal cords and paraglottic space.

- Epiglottis may be initially divided horizontally or sagittally, and then retracted into a plane tangential to the laser beam.
- The dissection can be done along the inner surface of thyroid cartilage, leaving the perichondrium in situ unless required as a margin.
- Resection done guided by depth of tumour and surface extent.
- Similarly, for resection of glottic cancers, tumour is held with aspirating forceps and retracted medially.
- The laser incision starts posteriorly or posterolaterally, with laser plume being aspirated simultaneously, while maintaining at least 1 mm margin.
- Ipsilateral false cord may be removed (ventriculotomy) in order to visualise the entire lesion.
- Dissection proceeds from posterior to anterior and resection of deep margin relies on appearance of vocalis muscle and vocal ligament in cases of true vocal cords.
- Contact endoscopy may be useful in mapping the margins.
- The surgical defect heals by secondary intention.

In cases of glottis carcinomas, the European Laryngological Society (ELS) has proposed eight types of cordectomies for partial resections depending on the degree of resection and to ensure better post-operative results (See Table 12.8).

Table 12.8 ELS Classification of Cordectomies

Type I	Subepithelial cordectomy	Resection of the epithelium
Type II	Subligamental cordectomy	Resection of the epithelium, Reinke's space and vocal ligament
Type III	Transmuscular cordectomy	Through the vocalis muscle
Type IV	Total cordectomy	Excision of vocal cord extending from anterior to posterior commissure
Type Va	Extended cordectomy	Encompasses the contralateral vocal fold and the anterior commissure
Type Vb	Extended cordectomy	Includes the arytenoid
Type Vc	Extended cordectomy	Encompasses the subglottis
Type Vd	Extended cordectomy	Includes the ventricle

Table 12.9 Conservation Laryngectomies

Type	Indication
I: Conservation Surgery for Glottic Cancers	
1. Vertical hemilaryngectomies	For primary tumours of the vocal cords that extend to involve anterior commissure, supraglottis or subglottis
1.1: Laryngofissure with cordectomy	Early glottis lesion, particularly midcord lesions of mobile true vocal cords, not extending to anterior commissure or arytenoids, thyroid cartilage, subglottis or supraglottis
1.2: Anterolateral vertical partial laryngectomy	Lesion of mobile cord extending to anterior commissure or involving vocal process and anterosuperior portion of arytenoids or less than 5 mm of subglottis or fixed vocal cord lesions not extending across midline. Unilateral transglottic lesion not violating beforementioned criteria
1.3: Frontolateral vertical partial laryngectomy	Tumour involves ipsilateral vocal cord, anterior commissure and up to 1/3 of contralateral vocal cord.
1.4: Anterior partial laryngectomy	Tumours only affecting anterior commissure
1.5: Posterolateral vertical hemilaryngectomy	All the endolaryngeal circumference except for one arytenoids region and posterior commissure are removed
1.6: Extended vertical hemilaryngectomy	Removes superior aspect of cricoid cartilage
2. Supracricoid partial laryngectomy with cricohyoidoepiglottopexy	For T1b glottis tumour that involves anterior commissure, selected T2 and T3 glottic carcinoma
3. Subtotal laryngectomy	Horizontal partial laryngectomy for glottis cancer
II: Conservation Surgery for Supraglottic Cancer	
Horizontal supraglottic partial laryngectomy	T1 or T2 lesions of the epiglottis, false vocal cords, aryepiglottic folds and T3 lesions involving pre-epiglottic space (Generally for <3 cm tumours, with both true vocal cords mobile, sparing of at least 5 mm margin at anterior commissure, no cartilage or ventricular involvement with interarytenoid, postcricoid and apex of PFS free and normal tongue mobility)
Supracricoid partial laryngectomy with cricohyoidopexy	For supraglottic lesions not amenable to supraglottic laryngectomy due to glottis involvement through anterior commissure or ventricle or pre-epiglottic space invasion, decreased cord mobility, limited thyroid invasion
Near total laryngectomy	For supraglottic cancer with fixed cord or glottis cancer with subglottic extension, for transglottic cancers, supraglottic cancers involving tongue base

Open Partial Conservation Laryngectomies

Prerequisites: good pulmonary function, node negative, age <70 years, well-differentiated squamous cell carcinoma, consent for total laryngectomy if required, patient choice, surgeon skill

Table 12.10 Selection Criteria for Supracriocoid Partial Laryngectomy

Indications	Contraindications
T1 and T2 supraglottic lesions with ventricle extension	Bulky pre-epiglottic space involvement
T2 infrahyoid epiglottis or posterior one-third of the false cord	Gross thyroid cartilage destruction
Supraglottic lesions extending to glottis or anterior commissure with or without vocal cord mobility	Interarytenoid/ bilateral arytenoids involvement/ fixed arytenoids
T3 transglottic carcinoma with limitation of vocal cord	Subglottic extension >10 mm anteriorly or >5 mm posteriorly
Selective T4 lesions invading thyroid cartilage	Inadequate pulmonary reserve

SURGICAL TECHNIQUES

Anterolateral Vertical Partial Laryngectomy

- Pre-operative tracheostomy performed and general anaesthesia induced.
- Skin crease collar incision, around 8 cm, placed at the middle of the vertical height of the thyroid cartilage.
- Subplatysmal flaps raised to expose strap muscles from thyrohyoid to cricothyroid membrane or second tracheal ring.
- Midline fascia incised, plane of thyroid cartilage reached and midline of cartilage exposed by retracting strap muscles on both sides. Sternohyoid is freed on involved side down its whole length but not detached. Similarly, sternothyroid and thyrohyoid are freed and cut from oblique line.
- Perichondrium incised in midline by electrocautery from thyroid notch to cricothyroid membrane.
- Using fine periosteal elevator, perichondrium is elevated from ala to posterior margin after detaching it from upper border of ala and inferiorly from cricothyroid membrane.
- Laryngofissure is performed through the anterior midline and divided cartilage alas retracted by hooks.
- The involved side of larynx is rotated forwards and another vertical cartilaginous cut made just in front of posterior lamina where the perichondrial flap is attached.

- Haemostat is inserted through the deficiency in subglottic mucosa and supraglottic larynx is retracted cephalad with a right-angled retractor.
- Soft tissues are divided at upper border and cricothyroid membrane at lower border of lamina.
- Mucosa of subglottic larynx incised up to posterior midline.
- Mucosal incision made in hemilarynx over false cord, arytenoids, posterior edge of true cord at midline to include the tumour with adequate margins and connected with the above incision.
- Surgical specimen including ipsilateral thyroid cartilage, true vocal cord, portions of subglottic mucosa and false cord is removed with angled serrated scissors after dividing superior horn of thyroid cartilage.
- Cricoarytenoid joint and attachment of inferior constrictor are divided.
- If growth reaches vocal process, arytenoids are removed; otherwise they are spared.
- The cut ends of thyrohyoid and sternothyroid are sutured together and everted into lumen opposite the remaining cord, and sutured to remaining mucosal edges anteriorly and posteriorly to form pseudocord.
- The sternohyoid muscle is brought in to add bulk.
- On both sides perichondria are sutured water tightly over the muscle flaps after feeding tube insertion.
- Drain is inserted and fixed over strap muscles.
- Skin wound closed.

Reconstruction can also be done with the following techniques:

- Advancement and rotation flaps of local mucosa (postcricoid mucosa, aryepiglottic fold, medial wall of PFS).
- Bipedicaled strap muscle flaps.
- Inferiorly based sternohyoid flap.
- Epiglottic flap for cartilage support and mucosal coverage if petiole is uninvolved.
- Free cartilage graft from contralateral ala.
- Revascularised free temporoparietal flap.

Open Cordectomy via Laryngofissure

When TLM facility or radiotherapy is not available, entire musculomembranous vocal fold with the vocalis muscle can be removed. Inner perichondrium can also be partially removed.

- Under GA, single transverse or vertical incision made.
- Vertical midline thyrotomy done after retracting skin, soft tissue and strap muscles.
- External perichondrial flap not developed, no cartilage removed.
- After laryngofissure, sound side is retracted, tumour margin defined and the involved cord removed with 1–2 mm mucosal margin. Generous portion of underlying vocalis muscle should be removed for deep margin.
- Superior laryngeal artery transfixed, mucosal closure done.
- Sternohyoid muscle slid inside the larynx on the inner perichondrium to replace the lost bulk.
- Closure done.

Frontolateral Partial Hemilaryngectomy

- Vertical cut in thyroid is performed 1 cm paramedian from anterior midline on contralateral thyroid ala.

Anterior Vertical Partial Hemilaryngectomy

- Pre-operative tracheostomy performed and general anaesthesia induced.
- Skin crease incision placed at the middle of the vertical height of the thyroid cartilage.

- Subplatysmal flaps raised to expose strap muscles from thyrohyoid to cricothyroid membrane.
- Midline fascia incised, plane of thyroid cartilage reached and midline of cartilage exposed by retracting strap muscles on both sides.
- Perichondrium incised in midline by electrocautery from thyroid notch to cricothyroid membrane.
- It is elevated approximately 6 mm to 1 cm on lesser involved side and up to half of ala or to posterior margin, depending on extent on primary involved cord.
- Thyrotomy is done on two sides at the markings. Lower border of cartilaginous component of surgical specimen retracted cephalad.
- Subglottis entered through cricothyroid membrane.
- Under direct vision, mucosal incisions placed in glottis, securing adequate margins.
- Scissors used to divide musculature and specimen is removed, leaving stumps of vocal cord on both sides and both arytenoids and supraglottic larynx intact.
- These stumps of vocal cords are sutured to remaining alas on both sides through holes drilled in cartilage and functional larynx is restored.
- Silastic keel is placed in midline and fixed by sutures.
- Strap muscles reapproximated, drain placed, skin wound closed.
- Keel removed after 5–6 weeks along with tracheostomy.

Supracricoid Partial Laryngectomy with Cricohyoidoepiglottopexy (See Table 12.10)

Resection of both true cords, both false cords, entire thyroid cartilage, paraglottic spaces bilaterally and maximum of one arytenoid unit.

- GA induced through orotracheal intubation. Endoscopic evaluation done.
- Transverse incision placed at the level of cricothyroid membrane.
- Subplatysmal flaps elevated and strap muscles exposed in midline superiorly to hyoid bone and inferiorly to isthmus and proximal trachea.

- Midline fascia incised, strap muscles retracted or divided, isthmus divided, low tracheostomy done and circuit switched.
- Larynx rotated and posterior edge of both thyroid lamina exposed one by one.
- Inferior constrictor detached from oblique line on both sides.
- Cricothyroid muscle divided and subglottis entered through cricothyroid membrane.
- Entire thyroid cartilage removed with superior horns. Inferior horns and cricoid are preserved to save recurrent laryngeal nerve (RLN), or a very careful disarticulation of cricothyroid joint is required.
- Supraglottis entered through thyrohyoid membrane just superior to false vocal cord.
- Mucosal incision made anterior to arytenoid to superior border of cricoid.
- On dominant side, incision can be made over arytenoids. Both vertical incisions meet with the incision in the cricothyroid membrane anteriorly.
- Full thickness resection of glottis in monobloc fashion.
- Redundant mucosa overlying arytenoids covers denuded cricoid.
- Two lateral sutures and a midline anterior suture traversing pre-epiglottic space and inferior edge of epiglottis, joins cricoid with hyoid, taking large portion of tongue base.
- Strap muscles and skin closure is done after placing drain.

CONSERVATION SURGERY FOR SUPRAGLOTTIC CANCER

Horizontal Supraglottic Partial Laryngectomy

Epiglottis, hyoid bone, pre-epiglottic space, thyrohyoid membrane, upper half of thyroid cartilage and supraglottic mucosa removed. Only one arytenoid may be removed.

- Pre-operative tracheostomy performed and GA induced.
- Endoscopic evaluation done.
- Preparation and positioning done.
- Skin incision made in neck crease at the level of thyrohyoid membrane from anterior border of left to anterior border of right SCM.

- Subplatysmal flaps raised superiorly to hyoid and attachment of suprahyoid muscles and inferiorly to thyroid cartilage.
- Strap muscles detached from hyoid bone to expose thyrohyoid membrane.
- Anterior commissure is marked at exactly the midpoint between thyroid notch and lower border of thyroid cartilage in midline.
- Perichondrial incision made over thyroid cartilage to excise upper third of alas, posteriorly curving cephalad.
- Suprahyoid muscles removed from central third of hyoid bone to skeletonise it and resect it for pre-epiglottic space excision.
- Holes are drilled on the remaining thyroid cartilage on each side of the midline for resuspension of larynx before dividing thyroid cartilage.
- Both thyroid cartilage and hyoid are divided.
- Under vision, soft tissue is divided below the upper part of divided thyroid cartilage.
- Central third of hyoid grasped and division of false cords is continued posteriorly.
- Specimen is mobilised cephalad.
- Oropharynx entered by dividing vallecula mucosa and connecting incision with that of same-sided false cord mucosal incision.
- Base of tongue is retracted cephalad and glosso-epiglottic fold divided, freeing the epiglottis to further mobilise the specimen.
- Taking adequate margins around the tumour, specimen is released.
- Mucosal edge of medial wall of PFS is sutured to remaining mucosa of false cord.
- Denuded false cord in posterior half is covered. No attempt made to approximate laryngeal mucosa to mucosa of base of tongue.
- Sutures passed through previously drilled holes and musculature of base of tongue
- All sutures tied at end sequentially. Detached strap muscles sutured to mylohyoid and base tongue in two layers.
- Drain placed, skin wound closed.

Supracricoid Partial Laryngectomy with Cricohyoidopexy

This involves resection of both true cords, both false cords, the entire thyroid cartilage, both paraglottic spaces bilaterally, only one arytenoid, thyrohyoid membrane and epiglottis.

- GA induced through orotracheal intubation. Endoscopic evaluation done.
- Transverse incision placed at the level of cricothyroid membrane. Standard apron flap incision can be placed if I/L or B/L neck dissection is required.
- Subplatysmal flaps are elevated and strap muscles exposed in midline superiorly to hyoid bone and inferiorly to isthmus and proximal trachea.
- Midline fascia incised, strap muscles retracted or divided, isthmus divided, low tracheostomy done and circuit switched.
- Larynx rotated and posterior edge of both thyroid lamina exposed one by one.
- Inferior constrictor detached from oblique line on both sides and PFS mucosa spared.
- Cricothyroid muscle divided and subglottis entered through cricothyroid membrane.
- Hyoid bone periosteum is incised and stripped from the deep surface of the bone.
- A tunnel is used to traverse the pre-epiglottic space and enter the pharynx just above the epiglottis.
- Tumour is visualised through pharyngotomy and the latter is connected to cricothyroid-otomy using heavy Mayo scissors on the lesser involved side and under vision on tumour-bearing side.
- Mucosal incision made anterior to arytenoid to superior border of cricoid.
- On dominant side, incision can be made over arytenoids. Both vertical incisions meet with the incision in cricothyroid membrane anteriorly.
- Entire thyroid cartilage removed with superior horns and epiglottis. Inferior horns and cricoid preserved to save RLN, or a very careful disarticulation of cricothyroid joint is required.
- Redundant mucosa overlying arytenoids covers denuded cricoid.
- Three submucosal 0 Vicryl sutures are looped around cricoid cartilage and passed around the hyoid bone, taking large portion of tongue base.
- Strap muscles and skin closure is done after placing drain.
- Reconstruction performed using hyoid bone, cricoid and tongue.
- A temporary tracheostomy and feeding tube will be required.

Treatment of Neck in Supraglottic Cancers

Due to high incidence of neck metastases (25–50%) with rate of occult metastasis being 20–40% and palpable 30–50%, if surgical treatment is selected, elective neck dissection (ND) on I/L side is recommended. Bilateral ND may be reserved for cases with high probability of occult metastasis, like central or bilateral tumours, or lateral tumours with clinically positive I/L nodes.

TOTAL LARYNGECTOMY

Indications

- Advanced (T4a) squamous cell carcinoma.
- Recurrent squamous cell carcinoma of larynx after radiation therapy or CCRT.
- Nonfunctional larynx with significant aspiration and low-quality voice.
- Poorly differentiated carcinoma of the thyroid with gross laryngotracheal invasion.
- Patients not suitable for partial laryngectomy.

Contraindications

- Tumour invades prevertebral space, encases carotid artery or invades mediastinal structures.
- Presence of distant metastasis.
- T1–T3 local disease amenable for radiotherapy, chemoradiation or partial laryngectomy.
- Selected T4 tumours with minimal thyroid cartilage.

Surgical Technique

The larynx should be removed in a block which includes the strap muscles, hyoid bone, pre-epiglottic space and at least a hemithyroidectomy on the side of the tumour.

Here we describe the detailed operative steps for total laryngectomy for a patient of laryngeal cancer having thyroid cartilage involvement (**Figure 12.3**).

1. Under GA, patient is laid supine with extension under shoulders and parts cleaned and draped.
2. A high tracheostomy at the beginning of the

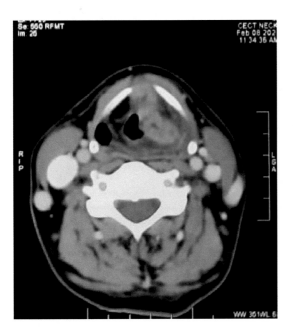

Figure 12.3 Axial CT scan of the neck showing tumour involving glottis and extending anteriorly to involve the thyroid cartilage.

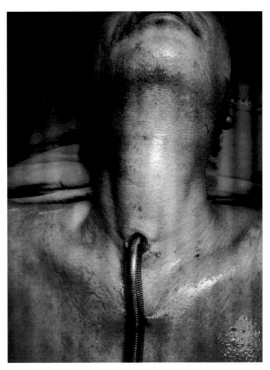

Figure 12.4 Patient placed supine with neck in extended position and flexometallic endotracheal secured to the chest.

surgery is preferred if patient was not previously tracheostomised.

3. Endotracheal tube is passed through stoma and fixed to chest (Figure 12.4).
4. Ryle's tube inserted and fixed.
5. Gluck-Sorenson U-shaped skin incision is made (most common). Horizontal limb of apron flap is 2 cm above sternal notch, incorporating stoma in the incision and vertical limbs starting at the level of hyoid bone, around 1 cm posterior to anterior border of SCM to the stoma (**Figures 12.5 and 12.6**). Collar incisions can be used, most commonly at level of thyrohyoid membrane with separate stomal incision in inferior flap. Incision may be modified if neck dissection is required or patient has been previously irradiated.
6. Subplatysmal flaps are elevated to hyoid bone with its attached suprahyoid muscles superiorly to suprasternal notch inferiorly (**Figure 12.7**).
7. Sternocleidomastoid muscles are retracted bilaterally after incising deep cervical fascia at the medial border of the muscle.
8. Bilateral paraglottic dissection is done and carotid tunnels are made to expose the great vessels. Bilateral omohyoid muscles are di-

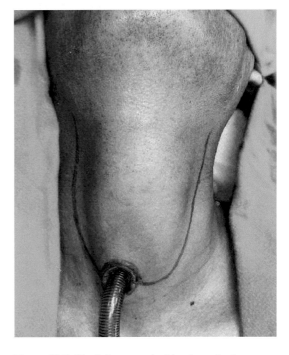

Figure 12.5 Gluck-Sorenson incision is marked.

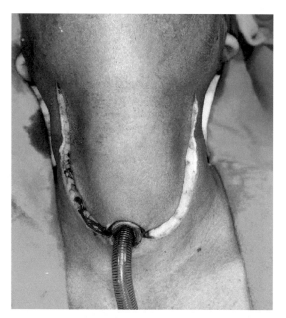

Figure 12.6 Incision deepened to the subcutaneous tissue.

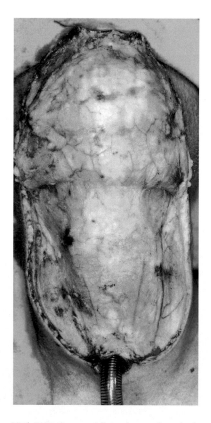

Figure 12.7 Subplatysmal flap elevated to the hyoid bone.

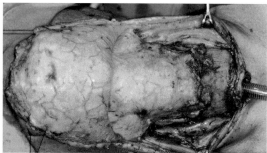

Figure 12.8 Bilateral paraglottic dissection done and strap muscles divided at the level of stoma to expose the thyroid gland.

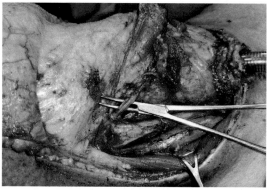

Figure 12.9 The superior thyroid pedicle identified and ligated.

vided at their tendons along with the ligation and division middle thyroid vein. Thyroid gland is exposed by dividing the strap muscles at the level of stoma inferiorly and hyoid bone superiorly (Figure 12.8).

9. Bilateral superior thyroid pedicles, inferior thyroid veins and ipsilateral inferior thyroid artery are identified and ligated. The inferior thyroid artery on the opposite side of the tumour is spared for blood supply to contralateral lobe (Figure 12.9).

10. Isthmus and recurrent laryngeal nerves are divided with sharp dissection at the ligament of Berry. Contralateral thyroid lobe is then reflected laterally after dissecting strap muscles over it. Ipsilateral involved lobe is left attached to the larynx and central compartment neck dissection performed.

11. The posterior border of thyroid ala is identified and made prominent by retracting the whole larynx on the opposite side (Figure 12.10).

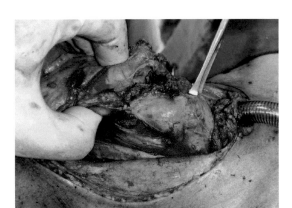

Figure 12.10 The posterior border of thyroid ala identified and made prominent by retracting the whole larynx on the opposite side.

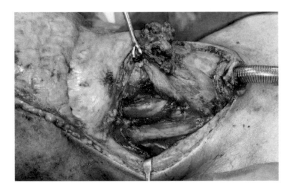

Figure 12.11 The inferior constrictor muscle divided at the posterior border of thyroid ala.

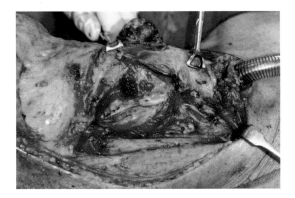

Figure 12.12 The posterior border of the thyroid ala is exposed and sharp dissection done to elevate the pyriform sinus mucosa on the uninvolved side. The same steps are repeated on the other side.

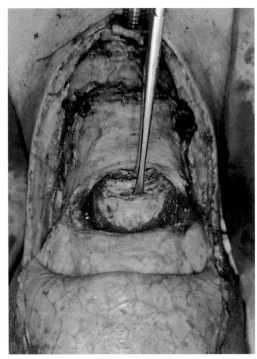

Figure 12.13 Hyoid bone identified and skeletonised.

12. Inferior constrictor is cut from thyroid cartilage at posterior border of lamina (Figure 12.11).
13. The posterior border of the thyroid ala is exposed and sharp dissection is done to elevate the pyriform sinus mucosa on both sides. PFS mucosa freed from thyroid cartilage by stripping the mucoperiosteum (Figure 12.12).
14. Next, the body of hyoid bone along with the greater cornu is identified, held with heavy forceps and skeletonised using monopolar cautery, taking care not to injure the hypoglossal nerve as an injury there will greatly reduce swallowing performance postlaryngectomy (Figures 12.13 and 12.14).
15. Pharyngotomy is done at level of hyoid bone on contralateral side of the tumour. Retracting the tongue base, the tumour is inspected. To perform optimal high pharyngeal entry just above the pre-epiglottic space, one can insert the blade of the laryngoscope in the vallecula, which can be identified easily to mark the site of pharyngotomy. This prevents a very high (base of the tongue) or low pharyngotomy (pre-epiglottic space entry) (Figure 12.15).

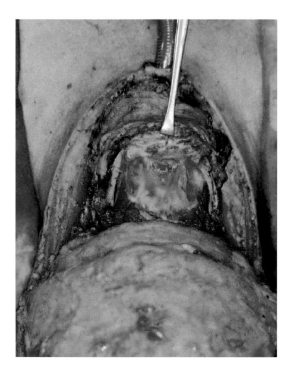

Figure 12.14 The greater cornu of the hyoid is also exposed on both sides.

16. Epiglottis is held with Allis forceps is pulled anteriorly and inferiorly. Standing at the head end, the surgeon cuts the pharyngeal mucosa on each side of the epiglottis, aiming towards superior cornu of thyroid cartilage and posterior part arytenoids to separate the larynx from hypopharynx, keeping as medially as possible and leaving at least 2 cm for closure. In the post-cricoid region, the mucosa is cut horizontally, inferior to cricoarytenoid joint, and this cut is joined with the previous two mucosal cuts. The space between the posterior wall of trachea and anterior wall of the oesophagus is entered (Figure 12.16).

17. The dissection is continued inferiorly between the wall of trachea and oesophagus to the stoma. Removing larynx from above downwards is preferred so that tumour is visualised while delivering the specimen (Figure 12.17).

18. Cervical trachea mobilised and trachea divided between two rings, depending on tumour extent. A new stoma is created inferiorly, endotracheal tube is inserted through it for ventilation and the larynx specimen is

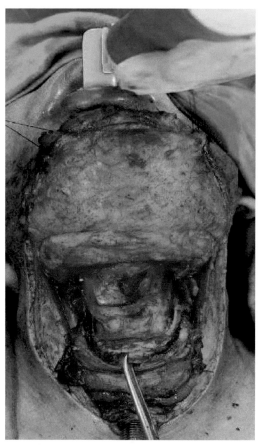

Figure 12.15 A high pharyngeal entry made after putting laryngoscope blade in vallecula to prevent entry into pre-epiglottis space.

delivered in toto along with thyroid gland/lobe (Figure 12.18).

19. A posterior midline cricopharyngeal myotomy is then performed (Figure 12.19).

20. A primary trachea-esophageal prosthetic device (TEP) is inserted next, if primary rehabilitation of voice is desired, after making a fistula between oesophagus and the tracheostome (Figure 12.20).

21. The sternal heads of sternocleidomastoid are cut on both sides. Neostoma is made in one or two layers to ensure airtight closure. One and a half suture technique with nonabsorbable suture (monofilament 2.0) is commonly used to approximate the subcutaneous tissue of lower subplatysmal flap to pretracheal fascia and tracheal cartilage (Figure 12.21).

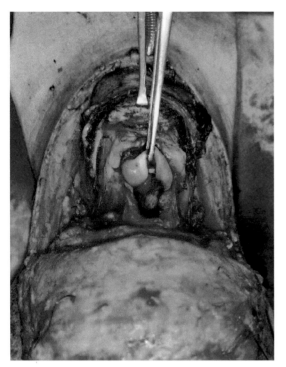

Figure 12.16 Epiglottis is held and pulled by Allis forceps and pharyngeal cuts made to separate the larynx from hypopharynx.

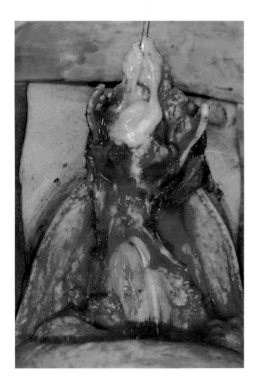

Figure 12.17 Dissection continues inferiorly between the wall of trachea and oesophagus to the stoma.

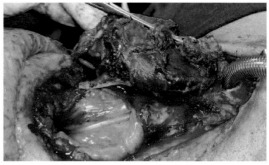

Figure 12.18 A new stoma is created inferiorly, the intubation tube is inserted for ventilation and the larynx specimen is delivered.

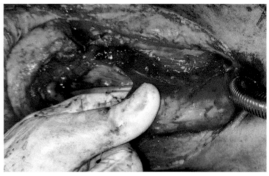

Figure 12.19 Cricopharyngeal myotomy.

22. Neopharynx is reconstructed, starting from below, by closing tidied edges of remaining pharyngeal mucosa using extramucosal, continuous and interlocking monofilament or braided absorbable synthetic sutures (running extramucosal to Connell stitch) (Figure 12.22).
23. The second layer of constrictor muscle is closed to provide further strength to the neopharynx repair (Figure 12.23).
24. Drains are inserted in bilateral paraglottic gutters, avoiding the neopharynx, and skin flap is sutured (Figure 12.24).
25. Skin wound closure is done in two layers and endotracheal tube is replaced with tracheostomy tube which is secured to the neck.
26. The specimen is split open in midline to look for the gross disease (Figure 12.25).

COMPLICATIONS

Early

- Drain failure
- Haematoma

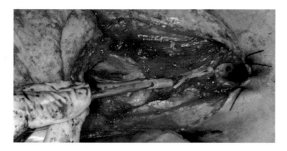

Figure 12.20 A primary TEP device is inserted.

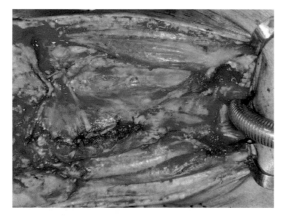

Figure 12.21 The sternal heads of sternocleidomastoid muscles cut on both sides.

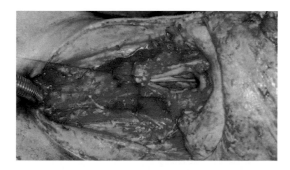

Figure 12.22 The neopharynx is created by closing the pharyngeal mucosa using extramucosal continuous interlocking sutures.

- Infection
- Pharyngocutaneous fistula
- Wound dehiscence

Late

- Stomal stenosis
- Pharyngoesophageal stenosis and stricture

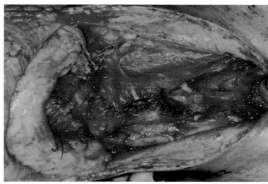

Figure 12.23 The second layer of constrictor muscle is closed to provide further strength to the neopharynx repair.

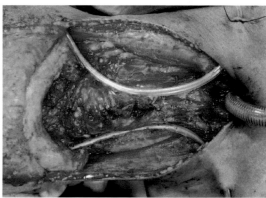

Figure 12.24 Drains inserted in bilateral paraglottic gutters.

- Hypothyroidism
- Hypoparathyroidism

Voice Rehabilitation

- Electrolarynx
- Esophageal speech
- Tracheo-esophageal voice using prosthesis
- Primary (at the time of laryngectomy) or secondary (after six weeks of laryngectomy) tracheo-esophageal puncture is between the posterior wall of tracheostome and the upper oesophagus into which a one-way silicone valve is inserted. Sound is produced by vibrating mucosa of pharyngoesophageal segment.

Stomal Recurrence

Recurrent disease may be secondary to the following.

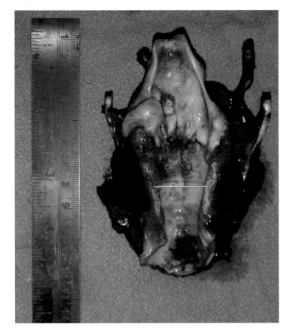

Figure 12.25 Specimen of total laryngectomy after midline split.

- Paratracheal node involvement.
- Invasion of the thyroid gland.
- Intraoperative tumour spill with implantation of tumour in the stoma.
- Incomplete excision of tracheal invasion by subglottic spread.
- Subglottic involvement of SCC is most commonly associated with stomal recurrence.

Adjuvant RT should be given, and treatment field should include the upper mediastinum in the following.

- Primary subglottic SCC
- Glottic SCC with greater than 1 cm of subglottic extension
- T4 glottic tumours

Treatment: Dissection of mediastinum and wide local resection for stomal recurrence.

Salvage Laryngectomy

- Laryngeal cancer that recurs after non-surgical treatment requires salvage laryngectomy.
- Prognostic factors in salvage laryngectomy include advanced recurrent AJCC stage, severe medical comorbidities and recurrent nodal disease.
- Most complications require operative interventions like locoregional or free flap reconstruction for pharyngocutaneous defects, revision of microvascular anastomosis, haematoma evacuation and carotid blowout.

FOLLOW-UP

This includes complete head and neck examination and fibre-optic examination.

- Year 1: Every 1–3 months.
- Year 2: Every 2–6 months.
- Years 3–5: Every 4–8 months.
- >5 years: Every 12 months.
- Routine annual imaging should be done in areas difficult to visualise on examination.
- TSH every 6–12 months if neck is.
- Dental evaluation.

13

Orbital Tumours

NITIN GUPTA AND RAVNEET R VERMA

INTRODUCTION

The orbit is a small anatomical space, surrounded by bone on all sides except anteriorly, containing a variety of important structures within. Tumours or tumour-like lesions may arise from these orbital contents.

The four rectus muscles form a muscle cone which divides the orbit into the intraconal and extraconal compartments. The intraconal compartment contains the globe, the optic nerve and sheath, orbital vessels and nerves. The extraconal compartment comprises the bony orbital walls, fat and the lacrimal apparatus. The orbital septum separates the anterior or pre-septal compartment from the intra-orbital contents. Localising orbital lesions to these specific compartments is an important diagnostic step and it helps to narrow down the list of differentials (See Table 13.1through 13.3).

Orbital tumours may arise primarily in the orbit or may invade the orbit from surrounding structures such as eyelids, paranasal sinuses, nasopharynx, bone or the cranial fossa. Orbital pathologies such as retinoblastoma (RB) and rhabdomyosarcoma (RMS) are typically seen in children, whereas lymphoma, malignant uveal melanoma and inflammatory orbital pseudotumours (IOP) are found in adults. The most common tumours that extend into the orbit are meningiomas, followed by sinonasal carcinomas.

Imaging plays a vital role in the management of these lesions. Understanding the presentation of various pathologies and clinical expertise can narrow the differential diagnosis and help to determine the appropriate imaging modality.

Intraconal tumours tend to cause early vision loss, impairment of ocular mobility, diplopia and proptosis. Extraconal tumours manifest early as proptosis, displacement of the globe and compression of the extraocular muscles and diplopia.

Classification
Orbital tumours may be classified, based on the region involved, as follows:

1. Intraconal tumours
2. Extraconal tumours
3. Multi-compartment tumours

Intraconal and extraconal tumours are subdivided based on the site of origin (Figure 13.1).

TUMOUR CHARACTERISTICS

The clinical features of orbital tumours vary according to site of origin and involvement of orbital and surrounding structures. These factors also determine the management of these tumours along with the histopathological grading of the tumour. These features have been summarised here for some of the common tumours.

Intraconal Tumours

1. **Retinoblastoma (RB):** It is a malignant tumour of retinal neoplasm and is the most

DOI: 10.1201/9780367430139-13

132

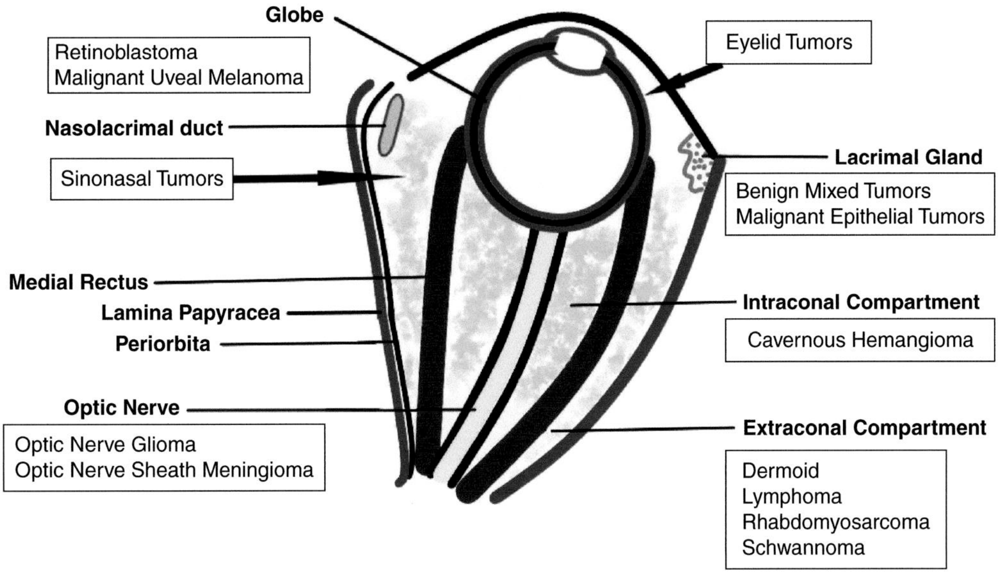

Figure 13.1 Schematic diagram of the orbit and associated tumours.

Table 13.1 Intraconal Tumours

Globe	Muscle cone and fat	Optic nerve and sheath
Retinoblastoma	Cavernous haemangioma	ON glioma
Hemangioblastoma		
Uveal melanoma	Pseudotumour	ON sheath meningioma
Choroid metastasis	Schwannoma (CN III, IV, VI)	

common intraocular tumour of childhood. It is caused due to mutation of the RB tumour suppressor gene on chromosome 13q14. Low-grade intraocular RBs are treated with chemotherapy, but advanced tumours need enucleation and/or radiotherapy.

2. **Malignant uveal melanoma:** It is the most common primary intraocular tumour in adults. Treatment options for smaller tumours are photocoagulation, radiotherapy, and globe-sparing surgery. Enucleation is used for larger tumours.

3. **Optic nerve glioma (ONG):** It is the most common primary optic nerve tumour. The low-grade form is more common and seen mostly in children, while the less common, aggressive form is seen in adults. Bilateral disease is pathognomonic of neurofibromatosis 1 (NF-

1). Patients present with decreased vision and painless proptosis. The role of chemotherapy and radiotherapy (RT) in the treatment is still controversial.

4. **Optic nerve sheath meningioma (ONSM):** It is the most common primary tumour arising from the ON sheath. It is a benign, slow-growing tumour with a tendency to recur. Primary ONSMs arise from the intraorbital and intracanalicular optic nerve. Secondary ONSMs are intracranial tumours extending to the orbit. The patients present with slowly progressive loss of vision and proptosis. Small ONSMs are often managed conservatively with follow-up imaging. Fractionated stereotactic RT is the treatment of choice.

5. **Cavernous haemangioma:** It is the most common benign orbital tumour-like condition

Table 13.2 Extraconal Tumours

Lacrimal apparatus	Eyelid	Others
Benign mixed tumours	Squamous cell carcinoma	Dermoid/epidermoid
Adenoid cystic carcinoma		Rhabdomyosarcoma
Adenocarcinoma	Basal cell carcinoma	Schwannoma and perineural
Mucoepidermoid carcinoma		spread—First and second
		division of trigeminal nerve
		(V1 and V2)
Carcinoma ex-pleomorphic adenoma	Melanoma	Osteoma
		Fibrous dysplasia
Pseudotumour	Lymphoma	Myeloma
Lymphoma, leukaemia		Metastasis

Table 13.3 Multi-Compartment Tumours: Tumours That Can Involve Any Part of the Orbit

Vascular malformations
Lymphoma
Rhabdomyosarcoma
Plexiform neurofibroma
Metastasis
Pseudotumour

in adults. Usually intraconal, it presents with diplopia and a slowly progressive, unilateral proptosis. Asymptomatic tumours are observed conservatively, while surgical resection is reserved for correction of visual disturbance and cosmesis.

Extraconal Tumours

1. **Dermoid:** It is the most common congenital orbital lesion. Epithelial sequestration at the zygomaticofrontal and frontoethmoidal sutures leads to dermoid formation. Dermoids are extraconal, supero-lateral, between the globe and the orbital periosteum. Small tumours do not require immediate treatment. Complete excision without rupture of capsule is necessary to avoid inflammatory reactions and recurrences.

2. **Lacrimal gland tumours:** They are classified as epithelial and non-epithelial tumours. Epithelial tumours constitute 40–50% of all lacrimal masses. About 50% these are benign mixed tumours (BMT), and the other half are malignant. Adenoid cystic carcinoma (ACC) is

the most common malignancy of the lacrimal glands.

a. Benign mixed tumours: They originate from the orbital lobe of the lacrimal gland. It presents as a painless, slow-growing mass in the lateral orbit. They are benign tumours, but recurrence and malignant transformation is known. Meticulous excision for complete removal and pathological identification of capsular invasion can help prevent recurrences.

b. Malignant epithelial lacrimal gland tumours: ACC is a high-grade malignancy and accounts for up to 50% of all malignant epithelial lacrimal gland neoplasms. It presents as a hard mass in the upper lateral orbit. Associated pain is caused by perineural spread or bony invasion. Radical resection is preferred for small, low-grade tumours.

3. **Rhabdomyosarcoma (RMS):** It is the most common malignant mesenchymal tumour of childhood. The orbit (40%) is the most common location in the head-neck region. RMS usually presents with rapidly progressive symptoms like proptosis, ptosis and signs of inflammation. It is an aggressive tumour and infiltrates into the sinuses, orbital fissures, cavernous sinus, and cranial fossa. Haematogenous spread is to the lungs. Surgery and chemotherapy used in combination can achieve good survival rates.

4. **Lymphoma:** It accounts for more than half of all adult malignant orbital tumours. They can be primary orbital tumours or secondary to systemic disease. The anterior extraconal space

and lacrimal gland are most involved. Low-grade tumours respond well to RT. Chemotherapy is required for high-grade or systemic disease.

5. **Fibrous dysplasia (FD):** It is a developmental disorder where the normal bone marrow is replaced by fibro-osseous tissue. Cranio-facial fibrous dysplasia involves the frontal, ethmoid or sphenoid bones. Orbital involvement causes hypertelorism, exophthalmos and visual impairment. Surgery is required to correct facial deformity or decompression of the optic nerve.

Multicompartment Tumours

1. **Venolymphatic malformation (VLM):** Also called lymphangioma, this is a congenital vascular malformation. It accounts for 5% of paediatric orbital tumours. They may present with proptosis, diplopia and optic neuropathy. Treatment is mostly conservative. Percutaneous sclerotherapy is useful in limited cases. Surgery is difficult due to the trans-spatial nature with high risk of recurrence.
2. **Orbital plexiform neurofibroma (OPNF):** It is a hamartoma of neuro-ectodermal origin. OPNF is diagnostic of NF-1. The sensory nerves of the orbit are usually involved. OPNF presents with periorbital masses, proptosis and visual impairment. Progressive glaucoma, optic nerve atrophy and blindness are eventual sequelae. There is a 10% risk of malignant sarcomatous degeneration. Although these tumours are not amenable to surgery, debulking is considered for preserving the vision or for cosmesis.
3. **Inflammatory orbital pseudotumour (IOP):** It is the most common cause of a painful orbital mass in adults. It is a benign, inflammatory condition without any discernible causes. The classic triad consists of unilateral orbital pain, proptosis and impaired ocular movement. The diagnosis is made after excluding other pathologies. Dramatic response to treatment with steroids helps to confirm the diagnosis.
4. **Immunoglobulin G4-related disease (IgG4-RD):** It is a chronic, systemic, autoimmune, fibro-inflammatory condition. Its most common presentation is autoimmune pancreatitis. Any part of the orbit may be involved. IgG4-RD has a dramatic response to steroids.

Secondary Orbital Tumours

1. **Lid tumours with orbital extension:** Common malignant tumours of the eyelid include squamous cell carcinoma, basal cell carcinoma, melanoma, sebaceous cell carcinoma and lymphoma. These tumours are aggressive and show frequent orbital involvement. Perineural spread along trigeminal nerve branches is also seen. Orbital exenteration is needed for local disease control.
2. **Sinonasal tumours with orbital extension:** It is more common for sinonasal pathology to affect the orbit than the opposite, and sinus pathology may present with predominantly orbital symptoms.
   a. Mucoceles: They result from sinus obstruction leading to expansion of the sinuses. Patients may present with diplopia and inferior (frontal) or lateral (ethmoid) globe displacement. When the contents become infected, mucopyoceles are formed. They can mostly be treated by marsupialisation via an endonasal route.
   b. Sinonasal neoplasms: Maxillary squamous cell carcinoma can invade the orbital floor and extend along the infraorbital nerve to the cavernous sinus. Neoplasms that originate in the ethmoid sinuses and the nasal cavity involve the orbit through the medial orbital wall. The goal of surgery is to obtain oncologic margins and maintain a functional eye. If the lamina papyracea is invaded but the periorbita is not, it allows for a more conservative surgical approach. If the periorbita has been breached, exenteration is required.
3. **Metastases:** These represent the most common orbital malignancy. Common primary sites for orbital metastases are melanomas, breast and lung cancers in adults and neuroblastomas in children. Painful proptosis is the most common presentation.

IMAGING

Imaging plays a vital role in the management of these lesions. Understanding the presentation of various pathologies and clinical expertise can narrow the differential diagnosis and help to determine the appropriate imaging modality (Table 13.4).

Table 13.4: Imaging Characteristics of Different Tumours of the Orbit

Tumour	Imaging Characteristics
Retinoblastoma	Necrosis and calcification with marked contrast enhancement.
Malignant uveal melanoma	CT is hyperdense with broad choroidal base. Calcification is rare. MRI is hyperintense on T1 and hypointense on T2 (due to high melanin content).
ON glioma	Fusiform/tubular enlargement and kinking of ON. OC widening. Hypointense on T1 and hyperintense on T2. Calcification rare.
ON sheath meningioma	Tubular thickening with calcification of ON sheath complex. OC widening. Hyperostosis. Isointense on T1 and T2. Tram-track sign and target sign.
Cavernous haemangioma	Well circumscribed. Separate from ON and EOMs. Phleboliths confirmatory. MRI T1 – Isointense to Hypointense and T2 – Hyperintense. Variable contrast enhancement.
Dermoid	Ultrasound shows sharply defined, capsular lesion. CT/MRI shows well circumscribed, cystic lesion. Occasional fat-fluid level and calcifications seen. Hyperintense on T1 and T2.
Benign mixed tumour – lacrimal glands	Well circumscribed. Cystic degeneration leads to inhomogeneous appearance. Lacrimal fossa deformation and calcifications. Moderate contrast enhancement.
Malignant epithelial lacrimal gland tumours	Infiltration of the surrounding orbital tissue and poorly defined margins. Calcifications more common than benign tumours. T1 hypointense and T2 hypo/hyperintense. Prominent contrast enhancement. Fat-saturated CE-MRI is ideal for tumour staging and identifying perineural spread.
Rhabdomyosarcoma	Isodense to muscle on CT and T1 images, hypo/hyperintense on T2. Significant enhancement on contrast. Necrosis and calcification are uncommon.
Lymphoma	CT shows hyperdense mass involving the lacrimal gland. Bony destruction or perineural spread suggests aggressive histology. High-cellularity tumours appear moderately hypointense on T1 and T2 images. Marked contrast enhancement. PET-CT used to detect systemic metastasis.
Fibrous dysplasia	Bony expansion and a "ground glass" appearance on CT. Narrowing of the optic nerve canal and impingement of the optic nerve. Hypointense on T1 and variable intensity on T2 images. Marked contrast enhancement.
Venolymphatic malformation	Poorly circumscribed, lobulated lesions. Haemorrhagic contents appear hyperdense. Fluid-fluid levels are common. Calcification and bony erosions are rare. Variable signal on T1 and T2 images.
Orbital plexiform neurofibroma	Defect in the greater wing of sphenoid on X-ray is called "Harlequin eye". CT and MRI show orbital and periorbital infiltrative soft tissue masses. On T2 MRI, target sign is seen. Post-contrast enhancement is variable.
Inflammatory orbitalpseudotumour	Enhancing orbital soft tissue, lacrimal gland, ON sheath and extraocular muscles and streaky fat stranding. Hypointense on T1 and iso- to hypointense on T2 images.
IgG4-RD	Hypointensity on T1 and T2 images with marked contrast enhancement. Diffusion-weighted MRI (DWI) can differentiate between IgG4-RD and lymphoma.
Metastasis	CT and MRI show enhancing infiltrative extraconal mass with bony destruction. DWI can help to differentiate it from lymphomas. PET-CT can detect the primary site and metastatic deposits to other organs.

CHOICE OF SURGICAL APPROACH

The orbit is a complex structure, with important neurovascular structures both within and around it. In selecting a surgical approach, the surgeon needs to find the best route to remove the whole tumour while preserving these structures. It is important is to avoid working across the neurovascular structures. In particular, the ON plane should not be crossed.

Tumours anteriorly in the orbit can be approached via an anterior orbitotomy via the eyelid crease or a sub-brow approach or transconjunctival/sub-ciliary approach. Larger anterosuperior lesions may need an additional craniotomy of the superior orbital rim. Lateral orbitotomy can provide excellent lateral access to the optic nerve and apex. A pterional or fronto-temporal orbital craniotomy can be used to approach tumours even with lateral intracranial extension.

Small and anteriorly placed lesions of the medial part of orbit may be excised via medial orbitotomy. Larger and more posteriorly located lesions are resected via a combined lateral and medial orbitotomy. Inferior and posterior lesions are tackled via an inferior orbital approach.

Extended endonasal approaches (EEAs) can be used to access tumours that are medial and inferior to the ON. EEA, with its anterior and medial trajectory, is ideal for skull base lesions that are anteromedial to critical neurovascular structures. Tumours that displace the optic nerve superiorly and laterally are usually the best targets for an endonasal approach.

APPROACHES TO THE ORBIT

There are three main routes to get access to orbital tumours: transorbital, transcranial and endonasal. An overview of the transorbital and transcranial approaches is provided and the endonasal endoscopic approach is discussed in detail.

1. Transorbital
   a. Anterior approaches:
      i. Sub-brow approach
      ii. Trans-septal anterior orbitotomy
   b. Lateral approaches:
      Lateral orbitotomy
   c. Medial approaches:

   i. Transconjunctival medial orbitotomy
   ii. Medial-lateral orbitotomy
   iii. Inferior orbital approach or posteroinferior orbitotomy
2. Trans-cranial
   a. Orbitofrontal craniotomy
      i. Medial approach
      ii. Lateral approach
      iii. Central approach
   b. Pterional (frontotemporal) craniotomy +/- orbitozygomatic extension
   c. Supraorbital keyhole approach

3. Endonasal
   a. Medial—inferior extraconal approach
   b. Transmaxillary extraconal approach
   c. Medial intraconal approach

Trans-Orbital Approaches

Anterior Approaches
1. Sub-brow approach

   An incision is made through the lower brow, parallel to the direction of the brow hair, down to the level of the orbital bone. The skin and subdermal tissues are retracted. The periosteum (periorbita) is incised and dissected from the orbital bone. The lesion is then identified, dissected and removed.

2. Trans-septal anterior orbitotomy

   Orbit is entered via the orbital septum of the upper eyelid via a superior lid crease incision or the lower eyelid via lid incision or a subciliary incision. Skin and muscle flaps are elevated to expose and open the orbital septum.

Lateral Approach
1. Lateral orbitotomy

   Used for extraconal and intraconal tumours that lie lateral and inferior to the optic nerve, including lacrimal gland tumours and retrobulbar tumours. The skin incision is S-shaped and extends from the lateral orbital rim to the upper border of the zygomatic arch. The orbicularis and deep fascia are cut to reach the periorbita over the orbital rim. The periorbita is incised just lateral to the rim and then elevated medially for 3–4 cm along the lateral orbital wall. Protecting the orbital contents, two transverse osteotomies are made over the lateral orbital wall and the bone piece removed. The sphenoid wing bone can be removed to reach up to the orbital apex. The periorbita is incised parallel to the lateral rectus muscle. The lateral rectus is retracted. Standard microsurgical methods are applied for tumour resection.

Medial Approaches

1. Transconjunctival medial orbitotomy

   The medial orbitotomy is used to remove small, medial orbital tumours. A conjunctival peritomy is done medially to expose the medial rectus muscle. Incisions are made superior and inferior to the muscle. It is then isolated and severed at its insertion site into the globe. Orbital fat is retracted. An additional lateral orbitotomy can provide more space for displacement of the globe. Standard microsurgical steps are carried out for tumour resection. The muscle is reattached at the original site, and the conjunctiva is sutured around.

2. Medial-lateral orbitotomy

   Medial orbital tumours which are large or in posterior places may be resected a combined lateral-medial-orbital approach. The lateral incision is made directly through the canthus extending 3 cm posteriorly and part of the lateral bony wall can be drilled away. This allows the globe to fall into the bone defect laterally, creating more room medially.

3. Inferior orbital approach or posteroinferior orbitotomy

   This approach can be used for posteroinferior orbital tumours. It utilises a standard Caldwell-Luc approach on the side of the tumour. The maxillary-sinus mucosa is removed, uncovering the orbital floor. The posteroinferior part of the floor is then removed, avoiding the infraorbital nerve. The inferior rectus muscle is retracted to one side. The tumour is removed and the inferior rectus is then placed back into position.

Trans-Cranial Approaches

1. Orbitofrontal craniotomy

   For lesions involving the optic canal and orbital apex, an orbitofrontal craniotomy provides easier access. Following a bicoronal incision, an orbitofrontal bone flap is removed.
   There are three routes to get access to the orbital contents.

   a. Medial approach between the superior oblique muscle and the levator and superior rectus muscles, which are retracted laterally, providing direct surgical access to the apical part of the ON.

   b. Lateral approach between the lateral rectus, retracted laterally, and the superior rectus and levator muscles, which are retracted medially. It provides a wider working space than the other orbitofrontal approaches. It is the best of the three routes for access to the lateral apical part of the ON. It can be combined with an orbitozygomatic craniotomy, for lesions extending to the middle cranial fossa.

   c. Central approach involves the levator muscle being retracted medially and the superior rectus retracted laterally. It is the most direct way to the midportion of the ON.

2. Pterional (frontotemporal) craniotomy +/- orbitozygomatic extension

   Particularly useful for tumours that have infratemporal fossa or a middle fossa extension. A curvilinear incision is made starting anterior to the tragus and ending near the middle of the hairline (Figure 13.2). Soft tissue flaps of the scalp and temporalis muscle are elevated. A frontotemporal craniotomy is performed, which may or may not extend to the zygoma. The greater wing of the sphenoid is made flush with the orbit. The orbital bone is freed from the dura and periorbita before performing the orbital osteotomies. Intraorbital tumour can be localised by direct visualisation, palpation, image guidance or intraoperative ultrasonography.

3. Supraorbital keyhole approach

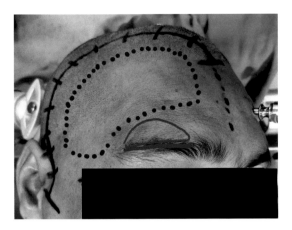

Figure 13.2 Pterional craniotomy: Skin incision (black) and craniotomy (red dotted line). Supraorbital keyhole approach: Skin incision (blue line) and craniotomy (pink line).

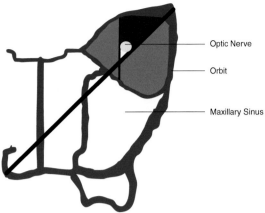

Figure 13.3 A plane propagated between a line drawn from the contralateral nostril (reflecting the trajectory of the trans-septal approach) and the long axis of the ON describes the plane of resectability. The green area, which lies lateral and inferior to this plane, can be approached by endonasal endoscopic approach. The red area lies medial and superior to this plane and is not amenable for endonasal approach.

The supraorbital keyhole is useful to access lesions that are located superior to the optic nerve. The skin incision is made over the eyebrow. Care is taken to preserve the supratrochlear and supraorbital neurovascular bundles. After elevating a peri-cranial flap, a craniotomy is made. The lower end of the craniotomy is flush with the orbital roof and it arches superiorly in a semi-circular fashion. Access is maximised by drilling the posterior part of the orbital rim flush with the roof of the orbit. Tumour is identified, dissected and removed using standard microsurgical techniques.

Endonasal Approaches

The endoscopic transnasal approach to the orbit is indicated for the following:

1. Medial extraconal space lesions.
2. Medial orbital apex lesions.
3. Radical removal or diagnostic procedures in the inferomedial intraconal space.
4. In combination with other approaches, to manage more complex lesions.

Pearls and Pitfalls

- The location of the lesion relative to the ON dictates the approach. Lesions located medial to the ON or below a plane of resectability (Figure 13.3), subtended by the contralateral nostril and the long axis of the ON,

are amenable to the exclusively endoscopic approach.
- Endonasal approach to the infero-medial part of the orbit avoids manipulation of the globe and ON required for external approaches.
- A bi-nostril, two-surgeon/four-handed approach is advocated, especially for lesions that are intraconal, involving the orbital apex or skull base. This approach allows bimanual dissection, greater access and wider working angles.
- A nasoseptal flap needs to be elevated for reconstruction.
- The medial intraconal space may be divided by the inferomedial muscular trunk of the ophthalmic artery and an imaginary line dividing the upper and lower half of the medial rectus muscle belly into three compartments (Figure 13.4).

- Retracting the medial rectus provides medial displacement and exposure of intraconal space. Access to intraconal zone A may be achieved by superomedial retraction of the medial rectus. Inferior retraction of the medial rectus provides exposure to zone B.
- Medial rectus muscle is within millimetres of the optic nerve in zone C.

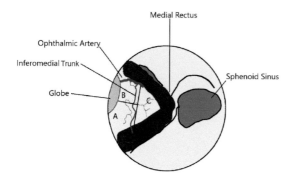

Figure 13.4 Schematic diagram of medial intraconal space divided into three zones. The inferomedial trunk of the ophthalmic artery and an imaginary line splitting the medial rectus divide the space into three zones. Zone A: Anterior to the artery and inferior to the imaginary line. It is the easiest zone to approach due to its direct access and the lack of neurovascular structures. Zone B: Anterior to the artery and superior to the imaginary line. It is more challenging due to proximity of the ethmoidal vessels. Zone C: Posterior to the artery. This region is the most difficult to address as the optic nerve and ophthalmic artery are closely related.

- The periorbita should be incised just anterior to the tumour to preserve the anterior part of the periorbita and avoid fat prolapse, which can impair visualisation.

Pre-Operative Checklist

- Evaluation by a multidisciplinary team is important. This includes an otorhinolaryngologist, an ophthalmologist and a neurosurgeon if a craniotomy may be needed or a dural breach is expected.
- A complete ophthalmologic examination should always be done.
- Radiological assessment by CT scan and MRI provides information regarding
  - Accurate estimation of the tumour volume and morphology.
  - Relationship between the lesion and the surrounding bony and neurovascular structures.
  - Course of the ophthalmic artery relative to the optic nerve.
  - Image guidance.

- Angiography is useful if a vascular lesion is suspected.

Steps of Surgery (Endonasal Endoscopic Approach)

- Positioning of the patient: Reverse Trendelenburg position improves endoscopic field of view and reduces intraoperative blood loss.
- Preparing the nasal cavity: Injection of local anaesthetic and epinephrine solution at the superior attachment of the middle turbinate and packing of nasal cavity with 1:1000 epinephrine pledgets provides vasoconstriction and decongestion. This results in a wider cavity to work in and helps to reduce bleeding and improve visualisation.
- Before embarking on any advanced transnasal endoscopic procedure, it is vital to establish and identify the surgical landmarks.
- Perform a complete ethmoidectomy, maxillary antrostomy and sphenoidectomy.
- Identify the frontal recess. Expose and remove the lamina papyracea.
- A septal window is created to allow the binostril approach.
- The nasolacrimal duct is given a sharp angulated cut if the approach demands.
- The anterior ethmoidal artery (AEA) is identified at the ethmoidal roof. The posterior ethmoidal artery (PEA) is usually harder to identify but runs about 12 mm behind the AEA within the skull base.
- The medial rectus can be identified under the periorbita in the posterior aspect, where the extraconal fat is less.
- At the level of the orbital apex, the annulus of Zinn is exposed, and the ON canal is usually identifiable posterior to it.
- The periorbita is incised. The extraconal fat is separated. It may be cauterised if it is prolapsed and obscures the view of the surgeon.
- Extraconal tumours can be identified and removed at this stage.
- Once the extraconal fat is separated, it exposes the medial and inferior rectus muscles. Between these muscles lies the window to the intraconal space (Figure 13.5).

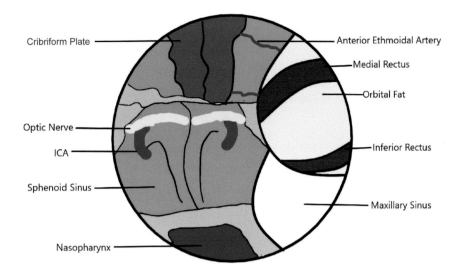

Figure 13.5 Schematic diagram of endonasal endoscopic view of the skull base and orbit.

- The medial rectus is retracted with the help of a probe superomedially or inferiorly, depending on the location of the tumour.
- Above the medial rectus, the ophthalmic artery with its terminal branches and the nasociliary nerve may be visualised. Lateral to them and on the medial side of the superior rectus muscle runs the superior ophthalmic vein.
- The ophthalmic artery as it enters the optic canal, lies inferomedial to the ON, then crosses over, superior to the nerve and onto the medial side. By splitting the annulus of Zinn between the medial and inferior rectus muscles, the inferior division of the oculomotor nerve with its branches and proximal part of the ophthalmic artery come into view.
- The lateral limit of dissection is the ON. The intraorbital tortuous course of the ON can be visualised by removing the medial part of the intraconal fat. In its anterior aspect, the ON is associated with a vascular network formed largely by the ciliary arteries.
- The posterior ciliary arteries can be seen in the posterior aspect of the orbit. It is possible to identify the central retinal artery, which enters the ON inferiorly.
- The tumour should be dissected bluntly. A two-surgeon four-handed technique is needed to hold the endoscope, retract the medial rectus muscle, dissect the tumour and suction the blood.
- The superior, medial and inferior attachments of the tumour are released first. The tumour is then gently retracted parallel to the ON and lateral attachment is separated.
- A nasoseptal flap is used for reconstruction. This prevents loss of orbital volume and the resultant enophthalmos and diplopia.
- Nasal packing should be placed with minimal pressure over the orbitotomy. This prevents rising of intraocular pressure due to post-operative bleeding and oedema.

Complications:

- Bleeding
- Diplopia
- Enophthalmos
- Visual impairment
- Ophthalmic artery or internal carotid injury
- Cerebrospinal fluid leak

Post-Operative Considerations

- Close monitoring with serial eye exams to look for any signs of nerve compression should be done.
- Post-operative corticosteroids may be useful to reduce the oedema.

- Pack removal can be done after 48–72 hours. Gentle saline cleaning should be started after pack removal.
- Careful endoscopic cleaning of the nasal cavity, away from the orbitotomy site, can be carried out between the 5–7 days post-operatively.

Medial-Inferior Extraconal Approach

This approach is used for sinonasal carcinomas extending to the orbit, meningiomas and juvenile nasal angiofibromas. The medial and inferior orbital walls are exposed and the lamina papyracea is removed. The tumour is identified and delineated from the orbital fat and muscles and removed.

1. Transmaxillary extraconal approach

   A medial maxillectomy is performed which allows direct visualisation of the floor of the orbit and the posterior part of the maxilla. Removal of posterior wall of maxilla, perpendicular plate of palatine bone and part of sphenoid bone allows the surgeon to remove tumours in the pterygopalatine fossa, infratemporal fossa and as far as Meckel's cave, in the middle cranial fossa.

2. Medial intraconal approach

   This approach is applied for infero-medial and posterior intraconal lesions. The dissection window is between the medial and inferior rectus muscles. To increase the size of this surgical corridor, the medial part of the orbital floor can be removed. Parallel to the medial rectus, the periorbita is incised. Looping the rectus muscles either endonasally or via a transconjunctival approach provides retraction and helps in tumour removal.

Various Approaches

Anterior Orbitotomy

- With osteotomy of the superior orbital rim: For larger lesions
- Without osteotomy: Superior mass

Eyelid supraorbital or sub-brow incision
   Inferior mass: Transconjuctival subciliary or lower eyelid incision

Incisions for Orbital Approaches

Superior Approach with Superior Osteotomy

- For larger extraconal superior orbital lesions.
- Incision: a sub-brow or a supraorbital with horizontal extent of at least 3 cm.
- The supratrochlear and supraorbital neurovascular bundles are preserved.
- The superior orbital rim is removed and is replaced and secured with titanium miniplates after tumour removal.

Anterior Transconjuctival Orbitotomy

- Medial conjuctival peritomy done.
- MR muscle is detached from the globe.
- Orbital fat is retracted from the anterior optic nerve.
- Optic nerve sheath (ONS) fenestration: posterior ciliary nerve and vessels dissected from the medial surface of the nerve sheath followed by fenestration to allow free egress of the cerebrospinal fluid (CSF).
- MR is reattached to the globe and conjunctiva closed.

Trans-Septal Orbitotomy

- Orbit is entered via the orbital septum of the upper or lower eyelid.
- Upper eyelid: Superior lid crease incision.
- Lower eyelid: Direct incision or a subciliary incision.
- Skin and muscle flap is elevated to expose the orbital septum, which is then opened.

Anterior Medial Orbitotomy

- The medial approach was described in 1973 by Galbraith and Sullivan to decompress the optic nerve and relieve papillo-oedema.
- Indicated for biopsy, decompression or removal of tumours of the medial intraconal space (area between the optic nerve and the MR muscle) such as cavernous haemangiomas, schwannomas, hemangiopericytomas and isolated neurofibromas.
- This procedure may be used in conjunction with a sinus procedure in cases in which both regions are involved.

Lateral Orbitotomy:

- The lateral approach was first proposed by Kronlein in 1889 for a large orbital and temporal fossa dermoid cyst.
- It was standardised in 1976 by Maroon and Kennerdell.
- The lateral orbitotomy is useful for retrobulbar lesions and it can be extended for more posterior lesions.
- The procedure involves temporary removal of the lateral wall of the orbit to gain access to the entire lacrimal gland and lateral, superolateral and inferolateral tumours, e.g., pleomorphic adenomas and cavernous haemangiomas.

Transcranial Approaches

- For tumours located in the orbital apex and/or optic canal, or involving both the orbit and adjacent intracranial areas.
- Divided into two types based on whether the orbital rim is or is not elevated in exposing the orbital lesion.
- Small frontal or fronto-temporal craniotomy, with removal of the orbital roof and/or lateral wall for limited lesions.
- Orbitofrontal or orbitozygomatic approach, with elevation of the orbital rim with the bone flap for larger lesions.

Orbitofrontal Craniotomy

- For lesions involving the optic canal and orbital apex.
- Bicoronal incision.
- Keyhole site burr hole which exposes periorbita on lower edge and frontal dura on its upper edge.
- The orbito-frontal bone flap includes the superior rim of the orbit and part of the orbital roof.
- The thin part of the roof of the orbit behind the orbital rim is opened to prevent fracture across the orbital roof.
- One-piece exposure: superior rim is elevated with the bone flap.
- Two-piece exposure: small frontal bone flap above the supraorbital rim is elevated as the first piece and the superior rim is removed as the second piece.
- In the one-piece approach, there is risk of fracture of the orbital roof between the medial and the lateral margins of the cuts, which may extend into the ethmoid air cells or cribriform plate.
- Three routes through an orbitofrontal craniotomy can taken to the orbital contents: medial, lateral and central.

Endoscopic Approaches

- Directed through the space between the SO muscle, which is retracted medially, and the levator and SR muscles, both of which are retracted laterally.
- It exposes the optic nerve throughout the interval from the globe to the optic canal.
- It is the most direct surgical approach to the apical part of the optic nerve.
- MC selected for tumours of the optic sheath oroptic nerve.
- Not suitable for lesions located on the lateral side of the optic nerve or for those involving the SOF and the cavernous sinus.

FURTHER READING SUGGESTIONS

1. Winn H. *Tumors of the orbit. Youmans and Winn Neurological Surgery.* 7th ed. Philadelphia: Elsevier; 2016.
2. Purohit BS, Vargas MI, Ailianou A, et al. Orbital tumours and tumour-like lesions: Exploring the armamentarium of multiparametric imaging. *Insights Imaging.* 2016;7(1):43–68. doi: 10.1007/s13244-015-0443-8
3. Goh PS, Gi MT, Charlton A, Tan C, Gangadhara Sundar JK, Amrith S. Review of orbital imaging. *Eur J Radiol.* 2008;66:387–95. doi: 10.1016/j.ejrad.2008.03.031.
4. Lee AG, Johnson MC, Policeni BA, Smoker WR. Imaging for neuro-ophthalmic and orbital disease—a review. *Clin Exp Ophthalmol.* 2009;37:30–53. doi: 10.1111/j.1442-9071.2008.01822.x
5. Kumar V, Abbas AK, Aster JC. *Robbins and Cotran Pathologic Basis of Disease.* 9. Philadelphia: Elsevier Saunders; 2014.
6. Chung EM, Specht CS, Schroeder JW. From the archives of the AFIP: Pediatric orbit tumors and tumorlike lesions: Neuroepithelial lesions of the ocular globe and optic nerve. *Radiographics.* 2007;27:1159–86. doi: 10.1148/rg.274075014.

7. Lemke AJ, Hosten N, Bornfeld N, et al. Uveal melanoma: Correlation of histopathologic and radiologic findings by using thin-section MR imaging with a surface coil. *Radiology.* 1999;210:775–783. doi: 10.1148/radiology.210.3.r99fe39775.

8. Becker M, Masterson K, Delavelle J, Viallon M, Vargas MI, Becker CD. Imaging of the optic nerve. *Eur J Radiol.* 2010;74:299–313. doi: 10.1016/j.ejrad.2009.09.029

9. Heran F, Berges O, Blustajn J, et al. Tumor pathology of the orbit. *Diagn Interv Imaging.* 2014;95:933–44. doi: 10.1016/j.diii.2014.08.002

10. Thorn-Kany M, Arrue P, Delisle MB, Lacroix F, Lagarrigue J, Manelfe C. Cavernous hemangiomas of the orbit: MR imaging. *J Neuroradiol.* 1999;26:79–86.

11. Chung EM, Murphey MD, Specht CS, Cube R, Smirniotopoulos JG. From the Archives of the AFIP. Pediatric orbit tumors and tumorlike lesions: Osseous lesions of the orbit. *Radiographics.* 2008;28:1193–214. doi: 10.1148/rg.284085013.

12. Jung WS, Ahn KJ, Park MR, et al. The radiological spectrum of orbital pathologies that involve the lacrimal gland and the lacrimal fossa. *Korean J Radiol.* 2007;8:336–42. doi: 10.3348/kjr.2007.8.4.336.

13. Eckardt AM, Lemound J, Rana M, Gellrich NC. Orbital lymphoma: Diagnostic approach and treatment outcome. *World J Surg Oncol.* 2013;11:73. doi: 10.1186/1477-7819-11-73.

14. Chung EM, Smirniotopoulos JG, Specht CS, Schroeder JW, Cube R. From the archives of the AFIP: Pediatric orbit tumors and tumorlike lesions: Nonosseous lesions of the extraocular orbit. *Radiographics.* 2007;27:1777–99. doi: 10.1148/rg.276075138.

15. Jacquemin C, Bosley TM, Svedberg H. Orbit deformities in craniofacial neurofibromatosis type 1. *AJNR Am J Neuroradiol.* 2003;24:1678–82.

16. Patnana M, Sevrukov AB, Elsayes KM, Viswanathan C, Lubner M, Menias CO. Inflammatory pseudotumor: The great mimicker. *AJR Am J Roentgenol.* 2012;198:W217–W227. doi: 10.2214/AJR.11.7288.

17. Pakdaman MN, Sepahdari AR, Elkhamary SM. Orbital inflammatory disease: Pictorial review and differential diagnosis. *World J Radiol.* 2014;6:106–15. doi: 10.4329/wjr.v6.i4.106.

18. Soysal HG, Markoc F. Invasive squamous cell carcinoma of the eyelids and periorbital region. *Br J Ophthalmol.* 2007;91:325–29. doi: 10.1136/bjo.2006.102673.

19. Loo JL, Looi AL, Seah LL. Visual outcomes in patients with paranasal mucoceles. *Ophthal Plast Reconstr Surg.* 2009; 25(2):126–29.

20. Iannetti G, Valentini V, Rinna C, et al. Ethmoido-orbital tumors: Our experience. *J Craniofac Surg.* 2005; 16(6):1085–91.

21. Llorente JL, López F, Suárez C, et al. Sinonasal carcinoma: Clinical, pathological, genetic and therapeutic advances. *Nat Rev Clin Oncol.* 2014;11(8):460–72.

22. Paluzzi A, Koutourousiou M, Tormenti M, Fernandez-Miranda J, Snyderman C, Gardner P, et al. "Round-the-Clock" surgical access to the orbit. *J Neurol Surg Part B Skull Base* 2012;73.

23. da Silva SA, Yamaki VN, Solla DJ, de Andrade AF, Teixeira MJ, Spetzler RF, et al. Pterional, pretemporal, and orbitozygomatic approaches: Anatomic and comparative study. *World Neurosurg* 2019;121:e398–403.

24. Park HJ, Yang SH, Kim IS, Sung JH, Son BC, Lee SW. Surgical treatment of orbital tumors at a single institution. *J Korean Neurosurg Soc* 2008;44:146–50

25. Signorelli F. Endoscopic treatment of orbital tumors. *World J Clin Cases* 2015;3:270.

26. Cockerham KP, Bejjani GK, Kennerdell JS, Maroon JC. Surgery for orbital tumors. Part II: Transorbital approaches. *Neurosurgical Focus.* 2001;10(5):1–6. doi: 10.3171/foc.2001.10.5.4

27. Kennerdell JS, Maroon JC, Malton ML. Surgical approaches to orbital tumors. *Semin Ophthalmol* 1989;4:209–18.

28. Bejjani GK, Cockerham KP, Kennerdell JS, Maroon JC. A reappraisal of surgery for orbital tumors. Part I: Extraorbital approaches. *Neurosurgical Focus.* 2001;10(5):1–6. doi: 10.3171/foc.2001.10.5.3

29. Srinivasan A, Bilyk JR. Transcranial approaches to the orbit. *Int Ophthalmol Clin.* 2018;58:101–10.

30. Kannan S, Hasegawa M, Yamada Y, Kawase T, Kato Y. Tumors of the orbit: Case report and review of surgical corridors and current options. *Asian J Neurosurg.* 2019;14:678–85

31. Tomazic PV, Stammberger H, Habermann W, Gerstenberger C, Braun H, Gellner V, et al. Intraoperative medialization of medial rectus muscle as a new endoscopic technique for approaching intraconal lesions. *Am J Rhinol Allergy* 2011;25:363–7.

32. Gregorio, LL, Busaba, NY, Miyake, MM, Freitag, SK, Bleier, BS. Expanding the limits of endoscopic intraorbital tumor resection using 3-dimensional reconstruction. *Braz J Otorhinolaryngol.* 2019; 85(2):157–61.

33. Dallan I, Fiacchini G, de Notaris M. Endonasal endoscopic-assisted intraorbital approach. In: Sprekelsen MB, Alobid I, editors. *Endoscopic Approaches to Paranasal Sinus and Skull Base: A Step by Step Dissection Guide.* Stuttgart: Thieme; 2017. pp. 144–53.

34. Miyake MM, Bleier BS. Endoscopic approach and removal of orbital tumors. In: Chiu AG, Palmer JN, Adappa ND, editors. *Atlas of Endoscopic Sinus and Skull Base Surgery.* 2nd ed. Philadelphia: Elsevier; 2019. pp. 165–70.

14

Sinonasal Tumour Surgery

JAGDEEP S THAKUR AND KARTIK N RAO

INTRODUCTION

Malignancies of the paranasal sinuses are rare. The incidence varies between 0.5 and 1.0 per 1,00,000 population, and it accounts for less than 5% of all head and neck cancers. Males appear to be affected twice as often as females, and this may be secondary to environmental or occupational hazards. Elderly population is more often affected by the disease, and risk increases after 50 years of age. The maxillary sinus remains the most common site of paranasal sinus malignancies (50–70%), followed by the nasal cavity (15–30%) and ethmoid sinus (10–20%).

The definitive treatment of paranasal sinus malignancies is difficult and often necessitates a multidisciplinary approach. Surgical resection is typically followed by adjuvant radiation or chemoradiation. For early T1 or T2 lesions, surgery alone is still an option, especially for low-grade lesions confined to the lower nasal cavity, septum or maxillary sinuses. Combined modality therapy is always required for more advanced lesions. Surgical planning entails assessing the bony and soft tissue structures that must be resected, devising the best approach to ensure proper exposure, and anticipating the patient's reconstruction and rehabilitation needs for function and cosmesis.

A complete resection with clear margins must be performed using either an open or endoscopic approach. Immediate post-operative rehabilitation is a crucial part of the recovery process. Preoperative impressions and preliminary prostheses are usually taken to determine this. Prefabricated obturators can help with post-operative packing and allow the patient to eat right away. After all treatment and healing has been completed, they can be adjusted or modified. The ideal obturator allows for complete restoration of function while also being removable to allow for recurrence inspection.

Microvascular soft tissue reconstruction is now used to repair larger defects, rather than traditional methods like skin grafting or prosthetics. Although covering persistent or recurrent disease is a potential risk, such flaps provide superior cosmesis and function. The fibula free flap, scapula flap, radius osteocutaneous flap, and deep circumflex iliac artery flap are all excellent midface reconstruction techniques for lower maxillary defects, closing the palate and allowing osseo-integrated dental implants to be placed later.

CONTRAINDICATIONS

It is important to recognise when surgical intervention is likely to be futile and will fail to extend meaningful life. Although some contraindications are relative depending on experience, various conditions make it unwise to attempt an endoscopic or open resection (see Table 14.1).

Tumour extensions that are beyond the reach of angled scopes and instruments, or that are so large that an open or combined approach would be more rational, are currently endoscopic contraindications. Patients with distant metastases, gross brain invasion, central skull base invasion and bilateral optic nerve or chiasm infiltration are anatomic contraindications. Significant trismus indicates

DOI: 10.1201/9780367430139-14

Table 14.1 Contraindications for Endoscopic and Open Approaches in Sinonasal Surgery

Approach	Contraindication
Endoscopic	Dura involvement beyond mid-pupillary line
	Anterior/lateral frontal sinus involvement
	Facial/orbital soft tissue extension
	Palatal involvement
	Gross brain parenchyma involvement
Open	Gross invasion of the brain
	Invasion of both orbits
	Carotid encasement
	Invasion of the cavernous sinus
	Significant comorbidities
	Extension to nasopharynx or pterygoid fossa

gross invasion into the pterygoid musculature, while extension through the sphenoid sinus walls often indicates involvement of the carotid arteries or penetration into the cavernous sinus. Primary chemoradiation, possibly in a palliative setting, may be the best treatment for such inoperable cases.

PRE-OPERATIVE MANAGEMENT

Clinical examination: Clinical examination is important to assess the extent of tumour and also helps treatment planning and counselling. Examination of skin, dentition and orbital wall with ocular movements is most important. Once origin and extent of the tumour is verified by nasal endoscopy, further examination is carried out. Skin infiltration carries poor prognosis, while trismus is a relative contraindication for surgical intervention as it indicates pterygoid infiltration until excluded radiologically. Dentition examination helps in prosthetic planning, while tongue deviation or palatal paralysis indicates parapharyngeal or skull base infiltration. Digital palpation of maxillary walls and infratemporal fossa should be done to exclude local infiltration. Visual acuity should always be performed to rule out orbital or optic nerve infiltration. Patients requiring orbital exenteration should have functional contralateral eye or vision should be corrected to the best before proceeding with surgery.

Neck nodes carry poor prognosis in these malignancies and decision for surgical intervention should be reviewed in a multidisciplinary meeting.

Ear and laryngeal examination also provide information regarding extent of the tumour. Any serous otitis media, earache and hearing loss needs thorough evaluation. Similarly, vocal cord paralysis indicates parapharyngeal or skull base infiltration.

Radiological examination: Computerised tomography (CT scan) is the investigation of choice in nose and paranasal tumours. Benign bony or intra-sinus tumours are easy to diagnose on CT scan. Bone erosion and local infiltration are hallmarks of malignant tumour, while widened osteomeatal complex indicates benign pathology. Sometimes slow growing, expansible tumours appear extended beyond a sinus on CT scan (Figures 14.1 and 14.2) and require careful evaluation or magnetic resonance imaging (MRI). Local infiltration should always be looked into as it usually contraindicates surgery, except anterior skull base infiltration that requires further evaluation by MRI. Any meningeal infiltration in anterior skull base also contraindicates surgery or carries poor prognosis if attempted in selected cases. Orbital infiltration requires thorough evaluation by CT scan and MRI. Orbital preservation is indicated in periorbital fascia involvement, while infiltration beyond this requires orbital exenteration, and apex infiltration contraindicates surgery as tumour-free margins are difficult to achieve, except in selected cases when frozen section facility is available. Distant metastasis is investigated as per standard protocol. PET-CT scan is indicated for follow-up cases with high clinical suspicion, negative or inconclusive CT scan or MRI.

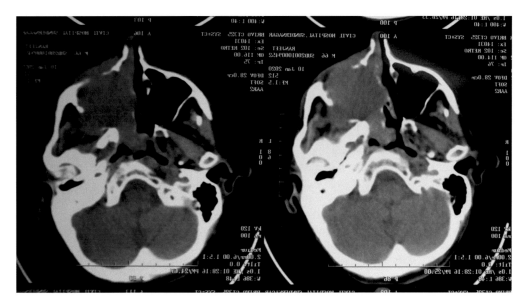

Figure 14.1 CT scan showing a tumour extending beyond maxillary bony walls.

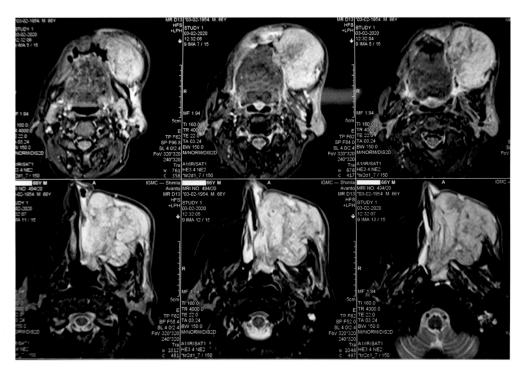

Figure 14.2 A big tumour extending beyond maxilla into subcutaneous space of the face.

Pathological examination: Tissue biopsy under endoscopic view should always be performed. Simple punch biopsy can be done in a large tumour visible externally, provided vascular tumours like juvenile nasal angiofibroma have been ruled out on clinical evaluation. Cytology is rarely required in these tumours, but patients refusing punch biopsy or suffering with bleeding disorders are the candidates where imprint cytology with gloved finger can be done. Aspiration cytology is required for neck nodes or sometimes for tumours presenting with isolated infratemporal swelling.

Prosthetic planning: As stated earlier, certain surgeries carry unavoidable facial, speech, eye and swallowing morbidities, and prosthetic rehabilitation planning should be carried out in consultation with surgeon and patient. Patient needs to be counselled and motivated regarding prosthesis. Advanced technology like 3-D printing has modernised the prosthetic implant. Custom-made implants are created to the satisfaction of the patient for better quality of life. Maxillectomy creates maximum facial disfigurement due to loss of cheek or malar prominence, orbital loss and voice and swallowing morbidity. In selected cases, reconstruction with composite free flap provides good quality of life, but the majority of such defects are managed by prosthesis.

Pre-operative preparation: Once the patient and attendants have been counselled and given consent for surgery, patient is examined by anaesthesia team for fitness for surgery. Reinforced nasotracheal tube should be used and kept to the contralateral side. Cases requiring anterior skull base resection and reconstruction need special consideration. Tracheostomy and intensive care must be kept ready as and when required and hence patient should be informed about the same.

External Nasal Surgery

Cutaneous carcinoma in terms of melanoma, basal and squamous cell carcinoma is the commonest tumour requiring surgical excision. However, this requires expertise in reconstructive surgery, as the nose is one of the most important facial sub-units. Primary closure after excision usually results in deformity, hence full thickness grafting and loco-regional flaps (forehead and nasolabial flap) are commonly used, although complete nasal excision needs free flap (radial forearm flap) (Figures 14.3 through 14.6). Sometimes, tumours from adjoining areas like eye, cheek and paranasal sinus may invade the nasal pyramid and require en bloc resection.

Sinonasal Tumour Surgery
Total maxillectomy

Indication

- Malignant maxillary tumour.

Contraindications

- T4b malignant tumours.
- Pterygoid plate invasion.
- Nasopharyngeal extension.
- Orbital apex invasion.
- Sphenoid invasion.

Surgical Approaches
Classic Weber-Ferguson incision

Absolute Indications

- T1–2 malignant maxillary tumours.
- Ethmoidal tumours.
- T3–4 malignant tumour.
- Cases requiring orbital exenteration or infra-temporal fossa clearance.
- In combination with skull base surgery.
- Maxillary swing approach for nasopharynx, pterygomaxillary fossa or infratemporal fossa.

Surgical Steps

- Nasotracheal intubation is done through contralateral nostril and head extended and positioned contralaterally.
- Incision site is infiltrated with freshly prepared 2% lignocaine or normal saline with adrenaline (1:1,00,000 or 1:2,00,000). Eyelids are closed with complete temporary tarsorrhaphy.
- After cleaning and draping, incision is marked. Special attention is given to lip and eyelid. The alar incision is curved inside the nostril and brought out laterally, not at midline of philtrum, to provide a better cosmetic result than incision at the midline.
- Incision is made with monopolar cautery in cutting mode except in eyelid area, where skin is quite thin and the orbicularis muscle can be damaged; therefore, the scalpel is preferred.
- Acute angulation near medial canthus is avoided due to risk of post-operative necrosis. Angular vessels are coagulated with bipolar cautery.

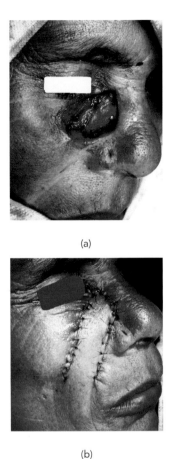

(a)

(b)

Figure 14.3a-b The defect after basal cell carcinoma excision and closure with advancement flap.

- Incision is made bone deep in lateral rhinotomy and gingival sections.
- Gingival incision is curved backward to last molar tooth and then curves medially over the hard and soft palate junction to midline, saving mucosa as much as possible (Figure 14.7).
- Now the midline incision over hard palate is made bone deep and brought anteriorly while curving towards the lateral incision, so as to save it depending upon oncological possibility.
- Cheek flap is raised over periosteum, depending upon tumour infiltration, where flap is to be modified and infraorbital neurovascular bundle is saved accordingly (Figure 14.8).
- Using Freer's elevator, periorbital periosteum is elevated.
- Osteotomy begins in naso-maxillary suture lines with osteotome or power saw towards medial canthus while retracting and saving orbital contents.

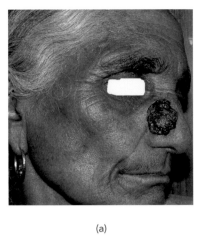

(a)

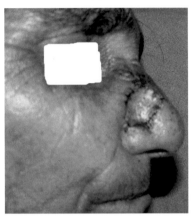

(b)

Figure 14.4a-b Wound closure with full thickness skin graft after excision of basal cell carcinoma.

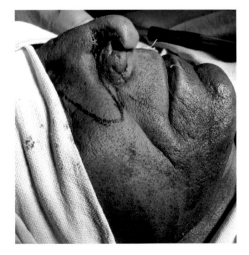

Figure 14.5 Nasolabial flap for reconstruction of alar defect that will arise with excision.

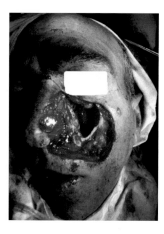

(a)

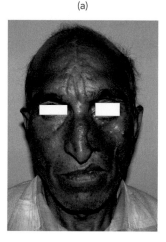

(b)

Figure 14.6a-b Reconstruction of large surgical defect with median forehead flap

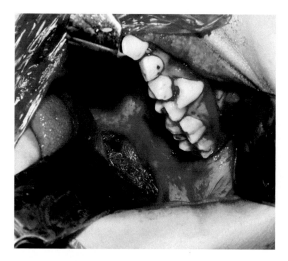

Figure 14.7 The palatal incision is made at the junction of hard and soft palate.

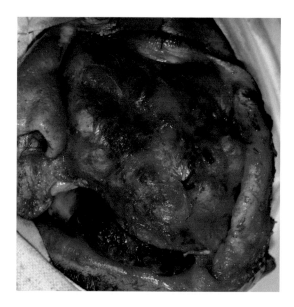

Figure 14.8 The skin flap is raised, taking care of extra-sinus tumour.

- Saw/osteotome is turned laterally about 1–2 cm to go backwards cutting lacrimal bone. Another bone, cut in the infraorbital margin about 2–3 cm lateral to the first, is taken backwards and meets the medial cut, making a triangle apex. This step can be modified according to involvement of orbital floor. As this is one of the most important aesthetic units, and due to availability of the power saw, the authors save as much as orbital margin as possible.
- Orbital floor is preserved as far possible, otherwise it requires reconstruction to avoid enophthalmos or ectropion.
- Now this cut is taken towards the orbito-maxillary-zygomatic arch while preserving malar eminence (Figure 14.9).
- Cut coronoid temporalis muscle tendon with electrocautery.
- Similarly, cut attachment of soft palate and hard palate.
- Take long haemostat clamp through ipsilateral nostril towards palate incision.
- Clamp Gigli's saw and perform palatal osteotomy slowly, as saw can break under excessive force.
- Power saw can also be used to do this osteotomy, but it requires expertise as midline breach and contralateral palatal fenestration can occur. Power saw is preferred for gingival cut (Figure 14.10).

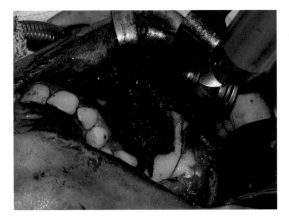

Figure 14.9 The zygomatic arch is cut with power saw, saving malar eminence if oncologically safe.

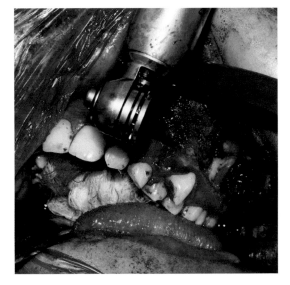

Figure 14.10 The midline osteotomy is made, saving lateral incisor.

- Pterygo-maxillary osteotomy typically requires heavy scissors, but authors prefer bipolar or coagulation mode monopolar cautery due to pterygoid plexus.
- Any bony fusion is displaced with chisel.
- As maxilla is pulled out, internal maxillary artery gets disrupted and is lamped and ligated.
- Complete haemostasis is achieved and cheek flap grafted with split skin thickness graft or flap (Figure 14.11).
- Temporary obturator is sutured to palate and contralateral arch.
- Cavity packed with medicated pack and incision closed in two layers with 3–0 or 4–0

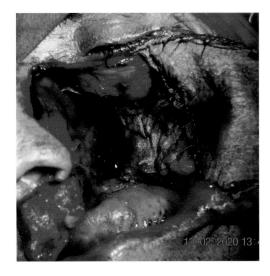

Figure 14.11 The soft tissue of surgical defect is covered with split skin graft.

sutures, taking special care with curves and the aesthetic units of nose and lips.
- Antibacterial ointment is applied to suture lines and tarsorrhaphy sutures removed.
- Nasogastric tube inserted and patient extubated.

FACIAL DEGLOVING APPROACH

Facial degloving incision is advantageous as it avoid external scars; however, it provides limited exposure (Figure 14.12a–c).

Indications

- T-2 malignant maxillary tumour.
- Inverted papilloma.
- Ethmoidal tumours.

Contraindications

- T3–4 sinus tumours as this approach has limited exposure.
- Infratemporal or skull base infiltration.

Surgical Steps

- Incision starts from lip frenulum and extends to last molar and then curves to midline, incising hard and soft palate junction (Figure 14.13).

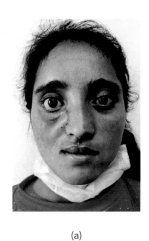

(a)

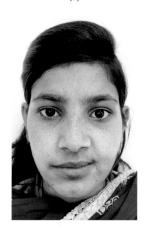

(b)

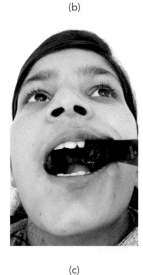

(c)

Figure 14.12 (a) The surgical scar visible after classical Weber-Ferguson incision. (b-c) The external surgical scar is avoided with facial de-gloving approach.

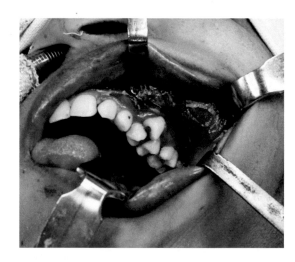

Figure 14.13 The sub-labial incision.

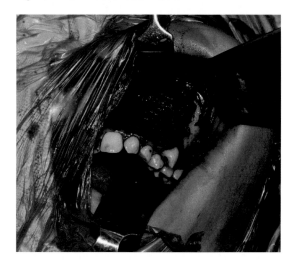

Figure 14.14 The flap is raised, exposing canine fossa.

- Musculo-periosteal cheek flap is raised depending upon tumour extent while exposing lateral nasal wall, infraorbital margin and malar eminence (Figure 14.14).
- Nasal cavity is entered through pyriform aperture while preserving external naris aperture (Figure 14.15).
- Infra-orbital neurovascular bundle is preserved as per oncology protocol.
- Further surgical steps are similar to open technique.

Post-Operative Care

- Antibiotic and anti-inflammatory are given as per institutional protocol.

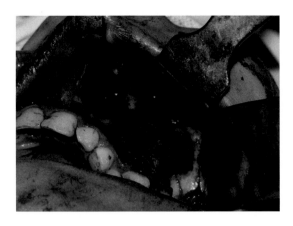

Figure 14.15 The ipsilateral pyriform aperture exposed fully. The classical facial degloving approach requires transfixion incision in septum and raising the nasal tissue.

- Nasogastric feeding continued till pack removal on fifth post-operative day.
- Nasal douching/irrigation are continued for six weeks till complete epithelisation of the surgical cavity.
- Interim prosthesis is provided and further management goes according to the pathological report.

REHABILITATION

The four major means of rehabilitation include the following:

1. **Dental prosthetic management:** A patient with a limited lesion of the alveolar ridge alone or the alveolar ridge and palate that does not involve more than half the hard palate can be rehabilitated relatively easily. Preoperative dental impressions are made and a surgical splint is fashioned and inserted at the time of resection, as described earlier. Prostheses are designed according to the Aramany classification. The permanent prosthesis will have teeth like a denture; it can be removed and cleaned by the patient. It is essential for the surgeon and prosthodontist to coordinate their efforts in restoring the patient's voice and ability for adequate oral intake. A removable denture that restores good oral-nasal separation and provides for a good cosmetic appearance is ideal.

2. **Local flaps:** The palatal island flap for reconstruction of palatal lesions is a single-stage mucoperiosteal flap that is a reliable source of regional vascularised soft tissue that obviates the need for prosthetic rehabilitation.
3. **Regional flaps:** The temporalis flap allows for immediate reconstruction with minimal morbidity for patients who have undergone total inferior maxillectomy. The temporalis muscle is an attractive option for reconstruction. Reconstruction of defects after inferior maxillectomy are well summarised under the theme of functional palatomaxillary reconstruction. Larger defects (classes III to VI) require reconstruction with composite free flap reconstruction to close off the defect and restore natural facial contour.
4. **The free flap:** must include vascularised bone and soft tissue from the radial forearm, fibula, iliac crest or scapula. Free tissue transfer is superior to prostheses in larger defects with regard to improved speech and swallowing; however, placement of dental implants may be delayed or impossible based on the type of flap used.

PARTIAL MAXILLECTOMY

Indications

1. Surgery is the first-line treatment for all benign and malignant tumours of the palate.
   a. Benign tumours may be removed without resecting bone and there is no requirement for reconstruction.
   b. Malignant tumours will require resection of part or all of the hard palate or maxillary alveolus (or both) to remove bone that is obviously involved, along with at least a 1 cm margin. These defects will require some form of reconstruction.
   c. Adjuvant chemoradiation is beneficial when there is bone invasion, perineural invasion, two or more positive lymph nodes or extracapsular spread.
2. Ipsilateral selective neck dissection, levels I to III, should be performed for tumours that do not involve the midline, especially in T3 and above tumours, 30% lymph node metastasis. Bilateral selective neck dissections should be performed for tumours involving the midline.

Contraindications

1. Presence of distant metastasis.
2. Very advanced local disease (T4b) involving the masticator space, pterygoid plates, skull base or encasement of the carotid artery.
3. Severe medical comorbidities.

Technique

1. Approaches to the surgical management of tumours limited to the hard palate and alveolar ridge include:
    a. Wide local excision-palatectomy-fenestration procedure.
    b. Partial lateral maxillectomy: Surgical approach for tumours of the hard palate that involve the maxillary sinus and nasal cavity.
    c. Inferior maxillectomy: Surgical approach for tumours of the hard palate that do not involve the floor of the maxillary sinus and nasal cavity.
    d. Complete maxillectomy.
2. Approach to benign mucosal tumours of the palate (biopsy-confirmed benign tumours involving only the mucosa (i.e., pleomorphic adenoma, etc.)
    a. Wide excision 0.5 cm margins of the lesion.
    b. The deep margin should be the periosteum of the hard palate.
    c. If there is concern for tumour involvement deep to the periosteum, the surface of the hard palate is drilled with a burr to remove the superficial layer of bone.
3. Reconstruction: A palatal island rotational flap or rotational flap based on either the greater palatine or ascending palatine arteries is used to cover the site of the defect.

Partial Lateral Maxillectomy

1. A self-retaining cheek retractor, a bite block or a mouth gag is placed to gain access to the oral cavity.
2. A tongue stitch along with a tongue depressor can be used to retract the tongue.
3. Mark the margins of the resection with a marking pen or electrocautery.
4. Margins should be at least 1 cm for any lesion suspicious for malignancy or biopsy-proven malignancy.

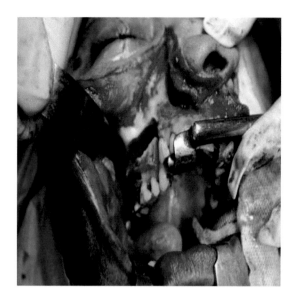

Figure 14.16 Completion of partial maxillectomy.

5. Elevate the soft tissue in the subperiosteal plane of the front and lateral walls of the maxillary antrum to the level of the infraorbital nerve with a Freer elevator.
6. Infraorbital nerve must be identified and preserved; this helps to prevent permanent anaesthesia of the soft tissues of the face.
7. Gingivobuccal incision is done, and anterior maxillotomy with visualisation of the maxillary sinus floor and infraorbital rim.
8. Enter the maxillary antrum using a small osteotome and remove the anterior wall with a Kerrison rongeur, sparing the infraorbital nerve.
9. This allows for sufficient visualisation of the maxillary antrum to evaluate the extent of resection.
10. A sagittal saw with reciprocating or sagittal blades is used to make osteotomies with at least 1 cm bony margins from the edge of the tumour along the anterior and lateral walls of the antrum (Figure 14.16).
11. Transect the palate into the maxillary sinus with care to avoid entering the nasal cavity.
12. If the nasal cavity is entered, the inferior turbinate is resected to facilitate fitting of the obturator made by the prosthodontist.
13. Posterior osteotomy created by aiming superomedially. Great care is taken not to violate the orbital floor.
14. Once the pterygoid plates are fractured, brisk

bleeding is expected from the pterygoid plexus and internal maxillary artery.

15. Use heavy curved Mayo scissors to complete transection of the soft tissues of the pterygo-palatine fossa and soft palate and remove the tumour en bloc.
16. The posterior osteotomy is the final cut due to risk of haemorrhage from the internal maxillary artery and its branches in the pterygopalatine fossa. Performing this cut last allows for removal of the tumour, and haemorrhage from the pterygopalatine fossa cannot be adequately controlled until the tumour is removed.
17. Control bleeding with clamp and ligature technique.
18. Obtain frozen section analysis from the left tissue margins of the specimen that are concerning for residual tumour or are too close to be oncologically sound.
19. Unfortunately, there is no way to evaluate bone margins by frozen section.
20. Remove the entire mucosa from the maxillary sinus to avoid contamination by oral cavity microorganisms and prevent resultant oedema and inflammation that can interfere with the fit of the oral splint.
21. Remove any sharp edges of bone with a drill or file.
22. A split-thickness skin graft is harvested at a thickness of 0.25–0.4 mm and is sutured into place to line the cheek defect.
23. The maxillary sinus mucosa is removed entirely.
24. Pack the defect tightly with xeroform gauze to close off dead space and compress the skin graft to the underlying tissue to ensure graft survival.
25. Place the previously formed surgical splint over the defect and secure it with a screw drilled into the remaining hard palate or suture it into place.
26. If there is any difficulty in the transoral procedure, upper cheek flap can be raised by a Weber-Ferguson incision.

Inferior Maxillectomy (Infrastructure Maxillectomy)

1. Retract the lips with a hands-free cheek retractor, a bite block or a side-biting mouth gag to gain access to the oral cavity.
2. Mark the margins of the resection with a marking pen or electrocautery.
3. Margins should be a minimum of 1 cm for any lesion suspicious of malignancy or biopsy-proven malignancy.
4. The maxillary sinus is entered, and the inferior aspect of the maxillary sinus is thoroughly evaluated.
5. A sagittal saw is used to make precise osteotomies.
   a. The osteotomy is usually completed with the osteotome at the level of the pterygoid plates.
6. The nasal cavity is entered, and the septum is transected with heavy curved Mayo scissors 1–2 cm superior to the floor of the nose.
7. The soft palate is transected with electrocautery, and any residual soft tissue attachments are transected with scissors.
8. After the mucosa of the maxillary antrum is removed as previously described, the inferior turbinate is also removed to prevent infection and oedema, which would interfere with the application of a palatal prosthesis.
9. More extensive tumours limited to the hard palate and alveolar ridge can be removed by simply extending the osteotomies.
10. Once the specimen is removed, it is sent to the pathology laboratory for frozen section diagnosis and assurance of clear surgical margins.

Common Errors in Technique

1. Inadequate exposure
2. Positive margins

MEDIAL MAXILLECTOMY

Indications

1. Medial maxillectomy is indicated for resection of tumours of the lateral nasal wall, nasal cavity, nasal septum or the medial wall of the maxillary sinus.
2. Medial maxillectomy may also be used for exposure of and access to the pterygopalatine fossa, pterygoid plates, nasopharynx, sphenoid sinus, clivus and the medial infratemporal fossa.
3. Medial maxillectomy can be combined with

resection of the floor of the nose, palate or upper gingiva (inferior maxillectomy).

4. Medial maxillectomy may also be combined with a transcranial approach for resection of the anterior skull base.

Contraindications

Medial maxillectomy is not adequate if the tumour extends laterally to the infraorbital nerve, palate or facial soft tissue.

Operative Technique

1. The patient is placed supine with a shoulder roll to extend the neck.
2. The head of bed should be elevated about 30 degrees. This reduces blood loss and allows better visualisation of the surgical field.
3. Soft tissue approaches:

   a. Lateral rhinotomy: The lateral rhinotomy is the standard incision for performing a medial maxillectomy. Lateral rhinotomy incision and its extensions can be utilised. A temporary tarsorrhaphy protects the ipsilateral eye. The basic lateral rhinotomy incision is outlined by connecting three surface points. The first point is marked halfway between the nasion and the medial canthus. The second point is where the alar crease begins, and the third point is at the base of the columella. The basic incision provides adequate exposure for a medial maxillectomy. The basic incision may be extended to include a lip splitting extension or a Lynch type extension if further exposure is necessary. The extended incision provides adequate exposure for a total maxillectomy (Figure 14.11).
      i. Elevation of the soft tissues of the cheek is done in a subperiosteal plane over the maxilla and around the inferior orbital. The periorbita is elevated over the anterior lacrimal crest to expose the lacrimal sac.
      ii. Dissection of the medial periorbita over the lamina papyracea reveals the anterior ethmoid artery at the level of the frontoethmoid suture line, which marks the level of the anterior cranial

floor. The artery is coagulated by bipolar electrocautery, clipped or ligated, then transected.

   iii. After the lacrimal sac is transected, it is marsupialised into the surgical cavity as a dacryocystorhinostomy. Silicone stents are placed through the upper and lower canaliculi and brought into the nasal cavity to prevent post-operative epiphora.
   iv. Osteotomies: (A) vertically medial to the infraorbital foramen, (B) horizontally above the level of tooth roots and into the pyriform aperture, and (C) obliquely along the nasomaxillary suture line. If the lateral nasal wall is to be resected, the lacrimal sac is transected and marsupialised into the nasal cavity.
   v. The attachment of the medial canthal tendon to the nasal bone is released.
   vi. The periorbita is elevated over the medial orbital wall, exposing the lacrimal crest, the lamina papyracea and the frontoethmoidal suture.
   vii. This suture serves as a landmark for the position of the floor of the anterior cranial fossa and, when followed posteriorly, leads to the anterior and posterior ethmoidal foramina.

   b. Midfacial degloving
      i. It involves a complete transfixion incision of the membranous septum.
      ii. This is joined endonasally with a bilateral intercartilaginous incision, with soft tissue elevation over the nasal dorsum as far superior as the nasal root. A gingivobuccal incision extends bilaterally across the midline to both maxillary tuberosities laterally.
      iii. The nasal skeleton is therefore "degloved" from overlying soft tissues as far laterally as the pyriform aperture.
      iv. Subperiosteal dissection is continued superiorly over the anterior wall of both maxilla to the level of the inferior orbital margins. The dissection joins the nasal degloving using sharp dissection over the pyriform aperture attachments.

v. Osteotomies and resection: Osteotomies are done as described previously. The anterior wall of the maxillary sinus above the level of tooth roots and medial to the infraorbital nerve is removed.

vi. Lateral to the infraorbital foramen, the anterior wall antrostomy may be enlarged to expose the zygomatic recess of the antrum. Resection of the lateral nasal wall begins with an inferior osteotomy along the floor of the nose below the attachment of the inferior turbinate, starting at the pyriform aperture, and carried posteriorly to the posterior maxillary wall.

vii. The orbital contents are retracted laterally and protected with a spoon. The lamina papyracea is identified and, if necessary, resected.

viii. Sphenoethmoidectomy is done as required, staying below the level of the frontoethmoidal suture to avoid injury to the floor of the anterior cranial fossa.

ix. Posteriorly, the lateral nasal wall osteotomies are connected with right-angled scissors behind the turbinates. The specimen is thus delivered and examined for adequacy of the margins using frozen section control.

x. Closure is begun by reattachment of the medial canthal tendon to the nasal bone in its anatomic position. Meticulous multilayered closure of the lateral rhinotomy is performed and usually results in excellent healing and acceptable post-operative appearance.

xi. Adequate nasal packing may be left in place for 1–2 days.

Endoscopic Medial Maxillectomy

- Oro-tracheal or naso-tracheal intubation is done.
- Nasal cavity decongested with 4% lignocaine or saline with adrenaline-soaked (1:50,000) (Moffatt's solution, if available) nasal packs for 10 minutes.
- Using zero degree nasal endoscope, injection 2% lignocaine or saline with adrenaline

(1:1,00,000/2,00,000) is infiltrated around sphenopalatine foramen using a long 18G needle, while a normal 20–22G needle is used in rest of the lateral wall supplied by ethmoidal, palatine and labial arteries.

- Endoscopic dacryocystorhinostomy is performed.
- Lamina papyrecia and floor of orbit are exposed by anterior ethmoidectomy.
- The uncinate incision is extended bone deep, downward towards anterior end of inferior turbinate and curved posteriorly in inferior meatus up to its posterior end.
- Power drill is used to cut the medial wall of the maxilla, which also involves part of anterior wall and floor of orbit.
- Usually, en bloc excision is not possible with powered instruments.
- Maxillary cavity is cleared of any disease.
- Complete haemostasis is achieved and surgical cavity packed with medicated pack.

Common Errors in Technique

1. Failure to properly drain the lacrimal sac after transecting the nasolacrimal duct.
2. Failure to properly reattach the medial canthal ligament.
3. Excessive traction on the infraorbital nerve leading to numbness of the cheek.
4. Failure to properly execute a complete sphenoethmoidectomy with adequate drainage and ventilation to avoid recurrent sinusitis.

Ethmoidectomy

Isolated ethmoid tumours are rare. Ethmoid commonly gets infiltrated by tumours of the nasal cavity or maxilla. Common ethmoid tumours are as follows:

- Epithelial tumours (e.g., squamous papilloma, squamous cell carcinoma)
- Salivary gland tumour (adenoma, adenocarcinoma)
- Fibrous dysplasia
- Osteoma
- Inverted papilloma
- Neural tumours (schwannoma, olfactory neuroblastoma)

Clinical Features

- Nasal obstruction
- Epistaxis
- Epiphora
- Swelling around medial canthus
- Telecanthus
- Proptosis
- Visual defects (diplopia, vision impairment)

Radiological Investigation

- CT scan: To find the extent and relation of the tumour to adjoining structures, e.g., orbit, extraocular muscles, cribriform plate, anterior cranial fossa and optic nerve.
- MRI scan: To assess soft tissue extension of the tumour, especially orbital content, optic nerve, carotid vessels, dura and brain.

Surgical Technique

- **Endoscopic:** Trans-nasal endoscopic resection can be done in all types and stages of tumours. It is the standard treatment for benign tumours. It results in faster recovery without any external scar.
- **Open Procedure:** Its application remains limited in the era of endoscopic surgery. Extensive tumours (T3–4) are the main conditions. It is usually combined with anterior cranial fossa clearance. Reconstruction with septal or Hadad flap is required.

Complications

- **Haemorrhage:** Massive intra-operative haemorrhage is rare. Injury to the internal maxillary artery is easily controlled through vascular clamp and suture. Ethmoidal arteries and sphenopalatine arteries injury are also controllable with bipolar electrocautery or vascular clip.
- **Nasal regurgitation/rhinolalia aperta:** This is an inevitable complication of maxillectomy that requires correct prosthetic placement. However, recent surgical techniques of cavity reconstruction with flaps avoids this complication.
- **Epiphora and ectropion:** This occurs due to failure to perform dacryocystorhinostomy at the time of maxillectomy. Fibrosis of orbicularis ocular muscle leading to ectropion can also lead to epiphora. Ectropion can be avoided with subcilliary, conjunctival or facial degloving incisions.
- **Enophthalmos:** This occurs due to removal of orbital floor and periorbital. This requires reconstruction of orbital floor with metallic or silicon plate or septal cartilage graft.
- **Nasal crusting:** This is occurs due to loss of secretory mucosa and grafting of maxillary cavity. It can be managed by nasal lubricants and saline spray or douching.

15

Bone Tumours

PAYAL KAMBLE AND SAURABH VARSHNEY

INTRODUCTION

Tumour masses of both mandible and maxilla usually arise from dental arches and can be broadly separated into tumours of dentition and bone proper. This division allows both approaches to differential considerations and the clinical decision-making process. The tumours of dentition can be further divided into odontogenic and nonodontogenic lesions. Tumours arising from bone proper can be subclassified as fibro-osseous lesions, reactive bone disease, giant cell lesions, bone tumours and others. The odontogenic and nonodontogenic tumours can be divided into cystic and solid groups. Cysts may be acquired and developmental. The solid group may demonstrate a mineralising matrix. Tumours and cysts of odontogenic origin may come from one of several cell lines that contribute to the formation of the tooth. These include the cells of the enamel, pulp, cementum, epithelium of the dental lamina, and fibrous and bony elements.

This chapter confines itself to an overview of the major odontogenic cysts and tumours, and other bone tumours are not discussed in detail. However, such lesions should be included in the differential diagnoses of a patient presenting with mandibular/maxillary radiolucency or swelling.

ODONTOGENIC MANDIBULAR CYSTS

Odontogenic cysts are defined as epithelial-lined structures derived from odontogenic epithelium. Most cysts are defined more by their location than by any histologic characteristics. They can be further divided into the following:

1. Periapical (radicular) cyst is the most common odontogenic cyst. The usual etiology is a tooth that becomes infected, leading to necrosis of the pulp.
2. Dentigerous cysts: The second most common odontogenic cyst is the dentigerous cyst, which develops within the normal dental follicle that surrounds an unerupted tooth. Discussed in detail later.
3. Primordial cyst.
4. Residual cyst.
5. Lateral periodontal cyst.
6. Gingival cyst of the newborn.
7. Gingival cyst of the adult.
8. Odontogenic keratocyst.
9. Basal cell nevus syndrome.
10. Glandular odontogenic cyst.

NONODONTOGENIC MANDIBULAR CYSTS

1. Stafne bone cyst is an unusual form of slightly aberrant salivary gland tissue wherein a developmental inclusion of glandular tissue is found within or, more commonly, adjacent to the lingual surface of the body of the mandible.
2. Traumatic bone cyst.

DOI: 10.1201/9780367430139-15

3. Focal osteoporotic bone marrow defect.
4. Aneurysmal bone cyst.

ODONTOGENIC TUMOURS

1. Ameloblastoma
2. Adenomatoid odontogenic tumour
3. Calcifying epithelial odontogenic tumour
4. Keratinising and calcifying odontogenic cyst/ calcifying odontogenic cyst
5. Odontogenic myxoma
6. Ameloblastic fibroma
7. Ameloblastic fibro-odontoma
8. Complex odontoma
9. Compound odontoma
10. Cementoblastoma

GENERAL DISEASE PATTERN

- In general, benign cysts and tumours will range from a unilocular cystic expansile appearance to a multilocular, septate mass, sometimes with an identifiable mineralised matrix.
- The odontogenic lesions are related to unerupted or impacted teeth in a predictable manner. The benign or low-grade malignant nonodontogenic lesions tend to have a narrow zone of transition and bulge, rather than infiltrate, into surrounding tissues, suggesting a lesion of low biologic activity.
- A more aggressive appearance with increasingly broader zones of transition and soft tissue infiltration pushes the differential diagnosis to a more malignant nonodontogenic lesion and one that also includes focal infectious and non-infectious inflammatory diseases.
- Such differentiation helps direct the most appropriate next step in the patient's evaluation and management.

CLINICAL PRESENTATION

The variety of clinical presentations of jaw masses often raises the possibility of lesions that arise outside the jaw.

- An asymptomatic mass, usually submucosal and seen by the patient, patient associate or health care provider
- Malocclusion or disordered mastication

- Jaw and/or temporomandibular joint or other facial pain and possibly trismus or otalgia and V2 or V3 sensory deficits or formications
- A cheek, parotid or submandibular region mass
- Devitalisation of teeth

DENTIGEROUS CYSTS

Dentigerous cysts are slow-growing benign and non-inflammatory odontogenic cysts.

Epidemiology

- Second most common cyst after periapical cyst.
- Seen in second to fourth decades of life; uncommonly seen in childhood.
- It develops within the normal dental follicle that surrounds an unerupted tooth.

Clinical Features

- Generally small, asymptomatic, and discovered during a routine radiographic examination.
- A few cases can grow exceptionally large and can move teeth and place the patient at risk for pathologic jaw fracture.
- Occasionally other, more ominous lesions arise within the walls of the dentigerous cyst, including mucoepidermoid carcinoma, ameloblastoma and squamous cell carcinoma.
- Dentigerous cysts are usually solitary. However, multiple cysts are recognised to occur in association with syndromes like mucopolysaccharidoses and basal cell nevus syndrome.

Pathology

- A dentigerous cyst is formed by the hydrostatic force exerted by the accumulation of fluid between reduced enamel epithelium and the tooth crown of unerupted teeth. Almost exclusively occurs in permanent dentition.
- More than 75% of all cases are in the mandible, with the most involved teeth being the following:

  - Mandibular third molar (most common)
  - Maxillary third molar (second most common)

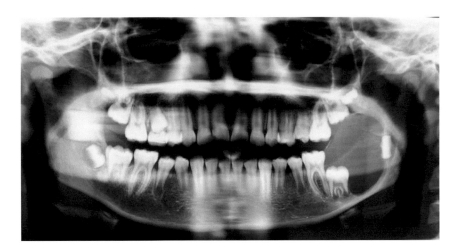

Figure 15.1 OPG showing dentigerous cyst of mandible.

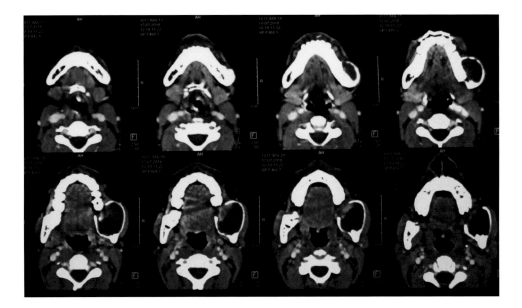

Figure 15.2 CT scan images of dentigerous cyst.

- Maxillary canine
- Mandibular second premolar

Investigation

- Radiological investigation: Dentigerous cysts are frequently identified on orthopantogram. CT and MRI may give additional information and help in distinguishing this entity from other cystic lesions of the mandible and maxilla.

- Orthopantogram appear as unilocular well-defined pericoronal radiolucencies centred on an impacted or unerupted tooth.
  - They have a thin regular sclerotic margin and expand the overlying cortex without cortical breach.
  - The roots of teeth are often outside the cyst (Figure 15.1).
- CT scan: The relationship to the unerupted tooth can often be better appreciated if the cyst cavity is filled with water density fluid (Figure 15.2).

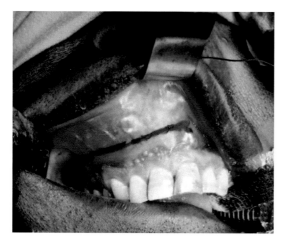

Figure 15.3 Incision for modified Caldwell-Luc approach.

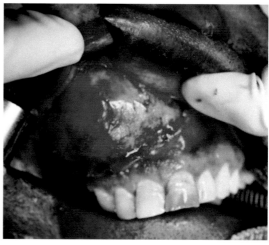

Figure 15.4 Raised mucoperiosteal flap.

- MRI: It helps distinguish these lesions from other cystic lesions of the jaw, when appearances are atypical.

TREATMENT AND PROGNOSIS

- Treatment involves removal of the entire cyst and the associated unerupted tooth. In patients with an exceptionally large lesion or who are unfit medically, marsupialisation is an option.
  - Enucleation and primary closure
  - Marsupalisation
  - Enucleation and packing open

Operative Steps (Three Different Case Scenarios)

- Under general anaesthesia.
- Prone position with head end raised.
- Marking the incision.
- Local infiltration – saline and adrenaline in 1:1,00,000 or 1:2,00,000 concentration.
- Cleaning and draping the patient.
- Approaches and incisions are marked based on the location and extent of the lesion (Figure 15.3).
- Raise mucoperiosteal flap (Figure 15.4).
- Remove bone and expose cyst completely (Figure 15.5).
- Avoid damaging the roots of the teeth and adjacent structures like inferior alveolar nerve.
- Aspirate the content of cysts.
- Complete enucleation/excision of the cyst with its epithelium.

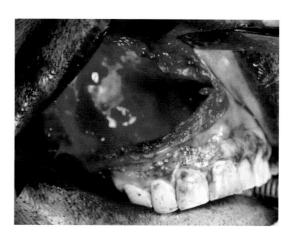

Figure 15.5 Enucleated dentigerous cyst.

- Remove the unerupted tooth.
- Wound care: wash the wound and reposition the flap and close the wound with sutures.

Complications

- Pathological jaw fracture if large.
- Very rarely it may develop into mural ameloblastoma.
- There is a potential for development of squamous cell carcinoma in the context of chronic infection.

AMELOBLASTOMA

Ameloblastoma is the most common epithelial odontogenic tumour arising from the dental lamina, Hertwig sheath, the enamel organ or the lining of dental follicles/dentigerous cysts.

Epidemiology

- They are slow-growing and tend to present in the third to fifth decades of life.
- The unicystic variant most often occurs in adolescents.
- The lesion is distributed equally between males and females.
- This lesion occurs in both the maxilla and mandible, but the posterior mandible is the most common location; only 20% of lesions are found in the maxilla.

Clinical Features

- Typically present as hard, painless lesions near the angle of the mandible in the region of the third molar.
- Usually seen along the alveolus of the mandible (80%) and maxilla (20%). When the maxilla is involved, the tumour is in the premolar region and can extend up into the maxillary sinus.
- Although benign, it is a locally aggressive neoplasm with a high rate of recurrence.
- Approximately 20% of cases are associated with dentigerous cysts and unerupted teeth.

Pathology

- Ameloblastomas arise from ameloblasts, which are part of the odontogenic epithelium and are responsible for enamel production and eventual crown formation.
- Four forms have been described in the literature: unicystic, solid (multicystic), desmoplastic and peripheral (extra-osseous).
- Ameloblastomas are locally aggressive benign tumours, and many have suggested that this lesion should be considered a low-grade or indolent malignancy.
- It generally does not metastasise but is slow growing, persistent and hard to eradicate.
- Chae et al. estimated that ameloblastomas have a mean growth rate of 87.84% per year, with solid, multicystic ameloblastomas having the highest growth rate and the peripheral form of the tumour having the lowest rate.

Investigation

Radiological

- Unicystic ameloblastomas are well-demarcated unilocular lesions that are often pericoronal in position.
- These are commonly seen in the posterior mandible, particularly at the molars.
- Multicystic ameloblastomas account for 80–90% of cases with classical expansile "soap-bubble" lesions, with well-demarcated borders and no matrix calcification (Figure 15.6).

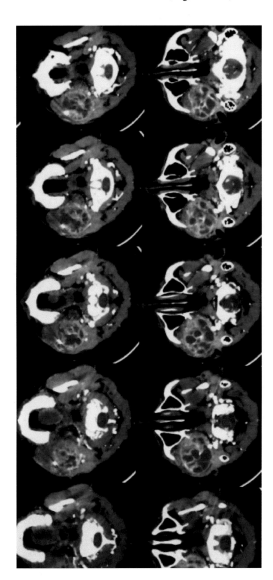

Figure 15.6 Soap bubble appearance of ameloblastoma.

- Resorption of adjacent teeth and "root blunting" is often seen.
- Larger lesions may erode through the cortex into adjacent soft tissues.

Treatment

- The treatment of ameloblastoma is surgical excision with wide free margins.
- All patients with ameloblastoma, regardless of surgical treatment method, or must be monitored radiographically throughout their lifetime.
- If excision is inadequate, recurrence is common.
- The maxillary ameloblastoma is not confined by the strong cortical plate found in the mandible. In addition, the posterior maxilla lies in close relationship to many vital structures. Thus, an aggressive approach is required for maxillary ameloblastoma.
- In the mandible, 1 cm clear margins are considered the standard. This may be accomplished with block or segmental resection.
- Unlike other types of ameloblastomas, unicystic ameloblastoma is lesion encapsulated and can be removed with enucleation/curettage procedures alone. These lesions may recur, and recurrences may require more aggressive treatment.
- For peripheral ameloblastoma, a more conservative excision with close clinical follow-up is the standard of care.
- Malignant behaviour is seen in three forms.
  - Ameloblastic carcinoma (frankly, malignant histology)
  - Malignant ameloblastoma
  - Metastases despite well-differentiated 'benign' histology

Operative Steps

- Under general anaesthesia.
- Prone position with head end raised.
- Marking the incision.
- Local infiltration: saline and adrenaline in 1:1,00,000 or 1:2,00,000 concentration.
- Cleaning and draping the patient.
- Approaches and incisions are marked based on the location and extent of the lesion (Figure 15.7a-b).

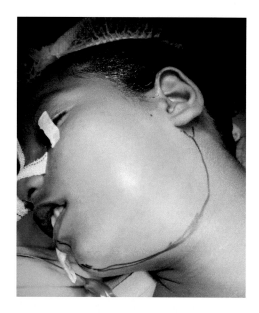

Figure 15.7a Incision for ameloblastoma of mandible.

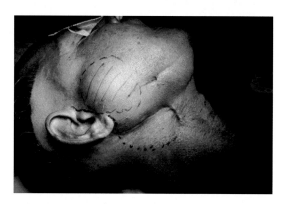

Figure 15.7b Incision for ameloblastoma developed in fibular free flap.

- Raise mucoperiosteal flap (Figure 15.8a-b).
- Complete exposure of cyst wall.
- Cyst is removed along with approximately 1 cm of normal mandible bone (Figure 15.9).
- Primary defect repaired with reconstruction plate.
- Reposition of flaps.
- Wound care and suturing.
- Treatment preferably includes resection with safety margins and immediate reconstruction whenever possible.
- The main success factor associated with the treatment is the early diagnosis, but to achieve a correct, definitive diagnosis it is crucial to correlate the histopathologic findings with

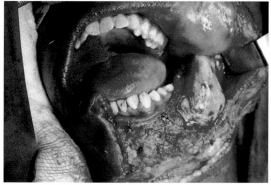

(a)

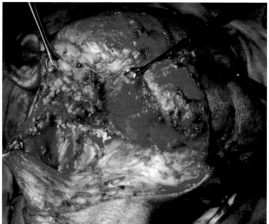

(b)

Figure 15.8a-b Mucoperiosteal flap is raised.

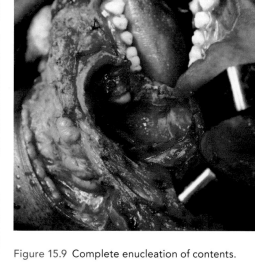

Figure 15.9 Complete enucleation of contents.

clinical and radiographic features. This is because all such lesions might have prognostically different biologic behaviours and the final diagnosis may alter the therapeutic decision significantly.

16

Neck Dissection

JAGDEEP S THAKUR

INTRODUCTION

Lymphatic drainage occurs through tissues and organs in a complex system in the body. Although intraoperative radionuclide scans can now delineate the draining lymph node, the pathway still remains elusive. There are about 600 lymph nodes in the human body of which 300 are located in the head and neck region, which gets maximum exposure to all types of disease-causing agents. Any head and neck disease is easily spread to other areas due to the rich lymphatic system while lymph nodes control the disease.

Head and neck cancer usually manifest with enlarged lymph nodes which carry a specific pattern of involvement. Jatin P. Shaw and co-workers of the Memorial Sloan-Kettering Cancer Center, New York, New York, did remarkable research on the lymphatic drainage in head and neck area which led to classification of neck nodes and modern neck dissection management strategies.

Neck dissection is the removal of the lymphatic system from the neck, achieved by excision of neck fascia and associated lymph nodes. Historically, George Crile classified neck dissection into two main groups which were further sub-grouped as the surgical evidence accumulated.

1. **Comprehensive Neck Dissection**
   a. **Radical neck dissection (RND):** In this neck dissection, sternocleidomastoid muscle, internal jugular vein and accessory spinal nerve of neck along with superficial fascia and part of deep fascia and lymphatic nodes in levels I–VII are removed.

   b. **Extended radical neck dissection:** This is the extended form of RND wherein other tissue, e.g., digastric muscle, parotid or lymph nodes is removed.
   c. **Modified radical neck dissection:** This is a modification of RND wherein one or more structures (sternocleidomastoid, internal jugular vein or accessory spinal nerve) are preserved. This is further classified by the structure(s) preserved:
      • Type I: Modified RND where accessory spinal nerve is preserved.
      • Type II: Preserves accessory spinal nerve and sternocleidomastoid muscle.
      • Type III: This is also known as functional neck dissection, as all structures except fascia and lymph nodes are preserved.
   d. **Selective neck dissection:** In this dissection, more than two groups or levels of neck node are removed. Traditionally, it is further classified into:
      i. **Central neck dissection:** Level VI is dissected.
      ii. **Postero-lateral:** Levels II–V are dissected.
      iii. **Supra-omohyoid neck dissection:** Levels I–III are dissected.
      iv. **Extended supra-omohyoid neck dissection** Levels I–IV are dissected.
      v. **Lateral dissection:** Levels II–IV are dissected.

   It is always better to mention the dissection levels rather than traditional classification in operative notes.

DOI: 10.1201/9780367430139-16

NECK DISSECTION CLASSIFICATION ON THE BASIS OF INDICATIONS

1. **Elective neck dissection**: This is performed in cases with primary cancer but clinically and radiologically absent nodal metastasis (N0). Surgical procedure involves a form of selective neck dissection which is discussed in other chapters. Specific indications are as follows.
   a. Oral cancers with N0.
   b. Extra-thyroidal differentiated thyroid cancer with N0.
   c. Medullary thyroid cancer with high serum calcitonin (>500 pg/ml).
   d. Selective high-grade cancers with N0.
2. **Therapeutic neck dissection:** This term is used in neck dissection performed in cases with metastatic neck disease (N1–3). Except for thyroid cancer, this usually mandates comprehensive neck dissection.

Until a classical neck dissection as mentioned above is performed, the surgeon should mention all neck node levels and any other structures removed in the operative record, as often a surgical procedure warrants removal of additional structure(s) which are not mentioned in the previously stated classification.

PRE-OPERATIVE MANAGEMENT

All patients planned for neck dissection should be evaluated thoroughly. Surgeon should have interactive and detailed discussion with patient and his/her near relatives. (Pre-operative counselling is discussed in chapter 1.) Surgeon should review clinical examination and all investigation before surgery. He/she should discuss any concerns with the associated team.

CLINICAL EXAMINATIONS AND INVESTIGATIONS

Clinical examination is the most important step in any pre-operative preparation of a patient. Evaluation should start from the primary tumour and its drainage pathway. Neck dissection is usually performed with resection of primary tumour but for a few exceptions where primary is managed by other nonsurgical modalities due to functional or anatomical considerations, e.g., hypopharyngeal cancers.

Neck should be properly and systematically examined to assess the nodal disease. Any nodal fixity warrants further radiological investigations. Nodal fixity to skin carries poor prognosis and neck dissection is contraindicated in a majority of cases, although en bloc resection with flap reconstruction can be considered in selective young patients. Similarly, restricted transverse movements of jugular nodes warrant non-surgical management as nodes have infiltrated to deep muscles or other structures of the neck and therefore tumour-free resection is not possible. Neck node in levels IV–VI should be specifically examined for movement and lower extent by palpations. Further detailed radiological evaluation is needed to rule out vascular or thoracic extension in case there is absence of space between node and clavicle bone.

Radiological Investigations

A general loco-regional and distant metastatic work-up is a prerequisite for any surgical intervention, although a majority of head and neck cancers are initially evaluated by CT scan, so nodal evaluation doesn't require further investigation. However, low-cost, high-frequency sonographic evaluation is a good option, especially in patients who are not candidates for a CT scan for primary tumour. Neck sonography has higher accuracy in detecting metastatic nodes in comparison to other radiological investigations. The radiologist relies on size, shape, vascularity and necrosis in the lymph node to find the disease.

The CT scan was formerly reserved for initial evaluation of the primary tumour and rarely required for neck evaluation, except post-irradiated cases where the first objective is to rule out residual primary tumour. Its role in primary tumour has been discussed in other chapters. CT scan has significantly better specificity than sonography in detecting metastatic lymph node, although sensitivity remains almost equal. It is always better to rule out neck metastasis after CT scan.

Absence of fat planes between node and carotid/thoracic vessels and more than 270-degree encasement of carotid on CT scan mandate further detailed investigation, like angiography and balloon occlusion test, in consultation with a vascular surgeon.

MRI is not performed routinely except initially for primary tumour evaluation, as it has comparable accuracy to CT scan. Similarly, pre-operative PET-CT scan is not performed for neck evaluation unless done chiefly for unknown primary tumour or high-grade tumours with negative nodal disease.

PATHOLOGICAL INVESTIGATIONS

Radiological metastatic lymph node needs to be validated through pathological evidence. The surgeon needs to be assured of a metastatic neck node(s) unless elective (prophylactic) neck dissection is planned. Fine needle aspiration cytology (FNAC) is the pathological investigation of choice in neck evaluation. Sonographic guided FNAC (US-FNAC) has higher accuracy but is reserved for small non-palpable lymph nodes. It is better to perform neck dissection in high-grade cancer even if US-FNAC doesn't reveal nodal metastasis.

PRE-ANAESTHESIA CONSIDERATIONS

Once neck dissection is planned, haematological and biochemical investigations are performed to assess the patient's fitness. Authors also seek cardiopulmonary assessment in all cases, as a majority of these cases are elderly and smokers. There are no specific pre-anaesthetic considerations for neck dissection unless any vascular or thoracic breach is anticipated. In such cases, a vascular or thoracic surgeon with a good amount of compatible blood replacement needs to be in the operating room. Other pre-anaesthetic considerations are related to primary tumour excision (discussed in another chapter). Antibiotic prophylaxis is as per the protocol for primary tumour excision.

OPERATIVE TECHNIQUE

- Once patient is intubated and cleared by anaesthesia team, neck is extended by putting shoulder bag at scapular level and towel roll is put below extended neck. Operating table is elevated about 300–450 degree at lumbar region, but the head end is dropped and made parallel to the lower end. This manoeuvre will decrease blood flow to neck intraoperatively.
- Once patient is positioned, the operative field is infiltrated with freshly prepared solution of 2%

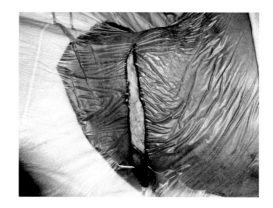

Figure 16.1 Transverse incision is used for neck dissection while modifying its length depending upon type of neck dissection and expertise.

lignocaine or normal saline with adrenaline (1:1,00,000 or 1:2,00,000) as discussed earlier.
- Surgical field is cleaned and draped and incision is marked. Numerous surgical incisions are used for various neck dissections, each with its own limitations and complications. The author uses a transverse incision in all types of neck dissection, which gives equal surgical field exposure but better cosmetic outcome compared to other incisions. Until primary tumour incision (e.g., parotidectomy) warrants, minor modification can be done in a difficult neck. Transverse incision is made with electrosurgery (taking care to avoid skin charring) and the site of incision is modified as per neck length and type of dissection (Figure 16.1).
- Subplatysmal flaps are raised to expose the anatomical boundaries of the nodal levels to be dissected. Surgical techniques beyond this vary according to type of neck dissection.

RADICAL NECK DISSECTION

Indications

- N3 nodal disease.
- Extra-nodal disease.
- Post-surgery or post chemoradiation nodal disease recurrence.

Contraindications:

- Poor general condition (e.g., cachexia, poor muscle mass, severe anaemia, uncontrolled diabetes and hypertension).
- Distant metastasis.

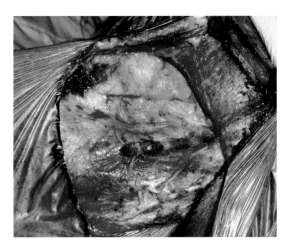

Figure 16.2 The flap (sub-platysmal) is elevated by keeping dissection level just below platysma.

- Selective extra-nodal skin, prevertebral, brachial plexus invasion.
- Common or internal carotid artery invasion or more than 270 degrees encasement of internal or common carotid artery with few exceptions, like young patients with good prognostic cancer where carotid resection and grafting is performed during neck dissection.
- Skull base and plural invasion by node.
- Oesophageal, pharyngeal or laryngeal nodal extension if they are not part of primary tumour excision.

SURGICAL TECHNIQUE

- Once superior and inferior sub-platysmal flaps are raised and secured for full exposure (Figure 16.2). Dissection starts with incision at the anterior border of the sternocleidomastoid muscle and it is dissected fully from the carotid sheath with fine haemostatic forceps and bipolar electrosurgery tongs (Figure 16.3).
- Two muscular tendons, omohyoid and digastric, are identified and exposed to know the exact extent and location of the carotid sheath. (Figure 16.4) Identification of internal jugular vein and carotid artery system is the most important step in neck dissection. This dissection extends inferiorly from sterno-clavicular joint to mastoid attachment of posterior belly of digastric superiorly.
- Once carotid sheath is identified, posterior end of sternocleidomastoid is exposed fully.

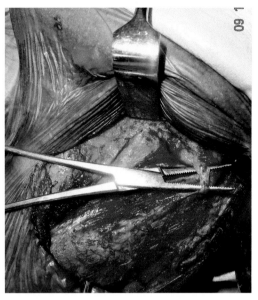

Figure 16.3 The medial border of the sternocleidomastoid muscle is exposed to reach the carotid sheath.

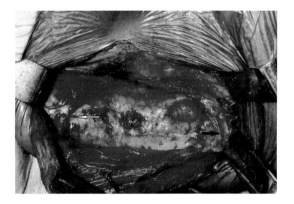

Figure 16.4 The posterior belly of digastric (large black arrow) and omohyoid (white arrow) crossing the internal jugular vein are exposed.

External jugular veins are saved when bilateral radical neck dissection is planned, as it decreases post-operative facial oedema. Otherwise veins are secured and cut.
- Lymph node dissection is started from level V by grasping fascial tissue with bipolar electrosurgery (Figure 16.5).
- Dissection starts at upper border of clavicle, encountering cutaneous branches of cervical plexus which are cut. These cutaneous branches can be saved to avoid post-operative sensory loss in the nerves, but this requires

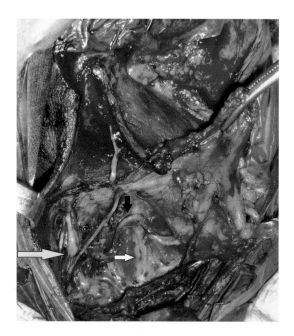

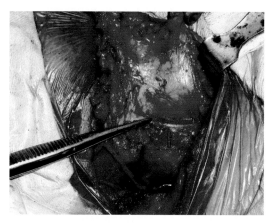

Figure 16.6 The phrenic nerve is identified with its typical curving course (arrow) near the posterior border of internal jugular vein.

Figure 16.5 The level V dissection remains just above the muscular sheath of the floor of supraclavicular fossa, saving brachial plexus roots (small white arrow). The branch of accessory cranial nerve supplying the trapezius branch is identified (large yellow arrow) with a contribution from cervical root. The black arrow indicates transverse artery.

surgical expertise so as not to leave behind any fascia or nodes.

- The clavicular end of sternocleidomastoid muscle is identified and exposed. The anterior border trapezius is exposed fully, which makes the posterior boundary of level V. As dissection proceeds, the deeper posterior belly of omohyoid is exposed, which is traced and fully exposed to the anterior belly.

- Identification of omohyoid is a crucial step, as all important neurovascular structures in level V lie below it (transverse cervical artery and brachial plexus roots) (Figure 16.5). Transverse cervical artery should be preserved especially if trapezius flap is planned as this flap is supplied by this artery.

- Dissection should remain just above the fascial planes of scalene muscles, i.e., floor of supraclavicular fossa. Brachial plexus roots lie just below this fascia and any breach will lead to nerve injury to upper limb (Figure 16.5).

- Cutaneous branches of cervical plexus are cut at a distance from their exit point so as

to avoid injury to phrenic and other contributory branches to brachial plexus and trapezius.

- Level V dissection is complete once posterior end of sternocleidomastoid is reached. Here the dissected specimen is divided, marked and kept aside for pathological examination.

- The phrenic nerve is identified just below the internal jugular vein posteriorly as it curves medially (Figure 16.6). Lymphatic channels draining to thoracic duct are visible at this site and care should be taken not to injure them, otherwise chyle leak is inevitable. It can further assured by positive intrathoracic pressure by anaesthetist.

- Carotid sheath is opened to the lowest point as it enters the thorax and all its contents (internal jugular vein, common carotid artery and vagus nerve) are identified and separated.

- Now a large haemostatic clamp is passed below sternal and clavicular head of the sternocleidomastoid muscle and cut with monopolar electrosurgery in blend mode, taking care of any brisk haemorrhage from the corresponding inferior muscular artery (Figure 16.7). Usually, the remnant inferior muscular cuff doesn't bleed, but it can be secured with ligature to avoid late haemorrhage.

- Now two haemostatic clamps are applied after separating the internal jugular vein from common carotid artery and Vagus nerve. Vein is divided about 5 cm above the lower end and 1–0 silk ligature applied on both ends.

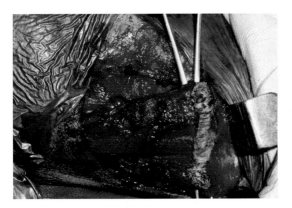

Figure 16.7 The lower end of sternocleidomastoid is cut with electrocautery.

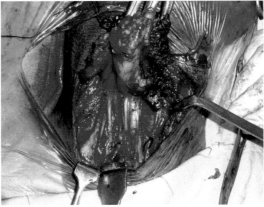

Figure 16.9 The internal jugular vein with associated lymphatic tissue and nodes are dissected just above the common carotid and vagus nerve.

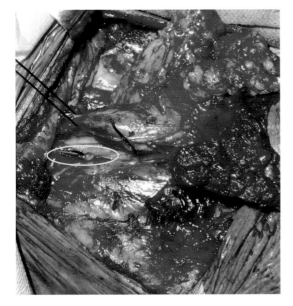

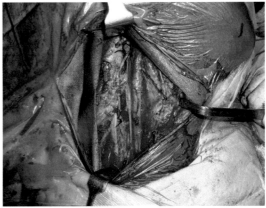

Figure 16.10 The superior end of internal jugular vein is also ligated with braided sutures.

Figure 16.8 The lower end of the internal jugular vein is ligated with at least two braided sutures and secured to the sternocleidomastoid stump. The lymphatic duct and channel (yellow circle) lies just below the posterior border of internal jugular vein.

Another 1–0 silk suture is applied through the vein above the previous ligature and secured to the lower sternocleidomastoid muscular stump (house surgeon/resident's ligature) (Figure 16.8).

- The internal jugular vein and sternocleido-mastoid cuff with associated lymph nodes is dissected superiorly, ligating or coagulating all draining venous branches (Figure 16.9).
- The mastoid end of sternocleidomastoid is cut and divided as previously. Accessory spinal

nerve with lymph node and fascia is dissected up to muscular planes.
- A branch of the posterior occipital artery is encountered as dissection proceeds cephalic over muscular planes, and secured with bipolar electrosurgery.
- Superior end of internal jugular vein is ligated and divided at the level of posterior belly of digastric, similar to lower end (Figure 16.10).
- This dissected specimen is marked according to lymph node levels and kept aside.
- Now dissection proceeds to towards level I. The common facial vein, ligated at the time of internal jugular vein dissection, is dissected with associated fascia up to the lower pole of submandibular gland.

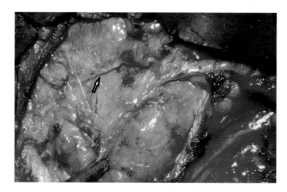

Figure 16.11 The marginal mandibular nerve (indicated by arrow) is dissected free from the fascia.

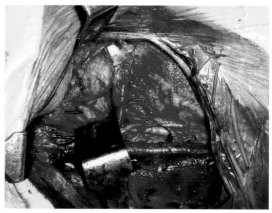

Figure 16.12 The facial artery (indicated by arrow) lies at the posterior border of the gland, just below the posterior belly.

- Marginal mandibular nerve is identified over the submandibular fascia and dissected and saved with loose sutures to hang it on the platysma (Figure 16.11). Sometimes, its identification is difficult, which is where the nerve monitoring system comes in handy. Rarely should the surgeon proceed without this identification in large metastatic facial lymph node dissection.
- Lower pole of submandibular is grasped, dissected and retracted cephalic, exposing anterior and posterior bellies of digastric.
- Facial artery is identified as it enters gland postero-superiorly, just below the posterior belly of digastric at the angle of the mandible. This artery is secured, ligated and divided so it can be saved if any local flap (nasolabial, mucosal-muscular buccal flap) is planned (Figure 16.12).
- The specimen is retracted antero-inferiorly and dissected from the lower margin of ramus, ligating and dividing the retromandibular vein with its tributaries as they exit the parotid gland inferiorly.
- As dissection proceeds anteriorly, facial vessels are encountered again, which must be ligated and divided.
- Dissection proceeds further anteriorly below ramus with bipolar tongs, and fascia, along with associated tissue over mylohyoid muscle, is dissected carefully by coagulating mylohyoid artery or its branches and exposing posterior border of mylohyoid. Mylohyoid artery and its branches must be coagulated satisfactorily, otherwise haemorrhage ensues, delaying further dissection.

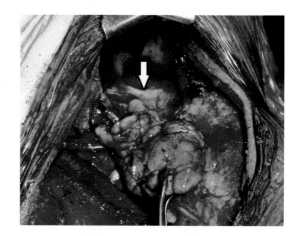

Figure 16.13 The lingual nerve (indicated by arrow) curves and appears hanging as gland is pulled.

- Now, mylohyoid muscle is retracted antero-superiorly while submandibular specimen is retracted inferiorly, thereby bringing into view the lingual nerve with submandibular ganglion (Figure 16.13). Submandibular gland specimen is retracted superiorly to dissect it over hyoglossus which also exposes hypoglossal nerve as it lies over this muscle (Figure 16.14).
- Once hypoglossal nerve is identified, specimen and mylohyoid are again retracted inferiorly and antero-superiorly, respectively, to expose the lingual nerve. Wharton's duct is identified and dissected to the floor of mouth and cut with bipolar tongs at 10–12W. A vein runs with

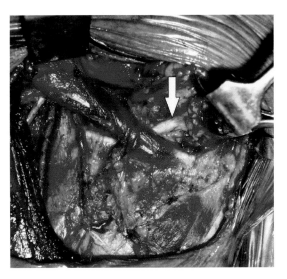

Figure 16.14 The hypoglossal nerve (indicated by white arrow) lies in the floor of submandibular fossa over the hyoglossus muscle.

this duct and must be coagulated carefully, otherwise a troublesome haemorrhage can occur later. The lingual nerve and ganglion are now divided with bipolar tongs to avoid injury to lingual nerve.

- Specimen is delivered and marked, completing level IB dissection. Currently submandibular gland preservation is advocated, but available data is debatable.
- Now dissection proceeds to level IA, again dissecting, preferably, with bipolar tongs. The dissection exposes muscular floor of the submental triangle while ligating and dividing the anterior jugular or its branches. The specimen is cut just below mandible genu in midline, being mindful of a few vascular branches which can result in brisk bleeding if not secured with bipolar tongs.
- Specimen is marked and kept aside. This completes the radical neck dissection. Once dissection is complete and all visible bleeding areas are coagulated and secured, anaesthetist is requested to maintain positive intrathoracic pressure to assess any bleeding or chyle leak. All areas should be examined thoroughly and especially without applying retractors, as they occlude bleeding vessels occasionally.
- Any vascular or chyle breach should be managed to the satisfaction of the whole surgical team.

- The surgical site is irrigated with about 0.5–1 litre of Ringer's lactate or normal saline for any clot or tissue debris.
- An appropriate size (12–16FG) suction drain is applied away from major vessels and secured. Platysma is sutured with absorbable sutures (3–0 or 2–0) and skin is closed with stapler or continuous sutures.
- Suction drain is checked before dressing and extubating patient.

MODIFIED RADICAL NECK DISSECTION

Indications

1. N1–3 nodal disease, except thyroid cancers with nodal disease where selective neck dissection is performed.
2. Anaplastic thyroid carcinoma even with N1 neck.

Contraindications

1. All indications of radical neck dissection.
2. Other contraindication of radical neck disease.

Modified radical neck dissection occurs where one or more structures (accessory spinal nerve, sternocleidomastoid or internal jugular vein) are preserved. Surgical technique remains similar to radical dissection except as follows.

- Surgical technique remains same as radical neck dissection up to exposure of carotid sheath and separation of sternocleidomastoid muscle.
- The accessory spinal nerve is identified in the upper part of sternocleidomastoid muscle where it passes below, above and (rarely) through the internal jugular vein from skull base towards sternocleidomastoid at an acute angle caudally. It is usually located about 2 cm below skull base and at the same distance above greater auricular nerve. It is dissected with 8–10W bipolar tongs as the superior sternocleidomastoid artery lies in close relation to this nerve. Digital palpation or nerve stimulator helps to locate the nerve in difficult situations.
- Now the trapezius branch of accessory spinal nerve is identified. It lies about 1 cm above the

greater auricular nerve on posterior border of sternocleidomastoid muscle and runs downwards and posteriorly, gradually merges with and innervates the trapezius about 5 cm above the clavicle (see Figure 16.5).

- Once this trapezius branch of accessory spinal nerve is identified and preserved, level V is dissected similar to radical neck dissection.
- After level V dissection is complete, sternocleidomastoid muscle is completely separated from fascial tissue and retracted.
- Fascial tissue is pulled and dissected from anterior scalene muscle towards carotid sheath.
- Phrenic nerve and lymphatic channels are carefully preserved, as mentioned earlier.
- Omohyoid muscle is retracted away and carotid sheath opened at the lowest ends.
- Fascia with lymph nodes over internal jugular vein is held with haemostatic clamps and retracted medially.
- This fascial tissue is dissected from vein, leaving no tissue over it. This dissection can be done with scalpel or bipolar electrosurgery at low power setting (15–20W) (Figure 16.15). Author prefers bipolar electrosurgery as it coagulates small venous channels draining into jugular vein. Any large venous tributary should be ligated and secured appropriately.
- As dissection proceeds upwards, the supraclavicular artery (branch of transverse cervical artery) or its branch is encountered and must be coagulated or ligated accordingly.
- In the upper end, once common facial vein has been secured, ligated and divided from internal jugular vein, further dissection needs extra care as numerous venous tributaries drain into the internal jugular vein near the posterior belly of digastric. Any injury to these channels will lead to profuse haemorrhage. Surgeon should not panic but apply digital pressure as blind application of any haemostatic clamp will injure the hypoglossal nerve which passes between these venous channels.
- Digital pressure for 2–3 minutes will stop or reduce the haemorrhage. Now, the bleeding vein(s) is clamped under vision with or without suction. This author coagulates the vessels with bipolar electrosurgery depending upon size of vein. Any breach in internal jugular vein is also managed by digital pressure initially and then applying the appropriate vascular clamp.

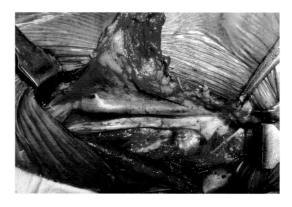

Figure 16.15 The carotid sheath is dissected free from the lymphatic, exposing its contents.

Head may be lowered to avoid air embolism which although quite rare until jugular breach is quite large or surgeon fails to occlude the vein. Vein is repaired with 5–0 round body non-absorbable monofilament suture. Positive intrathoracic pressure is maintained to verify accurate repair.

- The accessory spinal nerve is identified and dissected. The exposure of muscular floor below XI cranial nerve assures complete dissection of level IIB. The XI cranial should not be pulled unnecessarily as this may lead to paresis (Figure 16.16).
- The internal jugular vein, carotid artery and vagus nerve are completely dissected, free from the fascia and associated lymph nodes.
- This completes level II–IV dissection and the dissected specimen is marked as per lymph nodal levels.
- Further surgical techniques are similar to radical neck dissection.

SELECTIVE NECK DISSECTION

Type of selective neck dissection is based on lymphatic drainage of the primary site.

Indications

1. Oral carcinoma with N0 nodal disease (extended supra-omohyoid neck dissection).
2. Differentiated thyroid carcinoma with extrathyroid extension (central neck dissection).
3. Differentiated thyroid carcinoma with N1–2 nodal disease (antero-lateral neck dissection).

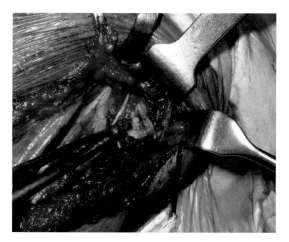

Figure 16.16 The accessory spinal nerve is identified and dissection is carried just above the muscular plane.

4. High grade carcinoma with N0 nodal disease (as per lymphatic system).
5. Submandibular, sublingual cancer with N0 nodal disease (level I–III dissection, known as supra-selective neck dissection).

SURGICAL TECHNIQUE

Transverse incision is also used for selective neck dissections except if being performed in association with parotidectomy. All surgical techniques are similar to comprehensive neck dissection, except dissection is kept to respective lymph nodal levels. Few types of selective neck dissection have less post-operative drain, hence glove drain instead of negative suction drain can be used. However, the author always prefers to use a negative suction drain of smaller gauge.

POST-OPERATIVE MANAGEMENT

Patient is kept on parenteral fluids as discussed in chapter 1. Pain and oral feeding are managed as per protocol. Patient is made ambulatory once anaesthesia effect wears off, usually after six hours. Skin flaps and sutures are observed for any discolouration or infection. Surgical drain is observed for volume and colour. Sometimes, surgical drain may exceed 150 ml over 24 hours, but it gradually decreases in the next 24 hours. Chyle leak needs to be ruled out if the drain is more than 300 ml (discussed in complications section). Usually, a drain of less than 20 ml over 24 hours mandates

suction drain removal. Surgical sutures or staples are removed after 5–7 days and further management depends upon final operative histopathology. Neck exercises are encouraged to avoid any post-operative fibrosis.

COMPLICATIONS

Minor complications like wound infection, removal of negative pressure and increase in drain volume can occur. Infection is avoided through pre-operative screening of anaemia, malnutrition and comorbidities (renal, hepatic, diabetes, HIV, etc.). Patients should be operated upon once these contributing factors have been managed. Antibiotics should be used as per the standard protocols.

Failure of negative pressure usually results from displacement of drain due to loose suture or its proximity to skin suture line. Suture should be applied again, ensuring proper placement of drain. Failure to maintain negative pressure despite these measures after laryngectomy is due to loose pharyngoplasty sutures. This situation is generally managed by applying pressure dressing over the suspected area.

Increased post-operative drain volume leads to an increase in hospital stay, increased cost or delay in further management (e.g., radiation therapy). Blood in drain indicates active haemorrhage and re-exploration may be required, depending upon its volume and purity in drain vacuum-assisted closure (VAC). Clear fluid may be chyle leak (to be discussed later). Light yellow fluid is due to excessive negative pressure in VAC that causes plasma removal from capillaries. Turbid fluid indicates infection and should be managed accordingly. Early removal of drain can lead to formation of seroma, which needs drainage through 18G needle and pressure. Antiplatelet drugs and NSAIDs need to be curtailed in such situations.

Haemorrhage: Haemorrhage is quite common in neck dissection but it is rarely fatal unless overlooked. Venous haemorrhage is more dangerous than arterial bleed, as veins collapse and haemorrhage stops, in comparison to an artery which keeps on bleeding and thus alerts the surgeon. Therefore, any venous bleed should be checked with positive intrathoracic pressure and veins should be ligated or repaired as per size. Internal jugular vein injury is common in neck dissection and can be managed as discussed earlier in the surgical technique of modified neck dissection. The surgeon should be extra careful at both ends of the jugular vein as any injury at this level will cause profuse haemorrhage and be difficult to repair. As stated earlier, the surgeon should not panic; rather, apply digital pressure and then apply a haemostat clamp. Inability to repair the vein may require intervention by a vascular surgeon. Sometimes, the internal jugular vein may be ligated in cases of profuse haemorrhage and reconstruction failure.

Carotid artery injury is rare unless the surgeon approaches overenthusiastically. This author always requests CT angiography in cases of any loss or decrease of fat planes between lymph node and carotid for better evaluation of carotid, internal jugular vein and circle of Wills.. Carotid artery repair can be done by surgeon with 3-0 monofilament round body suture; however, a vascular surgeon should be requested to do the repair, as it can worsen and may require grafting.

Nerve injury: Sensory and motor nerve injury is quite common. Severing of cutaneous branches does not lead to significant sensory loss, but a few patients may perceive it. In these patients, counselling and reassurance is the solution.

Motor paresis is usually due to thermal trauma by electrosurgery or overstretching. Marginal mandibular nerve injury is troublesome and can be avoided by thorough identification and meticulous dissection.

Cranial nerves are quite sensitive to retraction, hence care should be taken during level II dissection where accessory spinal nerve retraction is required even though it may not be clinically evident. However, shoulder pain is a common complaint and requires physiotherapy.

Hypoglossal nerve injury is uncommon until tumour is adherent at level II or level IB. Similarly, phrenic nerve injury is rare and may not be evident until bilateral.

Brachial plexus paresis occurs when dissection goes below the muscular fascia of supraclavicular fossa. Fixity of lymph node in the transverse plane favours its fixity to scalene or prevertebral muscles and neck dissection is contraindicated. In selected cases, surgery can be done after thorough counselling and informed consent.

Chyle leak: A meticulous dissection is performed near the lower end of the internal jugular vein and common carotid to avoid injury to the lymphatic channel and duct (see Figure 16.8).

Unchecked a chyle leak is a dreaded complication, so a careful examination of the lymphatic channel/duct area at the end of surgery should always be done without any excuse. Chyle is a colourless fluid in fasting patients, hence a leak should be suspected when the post-surgical drain is more than 300 ml in first 24 hours and serosanguinous. Later, it may be clear or turbid fluid in large volume. Once a chyle leak is suspected, management should start promptly, otherwise it will worsen. The author performs surgical re-exploration and repair within 72 hours, as a wait-and-watch policy in an obvious chyle leak will alter the appearance of the surgical site, making it difficult to find the leak. Conservative management in terms of pressure dressing is favoured in small volume leaks, but that decision requires experience, and hence re-exploration should always be considered. Rich fat diet or parenteral lipids may be required in prolonged chyle leaks.

Flap necrosis: Neck skin is supplied through platysmal muscle, hence flap necrosis is rare in transverse incision until platysma is debrided from the skin. However, radiation-induced fibrosis can increase the risk and therefore scalpel instead electrosurgery is preferred in flap elevation. Further, flaps should be regularly irrigated to keep them moist during surgery.

Skin should always be visible in the postoperative period to check for any change in colour and temperature. Change in colour or temperature requires exclusion of haematoma and infection. Patient should receive adequate parenteral fluids, haematoma removal and parenteral antibiotic in case of infection. Antiplatelet (low-dose clopidogrel or aspirin) or vasodilator drugs should be started once haematoma and infection are excluded.

FURTHER READING SUGGESTIONS

1. Robbins KT, Shaha AR, Medina JE, Califano JA, Wolf GT, Ferlito A, Som PM, Day TA; Committee for neck dissection classification, American head and neck society. Consensus statement on the classification and terminology of neck dissection. *Arch Otolaryngol Head Neck Surg.* 2008 May;134(5):536–8. doi: 10.1001/archotol.134.5.536. PMID: 18490577.
2. de Bree R, Takes RP, Shah JP, Hamoir M, Kowalski LP, Robbins KT, Rodrigo JP, Sanabria A, Medina JE, Rinaldo A, Shaha AR, Silver C, Suárez C, Bernal-Sprekelsen M, Ferlito A. Elective neck dissection in oral squamous cell carcinoma: Past,

present and future. *Oral Oncol.* 2019 Mar;90:87–93. doi: 10.1016/j.oraloncology.2019.01.016. Epub 2019 Feb 10. PMID: 30846183.

3. www.thyroid.org/professionals/ata-professional-guidelines

4. www.nccn.org/professionals/physician_gls/default.aspx#site

5. Gane EM, Michaleff ZA, Cottrell MA, McPhail SM, Hatton AL, Panizza BJ, O'Leary SP. Prevalence, incidence, and risk factors for shoulder and neck dysfunction after neck dissection: A systematic review. *Eur J Surg Oncol.* 2017 Jul;43(7):1199–218. doi: 10.1016/j.ejso.2016.10.026. Epub 2016 Nov 17. PMID: 27956321.

6. Agrawal N, Evasovich MR, Kandil E, Noureldine SI, Felger EA, Tufano RP, Kraus DH, Orloff LA, Grogan R, Angelos P, Stack BC Jr, McIver B, Randolph GW. Indications and extent of central neck dissection for papillary thyroid cancer: An American head and neck society consensus statement. *Head Neck.* 2017 Jul;39(7):1269–79. doi: 10.1002/hed.24715. Epub 2017 Apr 27. PMID: 28449244.

7. Sukato DC, Ballard DP, Abramowitz JM, Rosenfeld RM, Mlot S. Robotic versus conventional neck dissection: A systematic review and meta-analysis. *Laryngoscope.* 2019 Jul;129(7):1587–96. doi: 10.1002/lary.27533. Epub 2018 Oct 16. PMID: 30325513.

8. Borsetto D, Iocca O, De Virgilio A, Boscolo-Rizzo P, Phillips V, Nicolai P, Spriano G, Fussey J, Di Maio P. Elective neck dissection in primary parotid carcinomas: A systematic review and meta-analysis. *J Oral Pathol Med.* 2021 Feb;50(2):136–44. doi: 10.1111/jop.13137. Epub 2020 Dec 26. PMID: 33222323.

9. Gane EM, Michaleff ZA, Cottrell MA, McPhail SM, Hatton AL, Panizza BJ, O'Leary SP. Prevalence, incidence, and risk factors for shoulder and neck dysfunction after neck dissection: A systematic review. *Eur J Surg Oncol.* 2017 Jul;43(7):1199–218. doi: 10.1016/j.ejso.2016.10.026. Epub 2016 Nov 17. PMID: 27956321.

10. D'Cruz AK, Vaish R, Kapre N, Dandekar M, Gupta S, Hawaldar R, Agarwal JP, Pantvaidya G, Chaukar D, Deshmukh A, Kane S, Arya S, Ghosh-Laskar S, Chaturvedi P, Pai P, Nair S, Nair D, Badwe R; Head and Neck Disease Management Group. Elective versus therapeutic neck dissection in node-negative oral cancer. *N Engl J Med.* 2015 Aug 6;373(6):521–9. doi: 10.1056/NEJMoa1506007. Epub 2015 May 31. PMID: 26027881.

17

Thyroid Surgery

JAGDEEP S THAKUR

INTRODUCTION

Thyroid gland is one of the most important endocrine gland–regulating metabolisms of the body, functioning through pituitary-hypothalamic feedback mechanism.

Hypothyroidism is the most common thyroid disease, leading to goitre which is prevalent in certain geographical regions, like the sub-Himalayan area, due to deficient iodine in the water and diet. Hypothyroidism is managed by replacement therapy while large goitre requires surgical intervention. The incidence of thyroid cancers is increasing with dominance of differentiated thyroid cancers. These cancers have a good prognosis due to radio-ablation, provided surgery has been performed first. Over the years, management of thyroid cancers has been modified based on newly available clinical evidence. Various associations like the American Thyroid Association (ATA), National Comprehensive Cancer Network (NCCN), and British Thyroid Association (BTA) have formulated practice guidelines for thyroid cancers which are followed throughout the world. Certain local, geographical and economical factors influence management of thyroid cancers, but surgery remains the first line of treatment. Theodor Billroth and Theodor Kocher outlined basic thyroid surgical technique in the last decade of nineteenth century and since then surgical procedure has not changed significantly. Recently, however, endoscopic thyroid surgery has come into practice, but it carries numerous reservations and so open surgery is more widely accepted.

Beginners find thyroid gland surgery attractive, but complications like nerve palsy and hypoparathyroidism test even the experienced surgeons. Recurrent laryngeal nerve remains at highest risk of injury, leading to immediate hoarseness that may be unacceptable to the patient and can moreover lead to legal disputes for the surgeon. Similarly, parathyroid glands are also vulnerable in thyroidectomy. These complications can be avoided by good knowledge of clinical anatomy and meticulous dissection.

Clinical anatomy of the thyroid can be found in standard clinical anatomy textbooks. In general, each thyroid lobe has one artery, vein and nerve at superior and inferior pole that need to be identified before clamping or cutting. There are numerous surgical approaches to find superior or recurrent laryngeal nerves in both sides. However, the superior laryngeal nerve is rarely dissected out to locate its pathway, as the superior pedicle is ligated near the thyroid pole to avoid injury. However, recurrent laryngeal nerve should always be identified first before ligating any vessel in carotid-tracheal gutter. Parathyroid glands are found near the lower pole of the inferior thyroid artery and recurrent laryngeal nerve (Figure 17.1).

Thyroid tumour is common in certain geographical areas and may be classified as follows.

1. Benign tumours
   - Colloid goitre
   - Hyperthyroidism nodule/toxic nodule
2. Malignant tumours

DOI: 10.1201/9780367430139-17

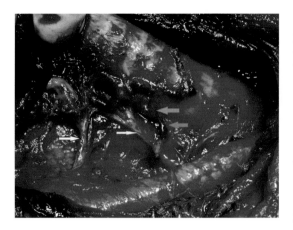

Figure 17.1 The recurrent laryngeal nerve (yellow arrow), inferior thyroid artery (white arrow) and parathyroid glands (green and blue arrows).

a. Differentiated thyroid cancer
   i. Papillary and its variants (tall cell, follicular variant, solid, etc.)
   ii. Follicular and its variants (Hurthle cell/ oncocytic, mucinous, clear cell)
b. Medullary thyroid cancer
c. Anaplastic
d. Poorly differentiated thyroid cancer, e.g., lymphoma, neuro-endocrine cancer

Thyroid tumours are managed surgically as per the guidelines/recommendations that are released from time to time by various thyroid and cancer associations (e.g. National Cancer Comprehensive Network, American Thyroid Association). General indications and contraindications of various procedures are discussed in the next section, but readers are advised to follow the most recent guidelines issued by these international and national associations.

PRE-OPERATIVE WORK-UP

Various international associations have formulated guidelines for thyroid nodules and the surgeon should keep himself/herself updated with latest guidelines. These are recommendations and one can modify them with patient counselling. Clinical examination is done to find the consistency, size, extent and mobility of the thyroid nodule and lymph node. Nodule is palpated in both extended and flexed position to find its extent. The fingers are insinuated between nodule

and sternocleidomastoid muscle and carotid is palpated to find invasion of carotid. Obliteration of the space between nodule and sternocleidomastoid muscle is indicated by CT scan. Obliteration of suprasternal space suggests retrosternal extension and a CT scan is warranted. Indirect laryngoscopy is done to find status of recurrent laryngeal nerve and subglottic space.

The patient is investigated for thyroid functions which need to be normalised as much as possible. Serum calcium and Vitamin D level are also estimated, as these will influence post-operative hypocalcaemia. All other general haematological and biochemical tests are done as per the institutional protocols.

Radiological Examination

Ultrasonography is the first choice of investigation. This should be performed before fine needle aspiration cytology, as the nodule's anatomy changes with intervention, failing the objective of ultrasonography. Ultrasonography looks for certain specific features that differentiate infective, benign and malignant nodules. It gives information on thyroid extent and nodal status. Any vascular, tracheal or mediastinal extension of thyroid nodule needs evaluation by CT scan. A few selective cases with extra-thyroidal extension and vocal cord palsy require CT scan too. Contrast-enhanced CT scan should always be performed in clinically bulky, hard disease, suspicious carotid and tracheal invasion and retrosternal/mediastinal extension. Contrast CT scan (Figure 17.2a-c) provides better evaluation and should always be performed where indicated (extrathyroidal extension, retrosternal extention, dysphagia, nerve palsy and vascular invasion). Contrast used in CT or MRI affects radioiodine scan after surgery as these contrasts are iodine-based and need three months to leave the body.

PATHOLOGY

Fine needle aspiration cytology/biopsy is the investigation of choice in thyroid nodule. It is more than 95% accurate and reaches 99% under ultrasonography guidance. Fine needle aspiration should be performed, preferably with a 22 FG needle. Cytology reporting is done as per the

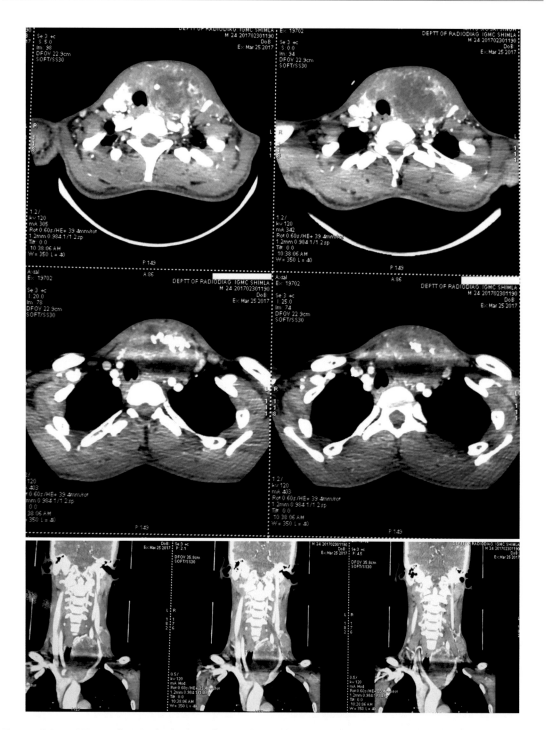

Figure 17.2a-c CT scan showing large thyroid tumour with extrathyroidal and retrosternal extension.

Bethesda system or the Thy classification of the Royal College of Physicians which guide the type and extent of the thyroid surgery. Open biopsy is not recommended until and unless inoperable or poorly differentiated thyroid cancer (lymphoma) demands histopathology confirmation.

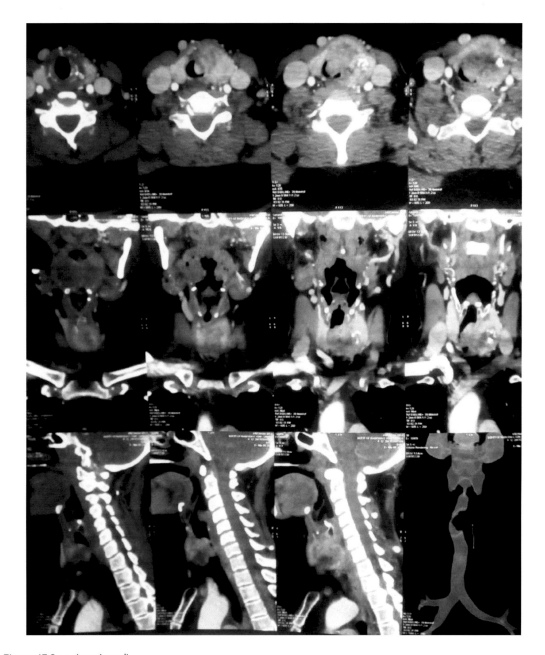

Figure 17.2a-c (continued)

ANAESTHESIA

Thyroidectomy is performed under general anaesthesia with endotracheal intubation. Patient should be euthyroid until surgery is being done for thyrotoxicosis, which requires preparation for a managed thyroid storm occurring after thyroidectomy.

Rarely, surgery can be performed in the hypothyroid state, but TSH should be brought to less than 10 micromole/litre for smooth anaesthetic recovery.

A nerve monitoring system requires a specific endotracheal tube with built-in electrodes. Muscle relaxant drugs must be controlled at time of nerve monitoring.

LOBECTOMY

Indications

1. Nodule with failed diagnostic cytology.
2. Follicular neoplasm.
3. Papillary carcinoma: Microcarcinoma/unifocal (T1–T2) without neck node/extrathyroidal extension.
4. Low to moderate risk differentiated thyroid cancer.

HEMITHYROIDECTOMY

Indication

1. As a part of total laryngectomy in selective cases.

Near-Total Thyroidectomy

1. Low risk DTC.
2. Graves' disease/thyrotoxicosis.

TOTAL THYROIDECTOMY

Indications

1. Papillary thyroid carcinoma with moderate- and high-risk individuals.
2. Anaplastic thyroid carcinoma.
3. Medullary thyroid carcinoma.

Contraindication

T4B Anaplastic thyroid carcinoma.

SURGICAL TECHNIQUE

- Once patient is intubated, the incision is marked, usually between the sternocleido-mastoid muscles depending upon the extent of tumour (Figure 17.3). Length can be about 5–7 cm in small tumours. (It is about 5 cm above the sternum in the non-extended neck, but can be higher depending upon disease bulk and neck nodes). Incision size should give proper exposure. The surgeon usually marks a small incision so as to achieve a good surgical scar (Figure 17.4), but smaller incisions have limited exposure and surgeons with limited experience may struggle for idle exposure leading to unnecessary retraction and contusions in flaps that may produce a bad scar. One should remember that besides the length of

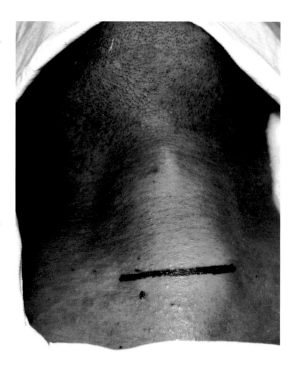

Figure 17.3 The Kocher incision for thyroid surgery.

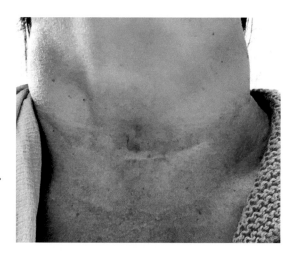

Figure 17.4 Cosmetically good thyroid incision scar.

incision, a number of other factors, like site of incision (skin crease and distant above sternum), tissue handling during surgery, type of needle, thread and sutures, racial and ethnic factors, inflammatory response of the body, and post-operative care of the incision scar, affect the aesthetic outcome.
- Once incision is marked, the neck is extended, especially in bulky and retrosternal tumours,

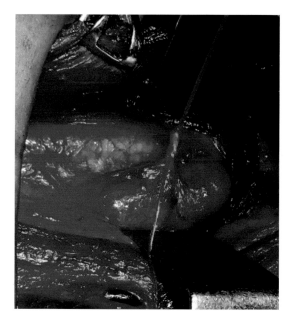

Figure 17.5 The ligated middle thyroid vein, which is present in less than 40% of cases.

so as to bring out superior mediastinum. Injection lignocaine 1–2% with adrenaline (1:1,00,000 or 1: 2,00,000) is injected in operative field.

- Operative field is cleaned and draped, and incision made with knife and later monopolar electrosurgery as described in chapter 1. Betadine is avoided in thyroid surgery as it may hinder radio-iodine scan post-operatively.
- Superior and inferior subplatysmal flaps are raised. Sometimes, especially with smaller incisions, a resident may have difficulty due to absence of platysma in the midline. In such cases, keeping dissection plane just above external jugular veins helps.
- Flap are retracted and secured. Neck midline (median raphae) is identified, which indicates fusion of strap muscles in midline. This step is quite important as deviation will lead to excessive haemorrhage. A small incision is made with electrosurgery and the midline dissected with haemostat forceps. Because the strap muscles are separated in midline, bipolar electrosurgery should be used, as vessels are encountered as one goes cephalad.
- Thyroid isthmus is exposed and identified. Strap muscles on either side are freed from the

isthmus and lobes, with bipolar keeping extra-capsular dissection.

- As strap muscles are dissected and lobes exposed, one can encounter the middle thyroid vein in some cases. This must be ligated as it directly drains into the internal jugular vein (Figure 17.5).
- Bulky thyroid disease has large dilated veins which bleed a lot, hence meticulous dissection with patience is required, and where necessary, veins should be ligated. Electro-coagulation of these dilated veins doesn't help every time, and quick access to thyroid arteries is required to decrease the vascularity.
- Strap muscles are retracted and dissection proceeds posteriorly, exposing internal jugular vein and common carotid artery.
- From this point, surgical steps differ according to which side of the thyroid lobe is dissected first. There are no guidelines on which lobe to dissect first in total thyroidectomy, but this author prefers to dissect the diseased lobe first as the nerve can be dissected better, with minimal risk of injury, at the start of surgery, before surgical fatigue takes a toll.
- The common carotid artery and internal jugular vein are retracted, and lateral and posterior border of right lobe is exposed and delivered out by ligating and cutting the middle thyroid vein, if present; as this vein may be absent in 30–40% cases (Figure 17.5).
- Strap muscles are retracted upwards and laterally by shifting single-hook retractors superiorly near the attachment of these muscles to thyroid cartilage. Superior pole of lobe is held with Babcock forceps and pulled downward and laterally.
- Superior pole is dissected free with bipolar from cricothyroid muscle, keeping dissection plane just adjacent to thyroid surface and applying Babcock forceps.
- With strap muscles still retracted, the superior pole is held with Babcock forceps near cricothyroid muscle.
- Superior vascular pedicle, consisting of superior thyroid artery and vein, is identified and ligated (Figure 17.6). This step doesn't require individual exposure of each vessel and they can be ligated together. Ligature should be placed first near the lobe so the vascular pedicle can be pulled down further and then double

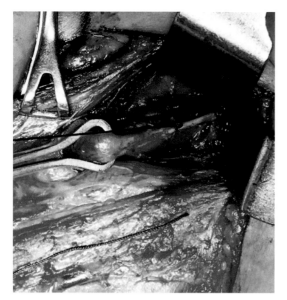

Figure 17.6 The superior pole is pulled down and secured.

ligature is applied on the superior end and tied tightly, keeping long tails so the vessel can be pulled in case of knot slippage as vessels retract beneath strap muscle.

- Superior thyroid nerve rarely comes in operative field as it gets retracted upwards with single hook retractors. Similarly, the external branch of the superior thyroid nerve does not usually need to be identified. However, dissection should be meticulous to avoid injury to these nerves.
- Once superior vascular pedicle is ligated and cut, lobe is pulled out and dissected from pharynx and oesophagus using bipolar, finger or swab. However, bipolar electrosurgery is kept at 8–10W setting to avoid nerve injury and monopolar use is contraindicated.
- Now dissection is shifted to the lower pole where many venous channels are encountered. These veins are electro-coagulated or ligated depending upon calibre. Ligation should always be preferred in case of doubt, as the bleeding vessel may get retracted to the mediastinum. Rarely, a very bulky disease displaces recurrent laryngeal nerve superficial within these veins and the surgeon should ligate and cut any structure carefully. A nerve monitor, if available, helps in these difficult cases; however, surgical acumen should prevail at any given time.

- As vessels are secured and divided, the trachea comes in view and is retracted to the left. Common carotid artery and internal jugular vein are retracted laterally and the thyroid lobe and trachea are retracted to the opposite side, exposing Beahr's triangle.
- Now the inferior thyroid artery, recurrent laryngeal nerve and parathyroid glands are encountered and must be identified and preserved to the best extent possible, as thyroid surgery is all about these three structures (see Figure 17.1).
- Sometimes, the inferior thyroid artery is easily identified as it comes posterior to the common carotid artery at an angle towards thyroid lobe, but is it not ligated until the recurrent laryngeal nerve is fully identified and traced.
- Recurrent laryngeal nerve is identified by blunt dissection away from the lower pole, preferably near lower end of the neck where nerve comes out of the thoracic cavity. This decreases the chances of nerve injury, as any attempt near the cricothyroid joint leads to haemorrhage from small arterial vessels. As a result, the surgeon will attempt coagulation or ligation to control it. Rarely, the nerve divides into two or more branches near the lower pole, subsequently increasing the risk of injury. As stated, in other difficult cases, a nerve monitoring system helps, but surgical acumen should always prevail. Monopolar electrosurgery should be avoided or switched off when a nerve monitoring system is in use.
- Recurrent laryngeal nerve is exposed fully, up to its entry in the cricothyroid joint. This requires ligation of the inferior thyroid artery and preservation of parathyroid glands (see Figure 17.1).
- Parathyroid glands are found in the course of recurrent laryngeal nerve and easily identified as small vascular structures which tend to change colour from dark red to caramel upon vascular insult (see Figure 17.1). All glands are preserved, except in difficult cases, where they are identified later in the excised thyroid specimen and removed, sliced into many parts, and then reimplanted into sternocleidomastoid muscles.
- Inferior thyroid artery is ligated near to the gland or trachea to preserve the arterial branches of parathyroid glands.

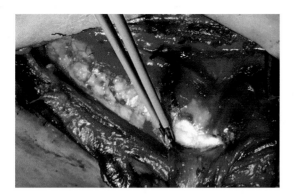

Figure 17.7 The thyroid tissue is dissected free from trachea with scalpel or bipolar electrocautery.

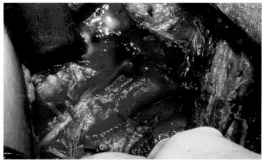

Figure 17.8 The left recurrent laryngeal nerve.

- At this level, small arterial twigs tend to bleed and should be controlled by applying pressure for 1–2 minutes and then performing bipolar coagulation at 8–10W. A small cricothyroid branch entering the joint with the recurrent laryngeal nerve may bleed heavily and test the surgeon's patience. One needs to identify this vessel after applying pressure as described above and then ligate meticulously. Any overzealous electrocoagulation will lead to nerve injury. Sometimes ligature may be difficult due to a shorter end that requires a vascular clip; or it can be left alone after sustaining pressure for 1–2 minutes as vasoconstriction will overcome this haemorrhage.
- Now the right lobe is dissected fully and can be excised by applying a large haemostatic clamp on the lobe isthmus junction and shaving off the lobe from the trachea with a scalpel or bipolar electrocautery (Figure 17.7). Silk 1–0 needle ligature is applied through the thyroid and secured at the isthmus end. This ligature should be dyed, braided and non-absorbable/ longstanding so the surgeon can find this thyroid end easily in case of completion thyroidectomy, and fibrosis makes dissection difficult in revision surgery.
- Lobectomy surgical procedure ends here. Surgical site is closed after complete haemostasis and drained (via glove or negative suction, depending upon haemostasis).
- The remainder of the surgical procedure can go ahead by pulling the lobe contra-laterally and dissecting out the isthmus. This requires excision of the ligament of Berry from the trachea,

which can be performed by scalpel or bipolar. Bipolar in lower power output (8–10W) is better if used cautiously, as minute trachea vessels cause bleeding.
- Excision of half of isthmus and lobe is called hemithyroidectomy and is performed by applying clamps similar to lobectomy.
- The surgical site is temporarily packed with gauze and left lobe dissection is started. This is similar to that of the right lobe except for the recurrent laryngeal nerve.
- Once the superior vascular pedicle has been ligated and divided, the recurrent laryngeal nerve is traced from where is enters the neck. Its course differs from the right nerve as it is found in the trachea-oesophageal groove and rarely shows any variations, although branching occurs near cricothyroid joint (Figure 17.8).
- Once the nerve has been identified and dissected, inferior vascular pedicle is secured, ligated and divided as on the right side, saving the parathyroid glands.
- Isthmus is freed by excising ligament from the trachea with bipolar or scalpel, similar to the right side, and this completes the total thyroidectomy (Figure 17.9).
- The surgical site is irrigated with normal saline or Ringer's lactate. Haemostasis is achieved by bipolar or ligation and any venous bleed should be ruled out through positive intrathoracic pressure.
- Integrity of bilateral recurrent laryngeal nerves is verified visually and/or with electro-stimulation.
- Excised specimen is checked for any parathyroid tissue, which is removed, sliced and implanted in sternocleidomastoid muscles.

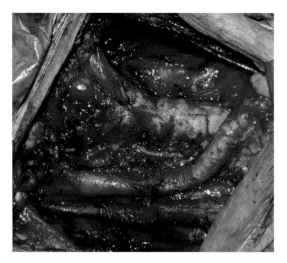

Figure 17.9 Total thyroidectomy with central neck dissection. Common carotid artery has slight aberrant course over trachea.

- Small-calibre negative suction drain or a glove drain is kept in in such a way that it covers both sides of the operative site and sub-platysma plane.
- Regional cervical or local anaesthetic block is applied for post-operative pain management.
- Strap muscles and platysma are closed in layers with absorbable 3–0 continuous sutures.
- Skin is closed with subcuticular 3–0 non-absorbable monofilament or absorbable braided sutures. Suture line is cleaned and medicated sterile dressing applied.

In cases of near-total thyroidectomy, a small portion of superior pole of one lobe is preserved without ligating and dividing the superior vascular pedicle.

Isthmectomy is excision of the isthmus only and, performed carefully, usually doesn't require dissection of lobe or recurrent laryngeal nerve identification, as the dissection plane overlies the trachea.

POST-OPERATIVE CARE

Patient is kept nil orally for 4–6 hours or till bowel sounds are heard, and ambulated once conscious.

Intravenous fluids are given as per protocol. Intravenous antibiotics and analgesic are given as per schedule.

Any change of quality of voice requires laryngoscopy examination and steroids are started early in case of any evidence of vocal paresis.

Drain is removed in case of less than 20 ml over 24 hours. Skin sutures are removed after 7–10 days.

Thyroxin supplementation is withheld in case of thyroid carcinoma for optimal post-operative radio iodine scan. Radioscan is performed when TSH reaches more than 30 micromoles/litre, while patient who had pre-operative CT scan requires at least three months must pass and TSH >30 micromoles/litre before an optimal post-op radio scan is performed.

COMPLICATIONS

Haemorrhage: Loose ligature in vascular pedicle can lead to haemorrhage intra- or post-operatively. It will require exploration and drainage of haematoma. Rarely, carotid or mediastinal vessels can lead to major haemorrhage, warranting intervention by a vascular surgeon.

Nerve injury: Right recurrent laryngeal nerve injury is common in thyroid surgery. Intra-operative nerve monitoring helps to confirm the integrity of the nerve at the end of surgery. However, sometimes nerve paresis occurs late due to oedema. Steroids are started immediately if nerve injury is diagnosed intra-operatively. If the nerve is engulfed in metastatic lymph nodes, they may be dissected grossly without injuring the nerve as residual lymph nodes can be managed by radio-iodine later.

Superior laryngeal nerve injury is rare and clinical diagnosis is difficult due to subtle change in quality of speech. Steroids, swallowing and speech therapy help in such cases. Injury to external laryngeal branch is rare as it runs below fascia over pharyngeal constrictors. Patient has subtle change in quality of voice, making diagnosis difficult.

Hypothyroidism: Patients with lobectomy may have hypothyroidism later. This usually occurs due to excision of the dominant nodule/lobe. This is managed by replacement therapy similar to the hypothyroidism protocol.

Hypoparathyroidism: Hypoparathyroidism is common in cases of total thyroidectomy with central neck dissection. Meticulous dissection and confirmation of parathyroid tissue with frozen section helps to avoid this complication.

Sometimes, vascular insult leads to hypopara-thyroidism beside preservation of glands. Patient should be observed for any clinical features of hypocalcaemia, which usually starts with a tingling sensation around the mouth and later positive Chvostek's sign. Serum calcium concentration and electrocardiogram are assessed and calcium gluconate is started. A few studies have advocated vitamin D3 prophylaxis to avoid post-operative hypocal-caemia, or addition of manganese with calcium gluconate. However, evidence remains low.

Oesophageal injury: Oesophageal injury is rare as gross invasion of the oesophagus is rare in thyroid carcinoma. Usually, the muscular layer is invaded by thyroid cancer which can be dissected, keeping mucosal layer intact. Any breach requires repair with inverted 4-0 sutures, similar to pharyngoplasty in total laryngectomy.

Tracheal injury: Tracheal injury is again rare and requires tracheoplasty or tracheostomy. Sometimes, shaving off the thyroid cancer from the trachea may lead to tracheomalacia, requiring elective tracheostomy.

FURTHER READING SUGGESTIONS

1. www.thyroid.org/professionals/ata-professional-guidelines/
2. Bible, KC et al. American Thyroid Association guidelines for management of patients with anaplastic thyroid cancer. *Thyroid* 2021 Mar;337–386. http://doi.org/10.1089/thy.2020.0944
3. www.nccn.org/professionals/physician_gls/pdf/thyroid.pdf
4. www.eurothyroid.com/guidelines/eta_guidelines.html
5. www.british-thyroid-association.org/current-bta-guidelines-and-statements

18

Parathyroid Surgery

RIPU DAMAN ARORA AND SUBINSHA A

INTRODUCTION

About 99% of parathyroid tumours are benign and commonly found in female. These tumours are usually present with hyperparathyroidism (HPT), most commonly primary hyperparathyroidism.

Primary hyperparathyroidism: characterised by hypercalcaemia in the presence of an inappropriate amount (unsuppressed) level of parathyroid hormone, most commonly due to adenoma.

Secondary hyperparathyroidism: occurs as a consequence of hypocalcaemia, where the glands increase the production of the hormone to mobilise the calcium from the bones to correct the condition.

Tertiary hyperparathyroidism: a condition that develops after a long period of increased parathyroid (PTH) secretion from the glands.

Anatomy

The parathyroid glands are usually located on the posterior aspect of the thyroid gland. They are flattened and oval in shape—situated external to the thyroid gland itself but within the pretracheal fascia. Blood supply of both superior and inferior glands is mainly from the inferior thyroid artery. Significant supply also comes from thyroid capsule but rarely from superior thyroid artery.

Most individuals have four parathyroid glands (Figure 18.1) although variation in number (from two to six) is common.

Superior parathyroid glands: The two superior parathyroid glands are derived from the fourth pharyngeal pouch. They are located at the middle of the posterior border of each thyroid lobe, approximately 1 cm superior to the entry of the inferior thyroid artery into the thyroid gland.

Inferior parathyroid glands: The two inferior parathyroid glands are derived from the third pharyngeal pouch. Although inconsistent in location among individuals, the inferior parathyroid glands are usually found near the inferior poles of the thyroid gland.

Ectopic location of gland is infrathymic, high in the neck, mediastanium carotid sheath, tonsillar area, lateral wall of nasopharynx and retropharyngeal areas.

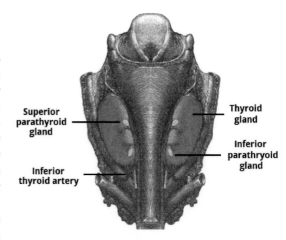

Figure 18.1 Anatomical location of parathyroid glands.

DOI: 10.1201/9780367430139-18

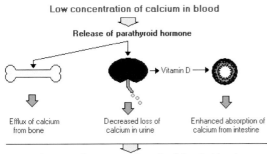

Figure 18.2 Line diagram showing parathyroid physiology.

Physiology

See Figure 18.2.

TYPES OF HYPERPARATHRODISM

There are three types of hyperparathyroidism: primary, secondary, and tertiary.

Primary Hyperparathyroidism

Primary hyperparathyroidism is a condition in which one or more parathyroid glands produce too much parathyroid hormone and the calcium level in the blood becomes elevated. It is commonly associated with parathyroid adenoma (usually single), parathyroid hyperplasia and (rarely) parathyroid carcinoma.

Secondary Hyperparathyroidism

Most cases of secondary hyperparathyroidism are due to chronic kidney failure that results in low vitamin D and calcium levels.

Tertiary Hyperparathyroidism

This type occurs when the parathyroid glands make too much PTH after the calcium levels return to normal and become autonomous. This type usually occurs in people with kidney problems.

Familial Hyperparathyroidism and MEN Syndrome

A positive family history should raise a suspicion of hereditary hyperparathyroidism or MEN syndrome.

Primary hyperparathyroidism is an autosomal disorder and all the parathyroid glands are hyperplastic.

In MEN syndrome type I, hyperparathyroidism presents along with tumours of pancreas or pituitary tumours.

MEN type II A presents with medullary thyroid carcinoma, pheochromocytoma hyperparathyroidism, lichen planus amyloidosis and Hirschsprung disease. MEN IIB presents with medullary thyroid carcinoma, pheochromacytoma, marfanoid body habitus, mucosal neuromas and ganglioneuromatosis on intestinal tract.

CLINICAL MANIFESTATIONS

As the saying goes, clinical manifestations include "painful bones, renal stones, abdominal groans, and psychic moans". Clinical features are mainly due to hypercalcaemia, which manifests in the following ways.

- Muscle weakness
- Muscle and bone aches and pains
- Depression
- Constipation
- Tiredness
- Peptic ulceration
- Pancreatitis
- Renal impairment
- Nephrogenic diabetes insipidus
- Nephrolithiasis
- Shortened QT interval
- Band keratopathy
- Thirst and polyuria

Work-Up

- Biochemical tests
  a) PTH
  b) Calcium
  c) Magnesium
  d) Phosphorous
  e) Vitamin D
  f) Creatinine
  g) 24-hour urine collection (40% of hyperparathyroid patients at diagnosis have hypercalciuria)

Diagnosis of hyperparathyroidism is generally suspected in patients with incidental finding of hypercalcaemia or symptomatic patients with increased blood calcium level. Further confirmation requires increased parathyroid hormone levels in primary hyperparathyroidism along with urine analysis for hypercalciuria. Further work-up of hyperparathyroidism consists of imaging studies.

- Imaging
  a) Neck ultrasound provides information about the location of the lesion and its structure. Advantages: it is easy to perform rapidly, well tolerated, and low cost. Disadvantages: poor localisation of the enlarged gland in retrosternal, retroesophageal and cervicothymic regions.
  b) 99mTc-sestamibi scan is the investigation of choice for localisation of parathyroid glands. Parathyroid cells have a large number of mitochondria which enables sestamibi to enter the parathyroid more intensely than surrounding thyroid tissue. In this method, the patient is intravenously injected with 20–25 mCi of Tc 99m sestamibi. Images are obtained at 10–15 minutes and then at 2–3 hours after injection.
  c) Computed tomography (CT) with contrast helps in location of the lesion, its relation to and invasion of surrounding structures and enlarged lymph nodes. It is also useful for localisation of the ectopic gland, a disadvantage being low sensitivity.
  d) Magnetic resonance imaging (MRI) gives the best detail on soft tissues of the neck. MRI is also superior to CT in assessing recurrent cases where surgical clips in the field can cause significant artefacts in CT studies. Useful for localisation of ectopic gland.
  e) Other imaging investigations are thallium technicium scintigraphy, selective arteriography or digital subtraction arteriography, intraoperative ultrasonography, and ultrasound guided FNAC.
- Conclusion: 99mTc-sestamibi scan along with ultrasound/CT or MRI should suffice for pre-operative localisation of parathyroid adenoma.

SURGERY

Surgical neck exploration is the treatment of choice, but selective parathyroidectomy should be considered for single parathyroid adenomas with good pre-operative localisation. For parathyroid hyperplasia, especially in cases of familial or MEN syndrome, for the choice is subtotal or total parathyroidectomy with autotransplantation.

In MEN type I syndrome recurrence rates are very high, while in MEN type IIA the course of disease is more benign.

Procedure: Left Inferior Parathyroidectomy

Surgical Steps

- Patient will be kept in supine position, intubated, and given general anaesthesia.
- Patient is positioned and the incision site marked with marker.
- Incision is two fingersbreadth above suprasternal notch, along skin crease, from anterior border of one sternocleidomastoid to another for multiple adenoma (single adenoma can be accessed with small incision made slightly lateral to trachea) (Figure 18.3a-b).
- Local infiltration is done with saline; adrenaline (1:1,00,000 or 1:2,00,000) is given over the planned incision site.
- Incision is made.
- Subplatysmal flaps are elevated.
- Soft tissue dissection is done.
- Linea alba is identified; strap muscles are separated and retracted.
- Right sternocleidomastoid muscle is cut horizontally and thyroid gland identified.
- Trachea is identified below thyroid isthmus.
- Small ~1.5cm diameter glandular tissue is located just inferior to right thyroid lobe and just lateral to anterior wall of trachea (Figure 18.4).
- Tissue dissection is done all around; blood vessels supplying the gland are identified and ligated.
- Gland is dissected out in toto along with the ligated blood vessels. Usually, parathyroid gland and lymph node float in saline but parathyroid tissue is conformed on frozen section.
- Haemostasis is achieved.
- Blood sample is sent for intact parathyroid hormone level 20 minutes after gland excision. If level decreases by more then half, there is no need for exploration of other glands; otherwise neck exploration should be done for other glands.

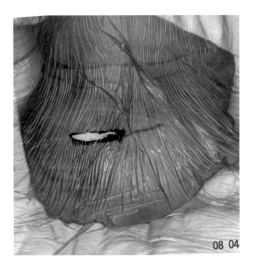

(a)

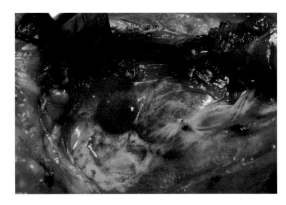

Figure 18.4 Enlarged parathyroid gland identified and excised.

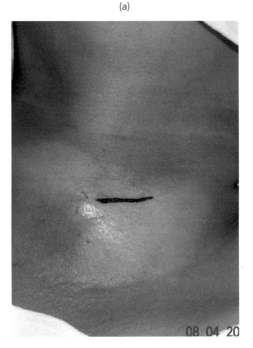

(a)

Figure 18.3a-b Midline incision is made for multiple adenomas while small lateral incision is sufficient for single adenoma.

- Right neck drain is placed and wound is closed in layers.
- Aseptic dressing is applied.
- Post-operatively, mobility of bilateral vocal cords confirmed by fibre-optic laryngoscopy.
- Patient is extubated.

Post-operative regular calcium monitoring is required and signs of hypocalcaemia should be looked for. Patient may go into "hungry bone" syndrome and may require calcium and magnesium supplements. Repeat parathyroid levels should be checked after three weeks.

SURGICAL COMPLICATIONS

a. Injury to the recurrent laryngeal nerve.
b. Bleeding or haematoma.
c. Damage to the remaining parathyroid glands with resultant problems in maintaining calcium levels in blood.
d. In some cases, surgical exploration fails to identify the abnormal parathyroid gland or multiple abnormal glands may be present; in these cases, further and more aggressive surgery may be needed.
e. Hungry bone syndrome.

19

Intraoperative Laryngeal Nerve Monitoring

KULDEEP THAKUR

"I am convinced that the best management of RLN injuries is of a preventable character."

Frank Lahey

INTRODUCTION

Unilateral vocal cord paralysis (VCP) presents as dysphonia, aspiration, ineffective cough, dysphagia and difficulty in performing manoeuvres requiring glottic closure, such as weight lifting, whereas bilateral vocal cord paralysis is a serious surgical calamity requiring urgent surgical interventions. The reported rates of temporary unilateral and permanent unilateral vocal cord paralysis are 6% and 3%, respectively, in patients undergoing thyroid and parathyroid surgery. Yet, when bilateral vocal cord paralysis occurs after thyroidectomy, it is found to be permanent in 45% of patients. The rate of tracheostomy in bilateral vocal cord paralysis averages 30%, with an additional 21% of patients requiring other varieties of airway procedures. That means some 50% of these patients require some form of airway surgical intervention. Moreover, some authors have observed that only 14% of temporary or permanent post-operative VCP was visually evident intraoperatively, emphasising the importance of loss of signal.

Certainly, recurrent laryngeal nerve (RLN) visualisation is required in thyroid surgery. However, neural monitoring adds a new functional dynamic during thyroid surgery. Another important benefit of monitoring is not only to identify

the RLN injury but also to identify the mechanism and the site of nerve injury.

MECHANISM OF RECURRENT LARYNGEAL NERVE INJURIES

The vast majority (83%) of nerve injuries are due to traction, and 60% of these traction injuries are neuropraxic in nature and localised to the ligament of Berry. The mechanism of nerve injuries in order of frequency is: traction > thermal > compression > clamping > ligature > entrapment > suction-related injuries > transection. Among these, thermal, clamping, and transection injuries are the most serious and are associated with poor long-term outcome.

CLINICALLY SIGNIFICANT APPLICATIONS OF INTRAOPERATIVE NERVE MONITORING

1. Neural mapping of the RLN even prior to visual identification of the nerve. This application not only speeds up RLN identification but also lowers the rates of temporary VCP.
2. Intraoperative nerve monitoring (IONM) also identifies the anatomical variants of normal RLN, such as extralaryngeal RLN branches.
3. IONM facilitates early and definitive intraoperative identification of non-recurrent laryngeal nerve.

DOI: 10.1201/9780367430139-19

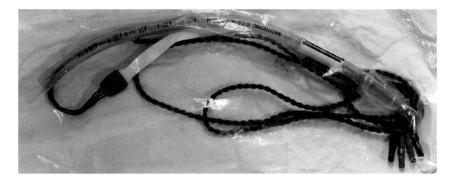

Figure 19.1 Surface electrode mounted flexometallic endotracheal tube.

4. In bilateral thyroid surgery, IONM reduces the rates of tracheostomy as intraoperative prediction of impending neuropraxic neural injury, allowing alteration of associated surgical manoeuvres.
5. It aids in identification of the SLN.
6. IONM is an important education adjunct and less experienced surgeons can have equivalent outcomes to those of experienced surgeons if they use IONM.

INDICATIONS FOR IONM

- Guidelines from the Intraoperative Neural Monitoring Study Group (INMSG) and the German Association of Endocrine Surgery recommend intraoperative neural monitoring in all patients who are undergoing thyroid and parathyroid surgery.
- Guidelines from the French Society of Oto-Rhino-Laryngology and Head and Neck Surgery recommend intraoperative neural monitoring only in difficult thyroid procedures such as surgery for recurrent cancer, locally advanced cancer or large hyperthyroid goitre.
- American Academy of Otolaryngology Head and Neck Surgery (AAOHNS) Clinical Practice Guidelines and Evidence-Based American Head and Neck Society (AHNS) Consensus recommend intraoperative neural monitoring in: 1) all bilateral thyroid surgery, 2) revision thyroid cancer surgery and 3) thyroid surgery on an only functioning nerve.
- ATA Recommendation 42B: Intraoperative neural stimulation (with or without monitoring) may be considered to facilitate nerve identification and confirm neural function.

METHOD AND BASIC SYSTEM SET-UP

The most common IONM format used and recommended by INMSG is the endotracheal tube-based IONM system.

- **Anaesthesia**
  Close partnership with the anaesthesiologist is an essential component of IONM and neuromuscular blockade must be avoided. Succinylcholine or a small dose of nondepolarising muscle relaxant can be used at intubation. During surgery, anaesthesia from nitrous oxide or any other inhalational agent must be sufficiently deep to avoid any other spontaneous movements of the vocal cords which would make it difficult to differentiate between evoked activity and spontaneous activity of vocal cords.

- **Tube Placement and Function**
  Patients are intubated with a specially designed, surface-electrode-mounted flexometallic endotracheal tube (Figure 19.1), positioned for surgery in the head extension. After positioning, adequate endotracheal tube position (i.e., adequate contact between vocal cords and vocal cord electrodes on endotracheal tube) must be assured (Figure 19.2). This can be done either by observing respiratory variations or by video-laryngoscopy in extended position. After positioning endotracheal tube, monitor must be sct and necessary connections made between recording side, interface box (Figure 19.3), stimulator probes (Figure 19.4) and monitor.

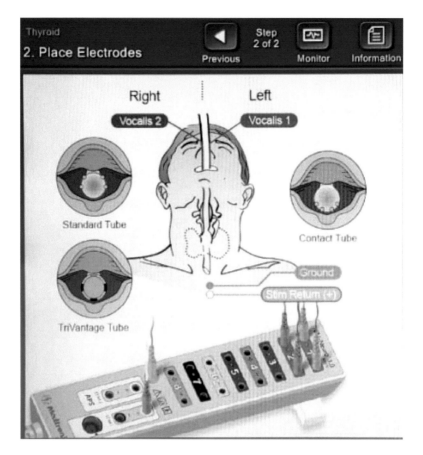

Figure 19.2 Adequate contact between vocal cords and vocal cord electrodes on endotracheal tube.

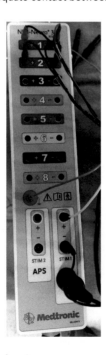

Figure 19.3 Interface box.

- **Important Precautions and Monitor Settings**
  1. Avoid lidocaine ointment or other tube lubricants on neuromonitoring endotracheal tubes.
  2. Pre-operative drying agents and intraoperative suction must be used to prevent pooling of saliva in glottis, which may result in alter signal.
  3. Check monitor settings: Stimulator probe, 0.8–1 mA, event threshold 100 microvolt, impedance value <5 kOhm and impedance imbalance of less than 1 kOhm.
  4. Electrocautery unit must be positioned greater than three meters away from the neural monitoring system.

- After the neuromonitoring set-up is complete (Figure 19.5) and at the onset of the surgery, strap muscles can be stimulated to confirm muscle twitch, thereby showing the lack of paralytic agents' effect and intact stimulator

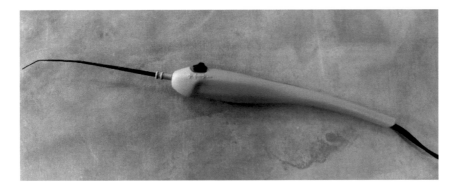

Figure 19.4 Stimulator probe.

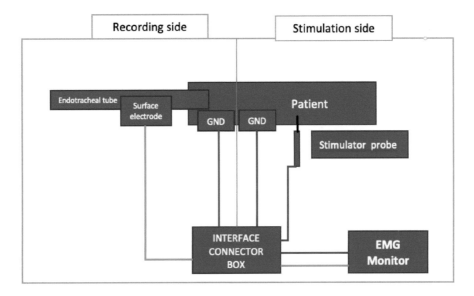

Figure 19.5 Patient and Monitoring Endotracheal Tube Scheme.

function. At the onset of dissection near the thyroid gland, the vagus nerve is stimulated high in the neck and robust EMG activity is obtained, which assures that the system is completely functional and RLN and branches can be safely searched through neural mapping. The normal neural evoked waveform is shown in Figure 19.6 and approximate normative neural monitoring parameters are shown in Table 19.1.

INTERPRETATIONS AND IMPORTANT DEFINITIONS

- **Optimal Normative Baseline**

A stimulation current of 1 mA and an initial waveform of 500 microV or greater amplitude, along with good laryngeal twitch at the beginning of the surgery, constitute optimal normative baseline.

- **Impending Adverse EMG (Combined Event): Impending Neuropraxia**

Combined event is combination of concordant amplitude decrease (50–70%) and increase in latency (>10%) and is an important early indicator of impending neuropraxic injury. These repeated combined events or a combined event lasting for 40 seconds or longer eventually leads to a more serious EMG event of loss of signal (LOS). INMGS (International Neural Monitoring Study Group) strongly recommends cessation of the surgical manoeuvre. The cessation of the surgical manoeuvre causing the combined event results in

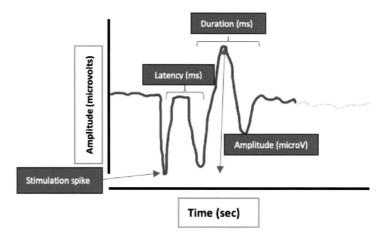

Figure 19.6 Normal neural monitoring evoked waveform.

Table 19.1 Approximate Normative Human Monitoring Parameters at Stimulation at 1 MilliA

	Amplitude (microV)	Latency (milliseconds)	Threshold (mA)
Right RLN	783 (+/−512)	2.47–4.25	0.25–1.4
Left RLN	604 (+/−504)	2.5–4.34	0.25–1
Right Vagus	717 (+/−479)	4.25–9.5	0.25–0.85
Left Vagus	420 (+/−255)	6.1–10	0.1–0.8
SLN	269 (+/−178.6)		0.4–0.6

70–80% recovery intraoperatively. The negative predictive value (NPV) and positive predictive value (PPV) of combined event are 97% and 33%, respectively.

- **Adverse EMG: Evolving Neuropraxia**

Loss of signal (LOS) has been variably defined, and INMSG define LOS as 100 micronV or less, typically associated with latency increase of > 10% of initial baseline. This caries a high risk of neuropraxia with PPV 83% and NPV of 98% with reduced chances of intraoperative recovery of 17–25% (see Flow diagram 19.1).

- **Final EMG**

Final EMG should be considered as recovery EMG at 20 minutes with recovery to >50% of baseline amplitude and an absolute amplitude value of >250 microV. Final EMG suggests extremely low risk of vocal cord paralysis. If the amplitude does not re-cover >50% of baseline value, the risk of early VCP goes very high (80%). Recovery of less than this amplitude caries a high risk of VCP and surgery should be staged.

FALSE POSITIVES (LOS WITH INTACT POST-OPERATIVE VOCAL CORD FUNCTION)

See table 19.1.

1. Endotracheal tube displacement.
2. Blood or fascia obscuring the stimulated nerve segment.
3. Neuromuscular blockade.
4. Vocal cord paralysis with early neural recovery.

FALSE NEGATIVES (GOOD EMG ACTIVITY WITH POST-OPERATIVE VCP)

1. Stimulation distal to injured segment (vagal stimulation).
2. Injuries subsequent to last testing stimulation, such as during wound irrigation and closure.
3. Delayed neuropraxia: Progressive oedema may affect RLN at an intralaryngeal location.
4. Posterior branch injury.

FLOW CHART 19.1:
TROUBLESHOOTING ALGORITHM

See table 19.1.

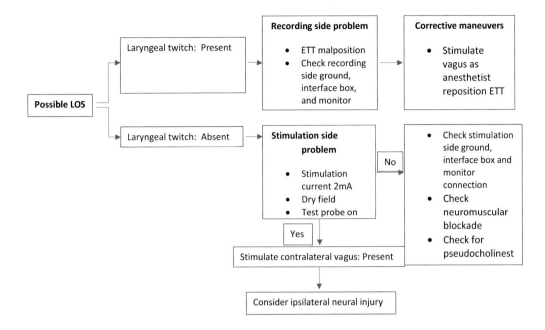

SAFETY OF COMPLETION SURGERY

The completion surgery is comparable to single-staged total thyroidectomy in terms of safety. However, total thyroidectomy has a statistically significant higher rate of transient hypoparathyroidism as compared to completion surgery.

TIMING OF COMPLETION SURGERY

Laryngeal recovery is a predominant and overwhelming consideration for safe timing of completion surgery, but oncologic treatment time frame in setting of malignancy must also be considered. Visual evidence of nerve function as documented by vocal cord exam should be used to denote functional recovery. Optimal timing of completion surgery is less than three days or greater than three months when attempting to minimise the risks related to completion thyroidectomy (see Flow diagram 19.2).

Oncologic Safety and Timing of Completion Surgery

When completion thyroidectomy is performed within six months of first surgery, there is generally no alteration of oncologic risk for most thyroid cancers in patients without evidence of residual tumour or distant metastasis. Studies on staged surgical strategy for extensive bilateral differentiated thyroid cancer showed that it was oncologically safe to delay second surgery by 4–25 weeks.

Laryngeal Recovery and Timing of Completion Surgery

Most neuropraxic RLN injuries generally recover within 2–6 months. At this time, it is vital to re-evaluate need for completion surgery through a multidisciplinary approach that considers disease and patient-related factors. Alternative nonsurgical management modalities such as observation, RAI and external beam radiation should always be considered as an alternative to completion thyroidectomy.

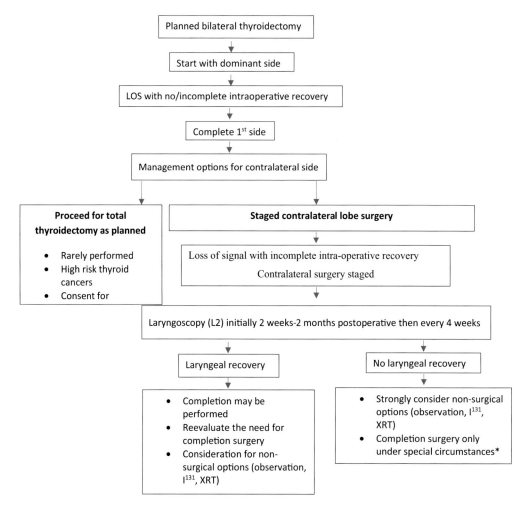

Flow diagram 19.2 Intraoperative management of loss of signal with incomplete intraoperative recovery in patients undergoing bilateral thyroidectomy. Asterisk indicates factors in favor of nerve sparing versus nerve sacrifice.

RECURRENT LARYNGEAL NERVE RISK-BENEFIT FACTORS

1. **Oncological Factors**
    - Possibility of complete resection of gross disease with nerve resection
    - Prognostic impact of leaving residual tumour on the nerve (amount and histology of tumour left, invasion site of subsequent visceral axis invasion)
    - Presence of distant metastasis in critical location
    - Perceived responsiveness of post-operative adjuvant non-surgical treatment: Radioactive iodine avidity, thyroxine suppression and external beam radiation

2. **Laryngeal Factors**
    - Pre-operative ipsilateral vocal cord status
    - Pre-operative contralateral vocal cord status
    - Impact of nerve resection on the patient, i.e., risk of aspiration or if patient is a professional voice user

Factors in Favour of Nerve Sparing

- Young patient, iodine avid papillary carcinoma thyroid
- Efficiency of adjuvant therapy (iodine or external beam radiation) judged to be good
- Elderly patients (increased risk of aspiration pneumonia in VCP)

- Patients who are voice professionals
- Contralateral vocal cord paralysis
- Known active distant metastases

Factors in Favour of Nerve Sacrifice

- Aggressive histological variants (tall cell, diffuse sclerosing type, solid variant)
- Iodine refractory disease
- Nerve invasion at the laryngeal entry point
- Normal contralateral vocal cords

OPTIMAL RECURRENT LARYNGEAL NERVE MANAGEMENT FOR INVASIVE THYROID CANCER

Local invasion occurs in about 13–15% of DTC cases and is more commonly seen in aggressive pathological variants and in elderly patients. RLN is the second most common invaded structure (33–61%), after strap muscle invasion, where the invasion may occur from either the thyroid primary or from paratracheal lymph nodes. The RLN invasion does not show significant negative impact on survival, and surgical resection of the invaded nerve uniformly lacks survival benefit when compared with the preservation of the invaded nerve.

Even after thorough pre-operative evaluation, up to 12% of patients presenting with invasive thyroid cancer may be asymptomatic. Few authors have observed that cases with pre-operative vocal cord plasy but with normal intraoperative EMG have better post-operative voice outcome if RLN is preserved during surgery. The management of RLN during thyroid gland surgery depends upon the pre-operative vocal cord status and intraoperative nerve invasion (Flow diagrams 19.3 through 19.6).

CONCLUSION

Intraoperative neural monitoring of RLN adds a new functional dynamic to thyroid and parathyroid surgery. Neuromonitoring helps in identification of the anatomically intact but physiologically non-functional nerve during surgery, thereby staging the planned single-stage bilateral thyroidectomy. Similarly, a nerve invaded by malignancy may maintain electric stimulability, or significant malignant invasion with preservation of glottal function may occur. In this resides the importance of the RLN neural monitoring. RLN neuromonitoring should be used in 1) all bilateral thyroid surgery, 2) revision thyroid cancer surgery, and 3) thyroid surgery on an only functioning nerve.

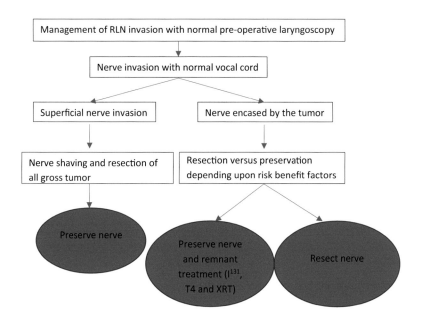

Flow diagram 19.3 Management of nerve invasion with normal pre-operative laryngoscopy.

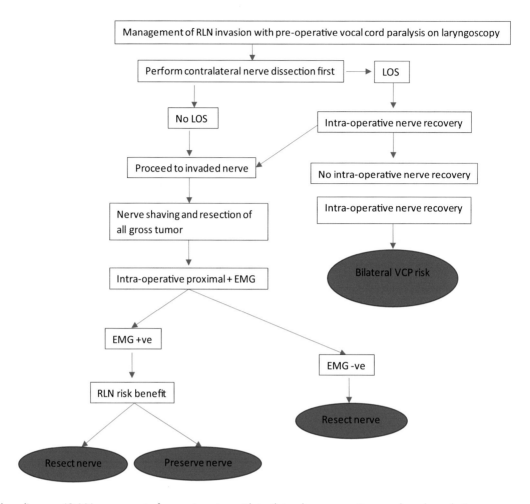

Flow diagram 19.4 Management of nerve invasion with ipsilateral pre-operative vocal cord paralysis on laryngoscopy.

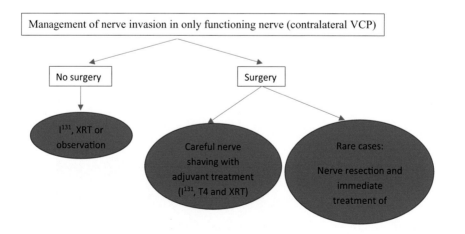

Flow diagram 19.5 Management of nerve invasion in only functioning nerve.

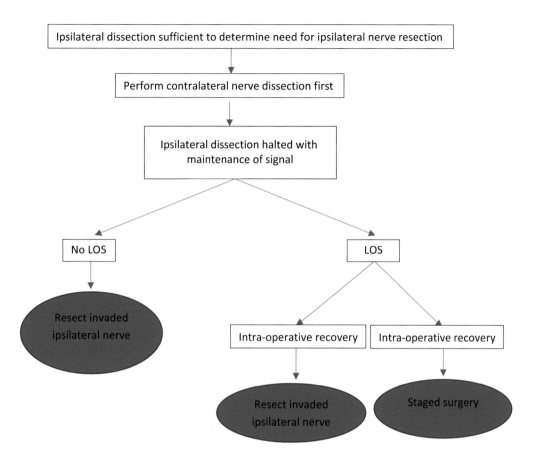

Flow diagram 19.6 Incorporation of intraoperative nerve monitoring to help reduce the risk of bilateral vocal cord paralysis when nerve resection is required.

20

Parapharyngeal Tumour Surgery

RIPU DAMAN ARORA, JAGDEEP S THAKUR

INTRODUCTION

Parapharyngeal space (PPS) tumours are rare and account for only 0.5% of all head and neck neoplasms. Surgical treatment of PPS tumours may be challenging due to the wide spectrum of both benign and malignant tumours and also due to the complex anatomic relationships and proximity of vital neurovascular structures within the PPS.

Anatomy

See Figures 20.1a and 20.1b.

The PPS sits lateral to the pharynx and can be viewed as an inverted pyramid with its base at the skull base and its apex reaching the greater cornu of the hyoid bone. Its superior boundary is the temporal bone and its inferior boundary is the junction of the posterior belly of the digastric muscle with the greater cornu of the hyoid bone. The lateral boundary is the mandibular ramus, medial pterygoid muscle and deep lobe of the parotid (through the stylomandibular tunnel). Medially, it is bounded by the buccopharyngeal fascia, which covers the superior constrictor muscle. The posterior boundary is the prevertebral fascia and muscles.

Since space-occupying lesions arising within the PPS are bound on three sides by bone – superiorly by the skull, laterally by the mandible and posteriorly by the spine – their growth proceeds either medially into the tonsillar and soft palate region or inferiorly into the retromandibular area.

The PPS is divided into two compartments by the styloid process.

- **Prestyloid**: Contains deep lobe of parotid, fat, and lymph nodes
- **Poststyloid**: Contains internal carotid artery, internal jugular vein, CNs IX–XII, sympathetic chain and lymph nodes

Tumours of the PPS

- Primary tumours
- Primary lymphoproliferative disease
- Metastatic lymph nodes
- Tumours extending from adjacent structures

Approximately 80% of primary neoplasms in the PPS are benign and about 20% are malignant. The most common primary tumours, accounting for 50% of PPS tumours, are salivary gland neoplasms that originate from the deep lobe of the parotid or from minor salivary gland tissue. Pleomorphic adenomas are the most common PPS tumour. Neurogenic tumours, primarily schwannomas or paragangliomas, are the second most frequent group of neoplasms.

Primary Tumours

1. **Salivary gland tumours**
   - Most common PPS neoplasms (40–50% of overall PPS tumours).
   - Pleomorphic adenoma (80–90% of salivary gland tumour).
   - Mucoepidermoid (most common malignant).
   - Less than 5% parotid tumours involve the PPS.
   - Located in prestyloid space.

DOI: 10.1201/9780367430139-20

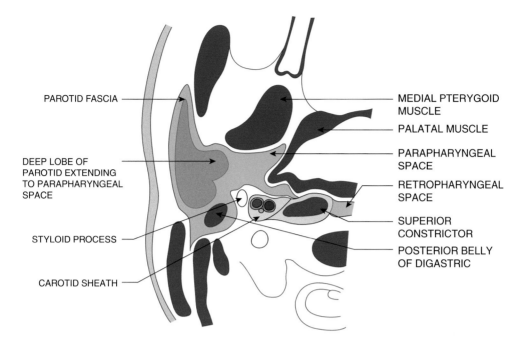

PAROTID FASCIA

DEEP LOBE OF
PAROTID EXTENDING
TO PARAPHARYNGEAL
SPACE

STYLOID PROCESS

CAROTID SHEATH

MEDIAL PTERYGOID
MUSCLE

PALATAL MUSCLE

PARAPHARYNGEAL
SPACE

RETROPHARYNGEAL
SPACE

SUPERIOR
CONSTRICTOR

POSTERIOR BELLY
OF DIGASTRIC

Figure 20.1a Anatomy of parapharyngeal space in axial plane.

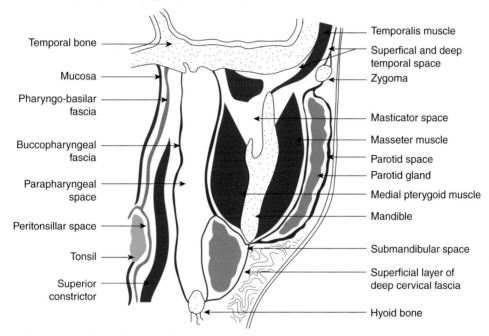

Temporal bone

Mucosa

Pharyngo-basilar
fascia

Buccopharyngeal
fascia

Parapharyngeal
space

Peritonsillar space

Tonsil

Superior
constrictor

Temporalis muscle

Superfical and deep
temporal space

Zygoma

Masticator space

Masseter muscle

Parotid space

Parotid gland

Medial pterygoid muscle

Mandible

Submandibular space

Superficial layer of
deep cervical fascia

Hyoid bone

Figure 20.1b Anatomy of parapharyngeal space in sagittal plane.

2. **Neurogenic tumours (17–25%)**
   - **Schwannoma**
     - Most common neurogenic neoplasm
     - Arising from vagus or sympathetic chain
   - Benign and slow growing
   - Less than 1% malignant
   - Displace internal carotid anteriorly
   - **Paraganglioma**
     - Second most common

- Highly vascular
- Arise from vagus, carotid body, jugular bulb
- **Neurofibromas**
  - Third most common neurogenic tumour
3. **Miscellaneous Tumours**
   - 20% of total PPS tumours
   - Lymphoma, haemangioma, teratoma, lipoma, branchial cleft cyst, arteriovenous malformation, internal carotid aneurysm, carcinoma

Clinical Presentation

- Asymptomatic most common
- Dysphagia/globus sensation
- Hoarseness
- Pain
- Airway obstruction
- Sleep apnoea
- Trismus
- Hypernasality
- Facial weakness/paralysis
- Horner's syndrome
- Tinnitus
- Hearing loss
- Aural fullness

Work-Up

- Detailed history
- Complete head and neck examination
- Pulse and blood pressure
- Cranial nerves
- Bimanual palpation
- Bruit, thrill
- Indirect laryngoscopy
  There is no standard staging system from American Joint Committee on Cancer or Union for International Cancer Control for tumours.

Investigations

a) Ultrasound guided FNAC
b) Special investigations:
   - 24 hour urine collection for catecholamines
   - Vanillylmandelic acid (VMA)
   - Metaiodobenzylguanidine scan (MIBG)
c) Imaging: CT, MRI, angiography, PET scan
   - CT

Locates tumour to prestyloid vs poststyloid
Fat plane between mass and parotid
Displacement of carotid artery
Enhancement of lesion
Bone erosion
Limited soft tissue detail
- MRI
Most useful study
Relationship of mass and other soft tissue
Carotid more easily seen than with CT
Characteristic appearance of tumour types on MRI allows pre-operative diagnosis in 90–95% of patients
- Angiography
Used for all enhancing lesions
Gold standard for relationship to blood vessels
Differentiate neurogenic and vascular
Main indication is planning for surgical treatment
- PET scan

Treatment

Mainly surgical excision
Surgical approach depends on location, size, suspicion of malignancy, relationship to neurovascular structures, surgeon experience
Goal is to achieve optimal exposure and vascular control without significant morbidity
Facial nerve may need to be dissected from Fallopian canal

VARIOUS APPROACHES

a) Transoral
b) Transcervical +/- mandibulotomy
c) Trans-parotid
d) Transcervical-parotid
e) Infratemporal fossa
f) Transcervical-transmastoid

Surgery: Excision of left side parapharyngeal space tumour
Approach: Transcervical + transparotid + mandibulotomy
Surgical steps:

- Patient was kept in supine position and intubation was done.
- Patient was positioned and incision site marked with marker; painting and draping done under all aseptic precautions (Figure 20.2).

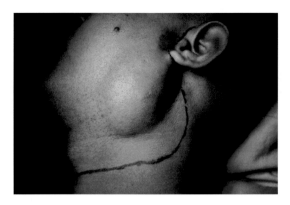

Figure 20.2 Classical approach to parapharyngeal space.

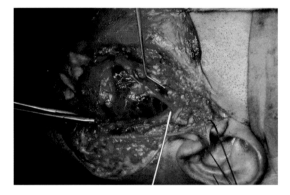

Figure 20.3 Cystic tumour with marginal mandibular nerve lying over it.

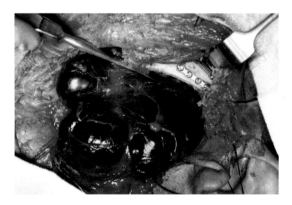

Figure 20.4 The parapharyngeal space approach with mandibulotomy. The mandible has been fixed with plates.

- Local infiltration with saline and adrenaline (1:1,00,000 or 1:2,00,000) is given over the planned incision site.
- An incision is made two fingers breadth below the left mandible, extending up to left side pre-auricular region (also known as a "lazy S" incision).
- Flaps are elevated superomedially up to the anterior border of masseter and inferolaterally up to the posterior border of sternocleidomastoid muscle.
- Soft tissue dissection is done.
- A soft, fluctuant, dark cystic mass is noted at left side parotid region which extended into left parapharyngeal space (Figure 20.3).
- Greater auricular nerve identified, anterior division of it sacrificed and posterior division preserved.
- Facial nerve trunk identified at 1 cm anterior and inferomedial to tragal pointer.
- Upper trunk of facial nerve identified as intact and preserved.
- Lower trunk of facial nerve splayed by left side parapharyngeal space tumour, which was stretched.
- Lower trunk of facial nerve is gently separated from the mass, cut at the periphery sites and placed in parotid region.
- Mass separated from left submandibular gland along with level Ib lymph node, and supracervical lymph nodes in parotid region are dissected and sent for HPE study.
- Facial vessels are ligated and cut.
- Anterior and posterior belly of digastric muscles and mylohyoid muscle identified.
- Hypoglossal and lingual nerve identified and preserved.
- Mandibulotomy was done for better exposure (Figure 20.4).
  - A paramedian cut is made anterior to mental foramen in between left side lateral incisor and canine.
  - Another cut is made at left side condyle of mandible.
  - Mandible is elevated superiorly without disturbing the medial mucosa of the mandible to preserve inferior alveolar nerve and vessels.
  - Entire left parapharyngeal space tumour gently separated from all surrounding tissues, tumour along with minimal parotid tissue is removed in toto and sent for histopathological evaluation (Figure 20.5).

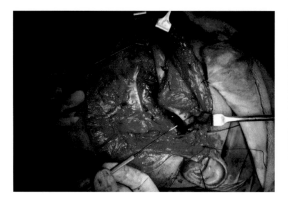

Figure 20.5 Complete excision of the tumour.

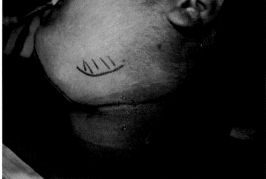

Figure 20.6 Transcervical approach for large parapharyngeal tumour.

- Styloid process and muscles attached to it identified.
- Mandible kept in initial position and fixed with 8 mm screws and 2 mm plates (see Figure 20.4).
- Suturing done at gingival site in between left incisor and canine with absorbable sutures.
- Haemostasis achieved, betadine-saline wash done.
- Cavity is filled with gel foam and surgicel (Oxidized regenerated cellulose).
- Drain kept and fixed.
- Incision sutured in two layers by Vicryl and Ethilon.
- Parotid dressing done.
- Patient was extubated and post-operative period was uneventful.
- Cranial nerves VII, IX, X, XI and XII examined and found functionally normal.

Left Parapharyngeal Mass (Pleomorphic Adenoma–Minor Salivary Gland)

Surgery: Excision by transcervical approach

- Patient positioned, parts cleaned and draped, skin marking done (Figure 20.6).
- Local infiltration with adrenaline and saline (1:1,000,00 or 1:2,00,000) given over marked site.
- An elliptical incision is made starting from left mastoid tip curving downwards 1 cm below the hyoid bone and reaching up to the mentum in midline.
- Subplatysmal flap raised superiorly to the lower border of mandible, inferiorly raised 1 cm from the incision line.
- Dissection proceeded further after identifying the left anterior belly of digastric.

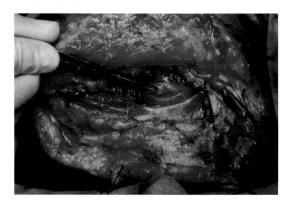

Figure 20.7 Tumour bulge visible in submandibular triangle.

- A bulge seen in submandibular triangle (Figure 20.7).
- Facial vessels identified and ligated.
- Left submandibular gland retracted laterally and myelohyoid muscle retracted anteriorly.
- Lingual nerve and hypoglossal nerve identified and preserved.
- Left submandibular gland duct ligated and gland removed.
- Left stylohyoid muscle identified and cut for better exposure.
- Left parapharyngeal mass identified in the submandibular triangle posteriorly (Figure 20.8).
- Overlying fat and fascia dissected.
- Finger dissection all around the mass is done to break all its adhesions to the surrounding tissues.
- Mass delivered out through submandibular triangle.
- Haemostasis achieved, cavity packed with Surgicel and gelfoam.

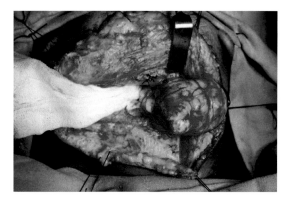

Figure 20.8 The tumour is dissected out from the parapharyngeal space.

- On intraoral examination, parapharyngeal bulge disappeared, uvula returned to midline.
- Vacuum suction drain No. 14 placed and secured.
- Neck incision closed in two layers.
- Dressing done.

CAROTID BODY TUMOUR

The insidious and progressive paraganglioma tumour is found in high-altitude residents. The location in the carotid artery bifurcation area and carotid pulsation in the swelling are diagnostic.

CLINICAL EXAMINATION

- Assess the dimension of the tumour.
- Complete auscultation for confirmation.
- Assess the higher cranial nerves, especially X and XII, which are commonly involved and also helpful for comparing the post-operative outcome.
- Ear examination should exclude jugular paraganglioma.
- FNAC or any other biopsy is contraindicated.

RADIOLOGICAL EVALUATION

- Doppler ultrasonography confirms the tumour and delineates the dimensions.
- Abdominal sonography is done to exclude other paragangliomas.
- CT angiography is the investigation of choice which will grade the tumour as per Shamblin's classification (Figure 20.9a-b).

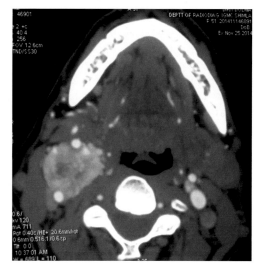

(a)

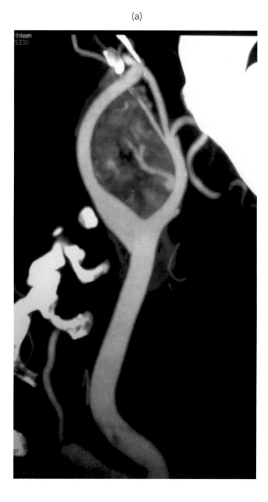

(b)

Figure 20.9 The CT angiography showing the carotid body tumour.

- MRI of the neck should be done in selected cases to assess the higher cranial nerves and soft tissue invasion.
- Balloon occlusion test in Shamblin grade II and III should be done to assess the flow in the circle of Willis as the carotid artery may require grafting.

PRE-OPERATIVE PREPARATION

- Counselling of the patient for carotid injury, risk of brain ischaemia, cranial nerve injury.
- Catecholamine assessment to exclude secretory paraganglioma.
- Arterial embolisation to reduce the vascularity.
- A good amount of cross-matched blood for replacement.
- Case discussion with vascular surgeon. Grade III definitely requires his/her intervention.

SURGICAL STEPS

- A transverse incision is made at the level of hyoid body in the skin crease.
- Subplatysmal flaps are raised up to mandible, saving marginal mandibular nerve and cricoid.
- Sternomastoid musculofascial plane is dissected out and sternomastoid muscle is dissected completely.
- The internal jugular vein is dissected free from the tumour, which usually has lymph node above it (Figure 20.10).
- Common facial vein is ligated and internal jugular vein retracted laterally to expose the tumour and carotid artery.
- Proximal and distal ends of common, external and internal carotid artery are dissected all around, allowing a vascular loop to be put around the vessels (Figure 20.11).
- Hypoglossal, vagus and superior nerves are identified and separated. Nerve electrodes are applied if nerve monitoring is being done.
- The tumour dissection starts from the caudal end in sub-adventitial plane with bipolar electrocautery at 10–20W.
- A non-embolised tumour bleeds profusely, and local compression and electrocautery help in such a scenario.
- Dissection is meticulous, taking care of any feeding vessel (usually the ascending pharyngeal artery).

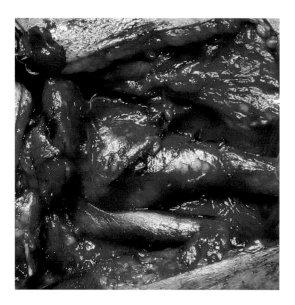

Figure 20.10 A lymph node is usually encountered over the carotid body tumour.

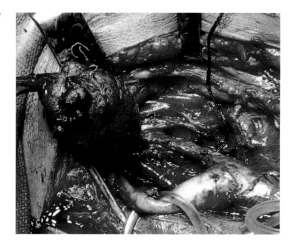

Figure 20.11. The tumour is dissected from the vessel. The internal carotid artery is gently retracted to avoid kinking which can lead to cerebral ischaemia.

- As dissection reaches carotid bulb, lignocaine is infiltrated in sub-adventitial plane to avoid bradycardia or cardiac arrest.
- Internal carotid artery is dissected completely. External carotid artery can be ligated and cut if its branches are engulfed by the tumour (Figure 20.12).
- Any carotid artery mural injury requires repair with propylene sutures or arterial grafting.
- Complete haemostasis is achieved. Nerve functions are confirmed through nerve monitoring.

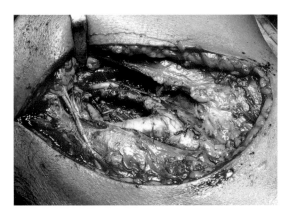

Figure 20.12 Surgical site after excision of the carotid body tumour.

- The wound is irrigated, a glove drain or small-calibre negative drain is placed and the incision is closed in layers.

POST-OPERATIVE CARE

- Antibiotics and NSAIDs are prescribed as per the protocol.
- Higher cranial nerves are observed for any paresis and steroids are started without any delay.
- Drain is removed on second or third day depending upon drain volume.

SURGICAL COMPLICATIONS

- **Carotid injury:** Surgeon should not attempt carotid body tumour excision if he/she is not well trained or the centre lacks vascular graft and repair facility. Meticulous planning and surgery helps in avoiding carotid injury. Any minor injury can be managed by primary repair, while a large defect or type III tumour requires grafting and vascular surgeon presence.
- **Neural injury:** Neural injury occurs when unnecessary traction is applied on nerves (vagus, hypoglossal or superior laryngeal nerve). Nerve dissection with electrocautery in high power also puts the nerve at risk. A nerve monitor helps to confirm the nerve integrity at the end of procedure while steroids and physiotherapy take care of any post-operative nerve paresis.
- **Seroma/haematoma:** Collection of blood or plasma leads to swelling in the operative site. Meticulous use of electrocautery and complete haemostasis at the end of the procedure avoids such complication.
- **Post-operative fibrosis:** This is quite a common problem faced by the patients. The operative site shows firm to hard swelling which takes weeks to settle down. Clinical examination should be performed to rule out any haematoma, which can be confirmed by high-frequency sonography.

21

Temporal Bone Cancer

KULDEEP THAKUR

INTRODUCTION

Carcinoma of the temporal bone is an extremely rare entity, with an annual incidence of less than one per 1 million and comprising only 0.2% of all head and neck cancers. Squamous cell carcinoma (SCC) can affect any part of the temporal bone: external auditory canal (EAC), middle ear or mastoid, or secondarily, from extra-temporal sites. The common extra-temporal sites that infiltrate the temporal bones include skin around the pinna, auricular skin, skull base and parotid gland (Figure 21.1a-d). Skin around the pinna and parotid gland malignancies infiltrate temporal bone more commonly than do the temporal gland malignancies.

Its anatomical location makes the extent of resection very problematic, because minimal surgical interventions threaten the oncological safety, whereas aggressive surgical excision with wide margins is associated with a high rate of complications.

The site of the tumour origin has important prognostic implications, e.g., primary tumours of the EAC have higher overall survival and disease-free survival rates as compared to periauricular, auricular and parotid primary tumours affecting temporal bone.

Most common age at diagnosis of SCC of the temporal bone is 60–69 years, and 60% of the patients are men.

ETIOLOGY

Unlike other SCC of the head and neck, temporal bone carcinoma does not appear to be strongly associated with tobacco and alcohol consumption. Established risk factors for temporal bone SCC within the epithelium of the temporal bones are chronic suppurative otitis media (CSOM) and previous radiotherapy. In CSOM, the chronic inflammatory process may lead to metaplastic and neoplastic changes. Up to 68% of patients in one series have been treated for CSOM prior to the development of temporal bone tumour. In a few studies, human papillomaviruses 16 and 18 were isolated in tissue and molecular levels in temporal bone carcinoma associated with CSOM. For radiation-induced temporal bone tumours, Lusting's criteria must be fulfilled, which are as follows:

- The second tumour must develop in the irradiated field.
- A latent period of several years must elapse between the radiation exposure and the development of a second tumour.
- The second tumour must be of a different histological type from that of the previously irradiated tumour.
- The previous tumour must show histological, radiological and microscopic evidence of neoplasm.

The latency period for radiation-induced malignancy ranges from 5 to 30 years. Radiation-induced tumours are very rare and tend to be aggressive and metastasise early. Common pathological types of radiation-induced malignancies include SCC, fibrosarcoma and osteosarcoma. The reported five-year survival

DOI: 10.1201/9780367430139-21

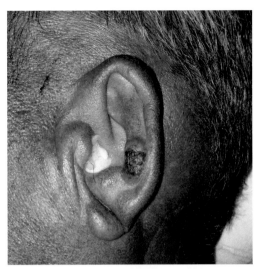
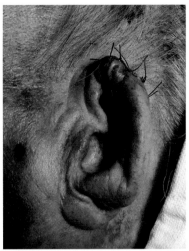
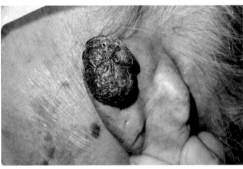
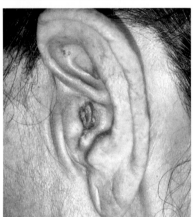

Figure 21.1a-d Tumour of pinna and external auditory canal.

rate in radiation-induced malignancies varies from 11 to 32%.

Exposure to ultra-violet light may be a risk factor for SCC of EAC, lateral concha and pinna. Ultraviolet-induced tumours are more likely in Caucasians, who are more prone to non-melanomatous skin malignancies in sun exposed areas. No strong evidence exists between occupational exposure to radiation or chlorinated disinfectant and temporal bone SCC.

PATHOLOGY

SCC constitutes 80% of all EAC tumours, whereas basal cell carcinoma and adenoid cystic carcinoma constitutes other less common entities involving temporal bone. Paraganglioma also constitutes a significant proportion of temporal bone tumours. Other rare entities include aggressive papillary middle ear tumour, haemangiopericytoma, chordoma, osteosarcoma and secondary tumours of the temporal bone (local spread of the tumour from an adjacent site such as the parotid gland, distant metastasis or manifestation of a haematological malignancy). The common temporal bone tumours in the paediatric age group include rhabdomyosarcoma and Langerhans cell histiocytosis. In this chapter temporal bone carcinomas will be discussed in detail.

WHO (2017) classify tumours of the ear into the following:

- Tumours of the external auditory canal
  - Squamous cell carcinoma
  - Adenocarcinoma

- Ceruminous adenocarcinoma
- Adenoid cystic carcinoma
- Mucoepidermoid carcinoma
- Ceruminous adenoma

- Tumours of the middle and inner ear
  - Squamous cell carcinoma
  - Aggressive papillary tumour
  - Endolymphatic sac tumour
  - Vestibular schwannoma
  - Meningioma
  - Middle ear adenoma

ORIGIN AND SPREAD OF TUMOURS

Tumours of the temporal bone can arise from any part of the temporal bone, including the external auditory canal, middle ear cleft, petrous apex and endolymphatic sac (Figure 21.1). The foramen of Huschke, the fissure of Santorini, petro-squamous suture line, stylomastoid foramen, the round window and oval window all provide a pathway for tumour spread. The temporal bone itself acts as a medium for microscopic diffusion of tumour cells through bony canals and intraosseous vessels. Apart from that, bones covering the jugular bulb, carotid vessels, tegmen tympani and antri, Fallopian canal and the bony labyrinth are thin and weak barriers for tumour spread. Tumours of the EAC extend anteriorly into the parotid gland and temporomandibular joint whereas tumours of the middle ear spread anteriorly to involve the Eustachian tube. Superior extension of the tumour can involve the middle cranial fossa while the otic capsule and labyrinth become involved in the medial extension of the tumour. Less frequently, the tumour may spread posteriorly to involve posterior cranial fossa. Tumour extension to petrous apex can involve or encase the internal carotid artery, but this is less likely due to the resistant bone of the otic capsule.

CLINICAL PRESENTATION

Patients usually present with symptoms of otitis externa or CSOM (otalgia, otorrhoea, hearing loss and vertigo), therefore early diagnosis is difficult and is often delayed until a relatively late stage, when other, more alarming features have developed, such as external swelling, facial palsy or bleeding. Pain associated with temporal bone malignancies is generally more severe than that experienced with other benign conditions. Invasion of the blood vessels gives rise to bloody otorrhoea. Other features of temporal bone malignancies may include the following:

- Trismus
- Progressive facial weakness
- Lower cranial nerve palsy (IX, X, XI and XII)
- Cervical metastasis

Cervical lymph node metastases are an infrequent finding in the early stage, but may occur in 10–20% of cases in locally advanced disease.

EXAMINATION

An exophytic or ulcerative lesion in EAC is likely malignant and needs urgent biopsy (Figure 21.1a-d). Meticulous facial nerve assessment, along with complete head and neck examination, is performed on particularly enlarged lymph nodes involving the parotid region, level II, level III and level IVa.

STAGING OF TEMPORAL BONE TUMOURS

Staging of the temporal bone malignancy is important for planning treatment and explaining prognosis and outcome of the treatment. The most useful staging system for temporal bone malignancies is modified Pittsburgh classification, but a standardised staging system has not yet been accepted universally.

MANAGEMENT

Pre-Operative Management

Management of the temporal bone carcinoma is controversial because of the paucity of the disease, very few large-scale studies and meta-analysis, and lack of randomised trials. Management therefore depends largely upon institutional practice.

A trans-canal biopsy is required to characterise the type of the lesion. Temporal bone malignancies rarely involve labyrinth; however, an audiogram is mandatory before commencing any major surgery.

Imaging is important in temporal bone malignancies as many patients have limited findings on

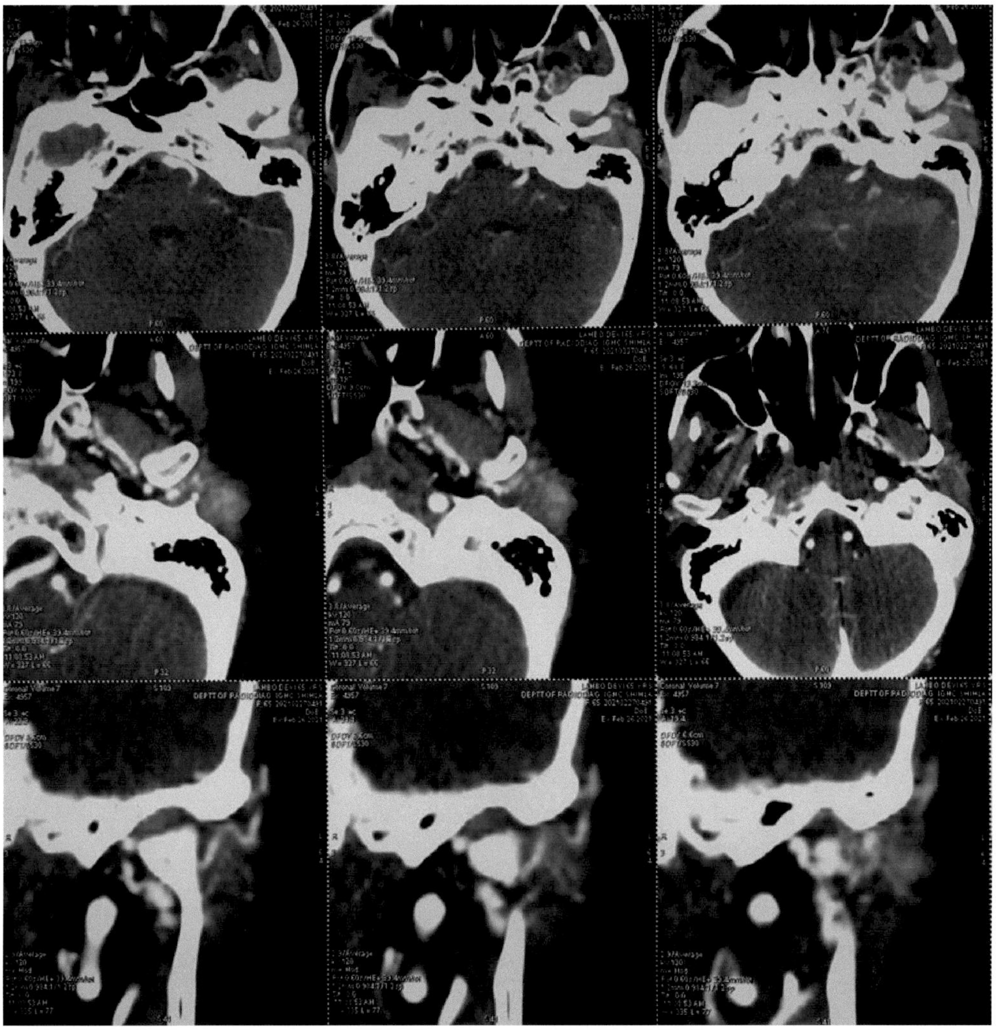

Figure 21.2 Contrast-enhanced computed tomography showing heterogeneously enhancing mass involving left external auditory canal with extent to the temporomandibular joint with normal middle ear and mastoid air cell system.

physical examination. High resolution computed tomography (CT) is the most accurate method for subtle bone erosion; however, it is unable to distinguish between tumour and fluid in the middle ear cleft (Figure 21.2). Magnetic resonance imaging (MRI) provides excellent differentiation between soft tissue tumour margins, muscle and soft tissue infiltration, and can also differentiate between tumour and obstructive inflammatory changes. Intracranial and infratemporal spread of the tumour is also better detected on MRI. If CT or MR raises the possibility of internal carotid artery (ICA) involvement, angiography with balloon occlusion should be considered. Similarly, the venous phase is also important if sacrifice of sigmoid sinus or internal jugular vein is anticipated.

SURGICAL TECHNIQUES FOR TEMPORAL BONE MALIGNANCIES

Surgery is the treatment modality of choice for temporal bone malignancies. Radiotherapy is used as an adjuvant therapy except in very advanced tumours requiring palliation.

General anaesthesia is achieved with orotracheal intubation, inhalational agent and intravenous narcotics. Neuromuscular blockades are usually avoided to permit monitoring of motor nerve activities; however, short-acting agents such as succinylcholine can be used at the start of the procedure for safe induction and intubation. During surgery, apart from the surgical site, other regions, including abdomen for fat; neck or leg for nerve grafts; and chest, abdomen or back for locoregional or free flaps, are prepared. A third-generation cephalosporin with cerebrospinal fluid penetration is administered peri-operatively.

- **Lateral temporal bone resection:**
  This is surgery of choice in T1 and T2 tumours of EAC and often combined with superficial parotidectomy, especially for T2 tumours. EAC is the anatomical unit removed in lateral temporal bone resection. The boundaries of resection include the mastoid cavity posteriorly, the infratemporal fossa inferiorly, the temporomandibular joint capsule anteriorly, the zygomatic root superiorly, the middle ear cavity medially and the concha and/or a portion of the pinna laterally.
  The lateral margins of the resection depend upon the site of the primary tumour. Lateral margins of the tumour limited to EAC include only the conchal bowl.

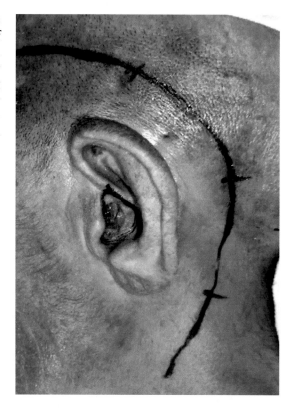

Figure 21.3 Post-aural and end-aural incisions marked.

Steps:

1. A circumferential incision is marked and incised around the conchal bowl for the tumours arising from EAC, leaving the tragus intact (Figure 21.3). If the subcutaneous tissue of the concha and tragus is involved, then more of the central portion of the pinna is removed with surgical specimen. The entire pinna can be removed if a significant portion of the pinna is affected by the tumour.
2. Post-auricular incision is marked 3 cm behind the post-auricular sulcus and extended superiorly to the temporal fossa. Inferiorly, incision is usually extended to the mastoid process; however, it can be brought more inferiorly if neck dissection is anticipated.
3. The skin flap is dissected in subperiosteal layer the posterior extent of the conchal incision is reached and a circumferential conchal incision is connected to the post-auricular incision. Care must be taken to avoid inadvertent entry into the EAC.
4. The lateral edge of the EAC is now sutured

in order to avoid tumour cell spillage and the external auditory canal is closed with a cul-de-sac suture on the residual skin of the conchal bowl.
5. The skin flap is further elevated, staying superficial to the sternocleidomastoid muscle inferiorly, parotid capsule to the posterior border of masseter muscle anteriorly and deep temporalis fascia superiorly. This manoeuvre will expose the entire parotid gland, temporomandibular joint (TM joint), EAC, and mastoid bone.
6. Complete mastoidectomy is performed and care must be taken to avoid entry into bony EAC.
7. Bone of the zygomatic root is drilled to expose tegmen tympani and epitympanum to the capsule of the TM joint. Drilling is directed antero-inferiorly towards glenoid fossa and drilling in anterior direction could breach dura of the middle fossa.
8. Now the vertical part of the facial nerve is identified from the second genu to the stylomastoid foramen and facial recess is opened

using small cutting burr, followed by a large diamond burr. Facial recess is extended inferiorly by sacrificing chorda tympani to expose the hypotympanum.

9. At this stage, the middle ear is inspected, incudostapedial joint is disarticulated and incus is removed.

10. Drilling is continued along with tympanic ring towards the anterior wall of the external auditory canal. Drilling is continued to the anterior limit of the dissection, i.e., periosteum between the temporal bone, the infratemporal fossa and the capsule of the TM joint, and care must be taken not to injure the internal carotid artery, which lies medial to the Eustachian tube. At this point, EAC is attached anteriorly by a small section of bone just lateral to the Eustachian tube and osteotomy can be performed with the help of gentle taps on the osteotome inserted through the extended facial recess.

11. Superficial parotidectomy, if required, is performed at this stage and EAC with superficial parotidectomy specimen is removed in continuity with the branches of the facial nerve under direct vision (Figure 21.4).

12. The posterior half of the temporalis muscle can be rotated into the surgical defect if the operative resection results in a large and deep defect.

13. Drains are placed superiorly and inferiorly in order to avoid trauma to the facial nerve and skin flap is returned to its original position.

14. Compression dressings are applied.

- **Subtotal Temporal Bone Resection:**
  This is indicated in T3 and T4 tumours that have invaded middle ear and mastoid cavities and is an extension of the lateral temporal bone resection. The medial extent of resection involves the otic capsule. This procedure is usually combined with either superficial or total parotidectomy and elective neck dissection. After lateral temporal resection, bone is removed over the sigmoid sinus and the dura. The strategy is to perform extradural and subperiosteal dissection, thereby exposing ICA anteriorly, middle fossa dura superiorly, sigmoid sinus and posterior fossa dura posteriorly, jugular bulb inferiorly and petrous apex medially. Care must be taken to drill adequate bone all around the tumour. The facial nerve is skeletonised from

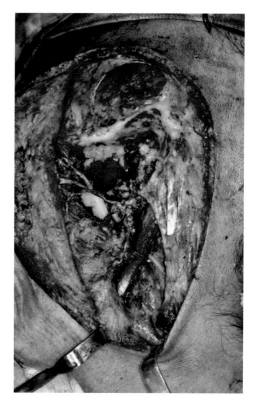

Figure 21.4 Operative field after en bloc resection of the tumour including EAC, superficial parotidectomy and basal resection of deep lobe of parotid with temporomandibular joint excision.

labyrinthine segment to stylomastoid foramen. Dura of the internal auditory canal can be opened for further mobilisation of the facial nerve. Bone dissection is continued to the vertical portion of the ICA medially and capsule of the TM joint anteriorly. The capsule of the TM joint and condyle of the mandible are resected when found to be involved (Figure 21.5). The middle and posterior fossa craniotomy might be necessary if dural involvement is suspected. If the cancer is infiltrating the jugular bulb, total removal of the tumour is achieved by resecting sigmoid sinus and jugular bulb, but if there is any doubt regarding clearance of the disease around the jugular bulb or lower cranial nerves, it is advisable to leave a vascular clip in situ for the site to be identified during adjuvant radiotherapy.

- **Total Temporal Bone Resection/Radical Temporal Bone Resection:**

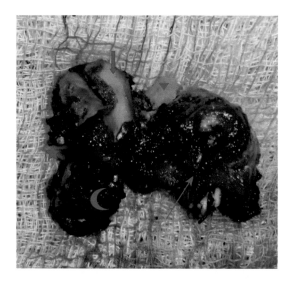

Figure 21.5 En bloc resection of the lateral temporal bone resection, with resection of the condyle. Arrow head: zygomatic arch. Star: condyle of mandible. Moon: masseter muscle. Thin arrow: sutured lateral end of the external auditory canal. Thick arrow: articular disc of the temporomandibular joint.

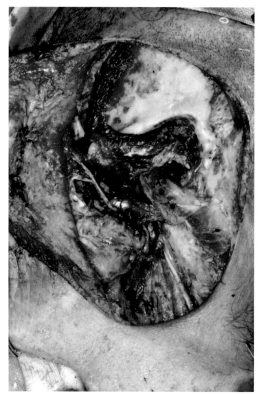

Figure 21.6 Obliteration of the cavity by using posterior half of temporalis muscle, posterior belly of the digastric and part of the sternocleidomastoid muscle.

This procedure is used in advanced T4 tumours when cancer extends to the petrous apex. After completion of the subtotal temporal bone resection, proximal (skull base of neck) and distal (floor of the middle cranial fossa via middle fossa craniotomy) control of the ICA is obtained. ICA is dissected free from its canal to the foramen ovale after removing the bone lateral to the ICA genu. After adequate exposure, the remainder of otic capsule and complete petrous bone until the apex is removed. The Eustachian tube is resected anteriorly to the level of the foramen ovale and the transected end of the tube is sutured to prevent CSF rhinorrhea.

RECONSTRUCTION

The goals of reconstruction include prevention of CSF leak, promotion of healing and alleviation of the cosmetic deformity, and these can be effectively achieved with a vascularised flap. The advantage of using vascularised flap is that it promotes adequate healing as most patients undergo adjuvant radiation therapy. The most commonly used vascularised flaps include locoregional (posterior portion of the temporalis muscles [Figure 21.6], pectoralis major muscle, sternocleidomastoid muscle) and free flaps (rectus abdominis, anterolateral thigh flap scapular or latissimus dorsi free flap). The facial nerve, if resected, can be reconstructed by using the greater auricular nerve. If the proximal end of the facial nerve is not available for anastomosis, hypoglossal-to-facial anastomosis is an alternate method of reconstruction.

POST-OPERATIVE CARE

The head end of the bed should be elevated 30 degrees and ambulation must be done as tolerated. The mastoid dressing is removed on the first post-operative day. The level of care is similar to that of trans-labyrinthine acoustic tumour surgery in cases of large dural defect created or significant brain retraction during surgery. All patients are monitored for CSF leak or signs of meningitis. Mouth opening exercises are initiated as soon as possible if mandibular condyle is resected so as to prevent fibrous ankylosis and maintain proper occlusal relationship. Patients with facial nerve paresis require proper eye care in the form of eye drops in daytime and ointments at night. A gold weight implant or temporary tarsorrhaphy can be done if recovery from facial nerve dysfunction is expected to take longer than 4–6 weeks.

COMPLICATIONS

- **Vascular complication:** Pre-operative evaluation in the form of CT and MRI and by angiography or balloon test occlusion should be performed if surgical intervention is required near the ICA. Intraoperatively, proximal control in neck and distal control in the horizontal portion of the ICA should be obtained before the manipulation of the ICA. The vein of Labbe is an important channel of venous outflow from the temporal lobe and its damage can lead to temporal lobe infarction or seizures. While ligating the sigmoid sinus, it is important to stay anterior to the insertion of the vein of Labbe into the transverse sinus.
- **CSF leak:** It occurs as a result of the inadequate closure of the dura. Usual sites are Eustachian tube, remnants of the EAC or incision site. All dural closures must be watertight and any dead space should be obliterated with vascularised tissue. Post-operatively, patient's head end is elevated 30 degrees and patient is instructed to avoid straining or performing the Valsalva manoeuvre.
- **Infection:** Brain infection occurs infrequently. More-feared complications are meningitis or brain abscess. All patients are closely monitored for symptoms of meningitis and diagnosis is made on lumbar puncture. Aspiration pneumonia is another fatal complication if lower cranial nerves are sacrificed during surgery.
- **Intracranial haemorrhage and hypertension:** These complications are seen when temporal bone resection involves intradural manipulation. The symptoms include altered sensorium or loss of consciousness, and signs include fixed and dilated pupils, bradycardia and hypertension. If intracranial hypertension is suspected, computed tomography is performed to confirm the diagnosis and the condition is managed accordingly.

EN BLOC VERSUS PIECEMEAL RESECTION IN SUBTOTAL OR TOTAL TEMPORAL BONE RESECTION

En bloc resection in temporal bone tumours involves more danger to the surrounding intracranial structures and cranial nerves. The alternative is to do piecemeal resection, which involves drilling around the tumour till healthy bone appears after gross tumour resection, and this modality is preferred in T3 and T4 temporal bone tumours. The advantage of piecemeal resection includes better exposure under microscope with fewer hazards to the cranial nerves. This technique does not compromise tumour clearance if adequate bone is removed around the lesion.

ROLE OF PAROTID SURGERY

Temporal bone cancers are very rare, hence little information is available regarding the management of parotid glands in surgically treated temporal bone carcinoma. In squamous cell carcinoma of the temporal bone, elective parotidectomy can be avoided in early stage lesions without radiological involvement of the parotid gland, whereas a total parotidectomy is advised in advanced temporal bone cancers. Some surgeons perform routine superficial parotidectomy for T1 and T2 cancer, especially tumours eroding the anterior wall of external auditory canal, but perform total parotidectomy for T3 and T4 cancers. The parotidectomy is typically performed in a retrograde fashion so as to maintain the continuity between the parotid gland and anterior wall of the EAC. In adenoid cystic carcinoma of the temporal bone, basal resection can be performed, rather than a superficial or total parotidectomy.

Site of the tumour in external auditory canal is an important factor regarding parotid gland management. Tumours originating on the anterior wall or floor of the EAC often invade parotid glands through the foramen of Huschke or the fissure of Santorini. Further, intra-parotid lymph nodes are first-echelon lymph nodes for tumours of EAC, therefore either the parotid gland or the parotid node could be involved in EAC carcinoma.

ROLE OF NECK DISSECTION

Lymph node metastasis is relatively rare (10–36%), though supra-omohyoid neck dissection is performed in most cases. An intraoperative frozen section of the level II lymph node can be performed, and one should proceed with neck dissection only when the frozen section shows evidence of lymph node metastasis. For N+ cases, comprehensive neck dissection is performed.

ROLE OF ADJUVANT THERAPY

Radiotherapy as single modality has not been very successful in any stage of temporal bone cancer.

It is generally believed that combined therapy (surgery followed by adjuvant therapy) provides the best chance to improve survival. Adjuvant therapy is indicated in T3 and T4 tumours and also in early stage tumours with evidence of bone erosion, positive margins and perineural invasion.

CONCLUSION

In view of the rarity of the disease, there is still a need to comprehensively study the temporal bone cancers and to standardise treatment protocols. Radical en bloc resection is the mainstay of treatment and adjuvant therapy is indicated in T2, T3 and T4 tumours and incompletely treated T1 tumours.

22

Reconstruction in Head and Neck Tumours

JITEN KUMAR MISHRA, SHAMENDRA ANAND SAHU AND MOUMITA DE

INTRODUCTION

Head and neck reconstruction is an important domain of reconstructive surgery. Reconstruction in post-onco-resection defects of head and neck region has a definitive role for functional rehabilitation in terms of chewing, speech, deglutition and retention of food inside the mouth. Reconstruction also addresses facial aesthetics and augments wound healing. Head and neck surgeons should be well aware of the vascular anatomy, indications of conventional flaps and choice of flaps for different defects. This chapter covers the basics of some conventional loco-regional flaps and free flaps that are commonly used for head and neck reconstruction.

DELTOPECTORAL FLAP

Deltopectoral (DP) flap remains the workhorse flap for reconstruction of the head and neck region. The DP flap, described by Bakamjian, was first used for oesophageal reconstruction in 1965.

Anatomy

It is known as the deltopectoral flap as it includes the skin over the pectoral region and the deltoid region. Skin over the pectoral part of the flap is the anatomical territory of the intercostal perforators, whereas the skin over the deltoid region is the dynamic territory supplied by the cutaneous perforators of the thoraco-acromial system

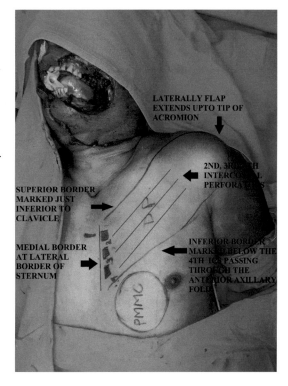

Figure 22.1 Marking of DP flap.

(Figure 22.1). Deltopectoral flap is harvested in single procedure, whereas flap extending beyond acromion requires two stages (delayed) due to the risk of distal end necrosis.

DOI: 10.1201/9780367430139-22

Vascular Anatomy

Conventionally the flap is based on the second, third and fourth intercostal perforators of the internal mammary artery. Although the flap can be raised on the second and third intercostal perforators only, the authors are of the opinion that all three perforators should be included in the flap, as this increases the perfusion pressure of the flap and improves the survivability of the distal end of the flap. The distal end of the flap can be narrowed as per the requirement of the defect.

The internal mammary artery (IMA) is a branch of the subclavian artery and it runs inside the rib cage about 1 cm lateral to the sternum. The 5–6 intercostal perforating branches arise from the IMA in the corresponding intercostal spaces. These perforating branches emerge about 10 mm lateral to the sternum, pierce the fascia of the pectoralis muscle and run superficial to the fascia of the pectoralis muscle and deltoid.

INDICATIONS

1. To cover the defect following tumour excision over middle and lower thirds of the face, oral cavity, neck and oesophagus.
2. To cover soft tissue defects of face and neck following trauma (vehicular accidents, ballistic or gunshot injury etc.).

PRE-OPERATIVE PREPARATION

Preparation of the whole chest on the side of the defect is essential to maintain hygiene and for easy post-operative dressings.

Position

Patient is positioned supine with slight neck extension and arm abducted by the side.

Anaesthesia Concerns

Patients are generally under nasal intubation as cases of post-carcinoma excision defect. After intubation, oropharyngeal passage is packed with ribbon gauze as there might be trickling of the blood into the throat while insetting.

Flap Markings

-   Medially, the lateral border of sternum is marked (Figure 22.1). Course of second, third and fourth intercostal perforators are marked in corresponding intercostal spaces 1 cm lateral to the sternum up to DP groove.
-   Superior border of the flap is just below the clavicle, starting 1 cm lateral to the sternum.
-   Inferior border parallels just below the fourth ICS, laterally crossing just anterior to the anterior border axilla into deltoid region.
-   Lateral boundary is up to the acromion over the deltoid region.

FLAP HARVEST

Incision is made at the lateral marking through skin, subcutaneous fat and deltoid fascia up to the deltoid muscle. Holding sutures are applied from the skin edges to the fascia, and cutting the sutures long helps in holding the flap while elevating the flap.

Flap elevation proceeds from lateral to medial side. Sharp dissection is done using scalpel to elevate the deltoid fascia completely, baring the deltoid muscle to the deltopectoral grove.

At the deltopectoral groove, as the deltoid fascia ends and pectoralis fascia starts, there is tethering, which should be carefully dissected out to preserve the cephalic vein lying in the deltopectoral groove.

Again continuing medially, sharp dissection is done using scalpel to elevate the pectoralis fascia, with the flap baring the pectoralis muscle completely.

Thoraco-acromial artery branches to pectoralis major at the lateral extent of flap are ligated/cauterised and divided.

Medial elevation of the flap is stopped about 2 cm lateral to the sternum to prevent injury to the perforators (Figure 22.2). The flap is generally interpolated over the supraclavicular skin for insetting (Figure 22.3). The donor area of the flap is split skin grafted (Figure 22.4).

GENERAL CONSIDERATIONS

-   For composite defect of oral cavity, the flap can be folded upon itself to form the mucosal lining and cover.

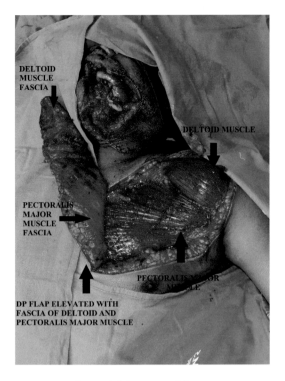

Figure 22.2 Elevated deltopectoral flap.

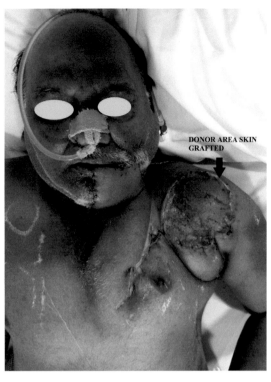

Figure.22.4 DP flap inset to cover composite lower lip defect.

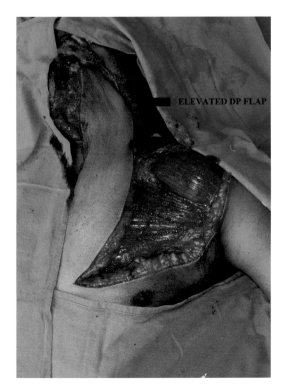

Figure 22.3 Elevated and interpolated DP flap.

- After transfer of the flap, the bridge segment can be tubed or it can be left open. On the second or third post-operative day, there is oedema and a chance of kinking when tubed, so tubing should be avoided. The bridge segment if left open requires daily dressing because there is secretion from the raw area beneath.
- The inferior margin of the flap is longer than the superior margin, so the pivot point lies at the medial point of upper margin.
- The actual length of the flap required is measured from the top of defect to the pivot point and the required length of flap is elevated. Practically, the flap is elevated in full length till the deltoid region. When flap is elevated in full length, flap elevation stops medially when adequate length is achieved.

DELAY

Delay is the surgical procedure done to increase the survivability of the distal end of the flap. The portion of the deltopectoral flap over the deltoid can be raised as a one-stage procedure. As per author's experience, the delay of the flap is required in the following circumstances:

- Extension of flap on the arm beyond the deltoid region.
- Portion of the flap beyond the deltopectoral groove over deltoid is delayed especially if the patient is a chronic smoker, obese or elderly, in which case the perfusion pressure of the intercostal perforators may be less.

Delay of the flap can be done in the following ways.

1. The deltoid portion of the flap can be elevated completely, dividing all the deltoid musculocutaneous perforators and cutaneous branches of the thoraco-acromial artery. The elevated flap is positioned back and loose tacking sutures are applied.
2. Margins all around the flap are incised and loosely sutured. Some surgeons also cut the cutaneous branches of the thoraco-acomial vessels in the infraclavicular fossa by limited under-mining (Figure 22.5). The delayed flap can then be safely transferred to the defect site after 7–10 days.

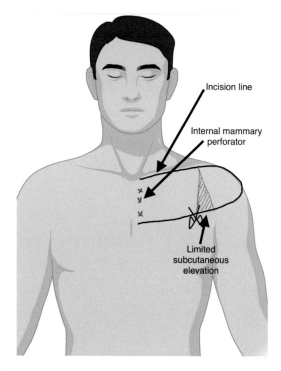

Figure.22.5 Delay of DP flap by making incision at the margins of the flap.

COMBINED DP AND PECTORALIS MAJOR MYO-CUTANEOUS FLAP

When both DP and pectoralis major myo-cutaneous (PMMC) flap are planned simultaneously, PMMC is used for lining and DP for skin cover. Often only PMMC is required for mucosal lining. Moreover, the vascularity of DP flap can be saved for future use. Therefore, while elevating the PMMC flap, the vascularity of DP flap needs to be safe-guarded. The following methods can be adopted to save the vascular territory of DP flap.

1. Completely elevate the DP flap and then elevate the PMMC flap (Figure 22.6). Afterwards, the DP flap can be sutured back if it is not to be used in the same setting. If required simultaneously, the DP flap is inset after the PMMC flap.
2. Fascia deep cut is made in the superior and inferior margins of the DP flap, and the flap is elevated off the pectoralis major muscle,

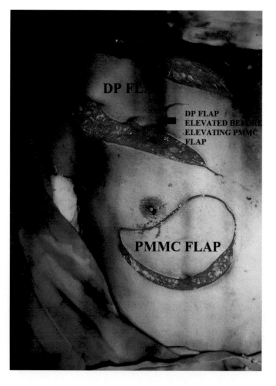

Figure.22.6 Simultaneous DP and PMMC flap elevation.

retaining its medial and lateral attachments. After that, the pectoralis major flap is elevated from beneath the DP flap.

Post-Operative Care

Post-operatively, minimal care is required. Pedicle is covered with paraffin gauze with antibiotic ointment to prevent it from desiccation. The rest of the flap and suture line are covered with paraffin gauze with a small surgical soft pad. The donor area is skin grafted and bolster/tie-over dressing is applied. This dressing is usually removed after 5–7 days and graft uptake is assessed. The donor area can be left open after 2–3 dressings if graft uptake is satisfactory.

Division and Inset of Flap

Division and inset of flap is planned after 14 days. The flap is divided and inset over the recipient area. The stump of the remaining flap can be reposited back to the donor area or the donor area can be split skin grafted (Figure 22.7).

Complications and Management

Flap failure is usually not a complication unless the pedicle is damaged or inadvertently not included in the flap. Epidermolysis, infection and suture dehiscence are minor complications. Facial disfigurement at the recipient site and scar from split skin grafting may sometimes be annoying to the patient.

PECTORALIS MAJOR FLAP

Introduction

Before the advent of microsurgery, the pectoralis major flap was the workhorse flap in head and neck reconstruction, especially in post-cancer extirpation surgery with intraoral defects. This robust flap has stood the test of time and in the present era of microsurgery, it is still a major flap in the armamentarium of the head and neck reconstructive surgeon. Its use in head and neck reconstruction was first described by Ariyan in 1979. Since then, many other surgeons have reiterated that, owing to its consistent anatomy and robust vascular supply, it remains a very reliable flap. In remote centres with limited scope for microsurgery, it is used as

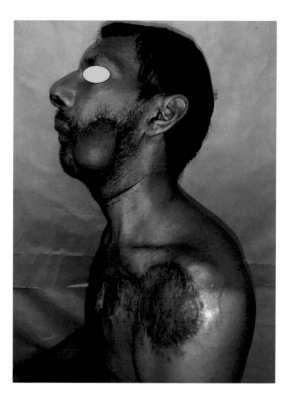

Figure.22.7 Post-operative image after inset of DP flap.

a primary flap for reconstruction. Even in microsurgical centres, it is often used as a salvage flap in cases of non-feasibility or loss of a free flap.

Indications and Advantages

Pectoralis major myocutaneous or costomyocutaneous or osteomyocutaneous flap are generally used for reconstruction of soft tissue defects in the head and neck region following cancer extirpation surgery such as intraoral buccal mucosal defect and defects in the laryngopharynx or upper oesophagus. It can also be used for coverage of chest wall defects.

For head and neck defects, the flap can reach to resurface defects up to the zygomatic arch as a pedicled flap. However, owing to its relatively short pedicle, it is not preferred for microvascular free tissue transfer.

The advantages of this flap are as follows:

- Relatively constant anatomy of the vascular pedicle. Also, the vascular pedicle is readily visible on the undersurface of the elevated muscle covered by the fascia, hence dissection is easy and safe.

- It provides good muscle bulk which can effectively cover important neck structures and also fill up soft tissue defects in the neck following cancer extirpation.
- Overlying skin paddle is well vascularised by multiple musculocutaneous perforators and survives well after transfer.
- No change in patient position is necessary as this flap is harvested in supine position.
- This flap remains well vascularised in patients who have received radiation therapy as the territory of the flap lies outside the usual irradiation territory for head and neck malignancy. Hence, even in irradiated and vessel-depleted areas, it provides healthy vascularised tissue.
- Pectoralis major is an adductor and internal rotator of the shoulder, hence its harvest causes some functional deficit. However, it is very minimal and patients usually tolerate this deficit quite well.
- It can be harvested along with costal cartilage as costomyocutaneous, or along with part of anterior cortex of sternum or part of ribs as osteomyocutaneous flap.
- It can be used as a salvage flap in case of failure of a previous free tissue transfer.

Contraindications and Disadvantages

Absolute contraindication to performing this flap is a patient with Poland syndrome with absence of muscle on the side of requirement. Also, in patients with prior chest wall trauma or chest wall surgery where the vascular pedicle to the muscle was violated, this flap should not be done.

Although it is one of the most reliable flaps available, there are some disadvantages owing to the nature of the tissue components.

- As it is a myocutaneous flap, it tends to be bulky. Especially in patients with substantial subcutaneous fat and in female patients in whom the breast fat comes into the flap, it becomes very bulky. For resurfacing small defects with less tissue requirement, the bulkiness of the flap becomes a problem.
- In female patients, harvesting pectoralis major myocutaneous flap distorts the shape and nipple areola position of the breast.

- As pectoralis major muscle forms the anterior axillary fold, harvesting this flap distorts the anterior axillary fold.

Anatomy of the Flap

The flap is composed of the pectoralis major muscle and the skin of the anterior chest wall overlying the muscle. This is a flat, fan-shaped muscle originating from the clavicle, sternum, costal cartilage of second to sixth ribs and the aponeurosis of the external oblique, and it inserts into the crest of the greater tubercle of humerus. The muscle and its overlying skin are supplied by mainly the pectoral branch of the thoraco-acromial artery. The axis of the pedicle lies grossly along a line joining the midpoint of the clavicle to a perpendicular dropped to the line joining the acromian process with the xiphisternum. The artery runs along the undersurface of the muscle about 2–3 cm medial to the lateral edge of the muscle, plastered to the muscle by its fascia (Figure 22.8).

The overlying skin paddle of the flap can be planned supero-medial or infero-lateral to the

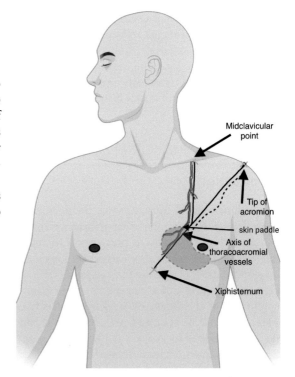

Figure.22.8 Vascular axis and flap marking of pectoralis major myocutaneous flap.

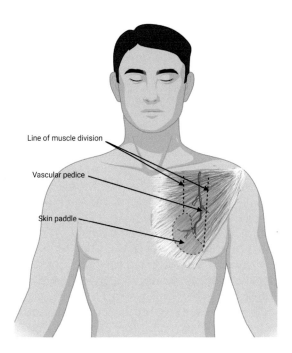

Figure.22.9 Skin paddle and muscle division marking.

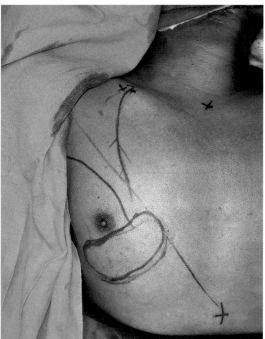

Figure.22.10 Marking of pectoralis major myocutaneous flap.

nipple areola complex (Figure 22.9). In the latter scenario, the flap reach is increased, but owing to paucity of musculocutaneous perforators, it is advisable to take part of the fascia covering the external oblique along with the flap.

The muscle also gets supply from lateral thoracic artery from the lateral side of the muscle and this may need to be sacrificed during flap elevation. The flap is usually tunnelled under the neck skin and delivered into the oral defect. Care must be taken to ensure that this tunnel is large enough to accommodate the bulk of the flap.

Pre-Operative Investigations

Clinical examination is done to rule out Poland syndrome or any previous chest trauma or surgery. History should be taken regarding presence of any cardiopulmonary disease or restrictive lung disease. As the flap donor site is mostly closed primarily, it can cause some restriction in chest movement which may rarely cause problems in such patients.

Pre-Operative Preparation

Overlying chest hair should be clipped. Flap marking should be done such that the skin paddle

reaches the defect without any tension. While flap marking, care should be given not to violate the territory of the deltopectoral flap as this flap may need to be used in future.

Operative Steps

- After prepping, draping and marking of the flap (Figure 22.10), first the incision is made laterally and lateral skin raised to identify the lateral border of pectoralis major. The lateral border of the muscle is delineated and dissected off the chest wall, dissecting between pectoralis major and pectoralis minor.
- Skin incision is made along the marking for skin paddle up to the fascia over the muscle. The fascia should be tagged to the muscle using sutures to avoid shearing between the muscle and overlying skin paddle. The incision is made along the anterior axillary fold in order to preserve the skin territory of the deltopectoral flap (a DP-sparing incision).
- The skin and subcutaneous tissue of the upper chest above the superior border of the flap paddle is elevated to expose the entire flat muscle.

- Care should be taken to not dissect more medially in the upper chest, especially in the second and third intercostal spaces, to preserve the internal mammary perforators that supply the deltopectoral flap.
- This skin flap elevation is continued over the muscle and into the neck to create a spacious tunnel for the muscle to reach the defect.
- The muscle is now incised a little beyond the skin paddle margin over the infero-medial part, using monopolar cautery to secure haemostasis.
- Now the muscle is elevated from below upwards and the pedicle is identified on the undersurface of the muscle.
- A cuff of muscle is kept on either side of the pedicle and the flap is raised with due care not to injure the pedicle. The medial and lateral pectoral nerve which supplies the pectoralis major muscle travels along the pedicle and must be divided for denervation of the muscle; this reduces unnecessary muscle contraction caused by dragging the skin paddle attached to the muscle, as well the atrophy of the muscle bulk.
- Haemostasis must be secured meticulously, as the pectoral branch of the thoraco-acromial artery communicates with branches from the internal mammary artery and also the lateral thoracic artery.
- After complete elevation, the flap is flipped and tunnelled through the neck and delivered into the defect in the head and neck (Figure 22.11).
- The skin margin is inset into the defect meticulously, making the suture line is water-tight. This is especially important in intraoral defects to prevent leakage of saliva.

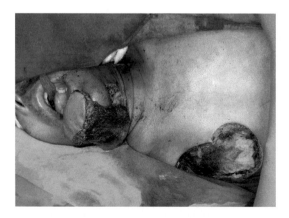

Figure.22.11 Flap tunnelled to reach defect.

- The lateral cut edge of the pectoralis major muscle can be over-sewn to secure haemostasis and also to avoid migration.
- Donor area is usually closed primarily. In cases where a very large skin paddle was taken, the donor area may need to be grafted.
- Suction drains are usually put in the chest.

Post-Operative Management

In the immediate post-operative period, the neck position has to be maintained. The neck can be kept in slight flexion; however, any acute flexion is avoided. Care must be taken to ensure that if there is a tracheostomy, the tie should not compress the pedicle. Post-operatively the flap has to be monitored clinically, and the neck should be monitored for any swelling that may compress the pedicle.

The donor area is usually closed primarily by mobilisation of local tissue. The suture line is inspected for any collection or haematoma. The wound can be left open after first dressing and suture removal can be done after seven days.

Complications and Management

Usually, the pectoralis major muscle is a reliable flap with robust blood supply. However, any inadvertent injury to the pedicle or previous trauma or injury may cause partial or total flap necrosis. If partial, it may be treated with debridement and flap re-advancement and adjustment. In case of a total flap necrosis, other local flaps like DP or lateral forehead flap can be considered.

Usually, patients develop a band across the neck where the muscle is tunnelled. This becomes evident especially after radiotherapy and patients complain of tightness on extension of neck and sometimes of dull aching pain. In such cases the pedicle may need to be divided to relieve the symptoms.

Due to its bulk, inset of the flap is difficult, especially over the posterior aspect of the defect. Orocutaneous fistula is a nagging complication which may develop in cases where proper inset could not be done.

Donor site complications like infection or dehiscence can occur. Chest wall deformity, especially breast and nipple areola malposition, can be prominent in female patients.

MEDIAN FOREHEAD FLAP

Introduction

The oldest records of median forehead flap date from c. 600 BCE, described in *Sushruta Samhita*. There is still doubt about the method used by Sushruta, as some research points towards the use of a full thickness skin graft from the cheek. Still, the rhinoplasty performed by Sushruta was very advanced for his time. Sushruta is called the father of surgery due to his surgical procedures and instruments which were far ahead their time. He is also known as the father of plastic surgery because he performed the first known plastic surgery procedure: the rhinoplasty. Today's rhinoplasty is adopted from the famous Indian rhinoplasty method as practised by the Maratha potter clan in the 17th century. The procedure was later popularised in the Western world following publication of this technique in the *Gentleman's Magazine* in 1794. Then in the early 19th century, the median forehead flap was mastered by Kazanjian and Converse. Later, the knowledge of precise vascular territories of the body led to the development of the paramedian and other types of forehead flap.

Anatomy

The midline forehead flap or classic forehead flap is ideal tissue for complete or subunit reconstruction of the nose. Knowledge of the vascular anatomy of the forehead helps in planning of the flap and pedicle placement.

The forehead is supplied by branches of internal carotid artery (supratrochlear and supraorbital artery) and external carotid artery (superficial temporal artery).

Vascular Anatomy of Mid-Forehead Region

The supraorbital notch/foramen lies an average 20 mm from the midline (range 13–25 mm). Ophthalmic artery terminates in three branches: the supratrochlear artery (usually the largest), the medial palpebral artery and external nasal artery. After intracranial origin from the ophthalmic artery in the superomedial angle of orbit, the supratrochlear artery assumes a somewhat midline course and ascends about 1.7–2.2 cm in the forehead, lateral to midline in the vertical vector,

roughly corresponding to the medial end of the eyebrow. Understanding the plane of the supratrochlear artery is important for elevation of the forehead flap. After its exit from the frontal notch, the artery pierces the orbital septum and passes superficial to corrugator superciliaris deep to the orbicularis oculi. The supratrochlear artery then runs upwards, and at about mid-forehead level, about 15–25 mm above the supraorbital rim it pierces the frontalis muscle and becomes subdermal. Thus, the artery runs from a subperiosteal plane at the start to submuscular up to the midline and ends in subdermal plane. The branches of the supratrochlear artery anastomose with the branches of the supraorbital artery and dorsal nasal artery of the same side and supratrochlear artery of the opposite side (Figure 22.12).

Classical midline forehead flap is not always based on the axial supply of the supratrochlear artery. A median forehead flap with wide-based pedicle incorporates one side or both of the supratrochlear arteries. Also, Millard, through his rhinoplasty procedures, showed that the midline forehead flap can be based on a single unilateral supratrochlear vessel.

But it is not so when the base of the median forehead flap is narrow and the supratrochlear artery is

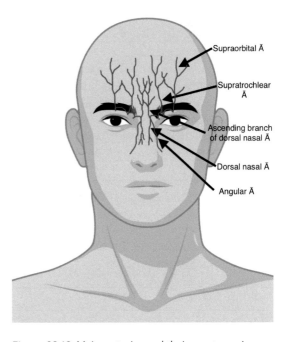

Figure.22.12 Major arteries and their anastomosis across forehead.

cut. Also, it was observed that the median forehead flap survived in an operated case of hypertelorism and orbital exenteration in which the supratrochlear vessels were damaged. Theoretically there was no named artery to support this, but through anatomic study it was postulated that the terminal branches of the facial artery (angular artery) present at the base of forehead flap have sufficient caliber to ensure the flap viability. The flap vascularity was reinforced by the branches of the rich anastomotic plexus around the medial canthus formed by dorsal nasal artery and angular artery.

Lately, a new theory for vascular supply of the median forehead flap has been proposed. The dorsal nasal artery, after perforating the orbital septum, travels along the side of nasal bones inferiorly. The dorsal nasal arteries constantly provide two longitudinal paramedian branches which freely communicate in the midline. These branches are responsible for the blood supply of the median forehead flap in those cases in which both supratrochlear arteries are cut.

The supratrochlear nerve does not accompany the supratrochlear artery. It arises from the frontal division of the trigeminal nerve in the orbit and runs in the medial orbital wall above the trochlea of the superior oblique muscle. It then exits through the frontal notch. After exiting, it does not accompany the supratrochlear artery but runs lateral to the artery.

General Consideration

Staged procedure: Unless islanded, this is a two-stage procedure. Stage 1 is transfer of the flap and stage 2 is division and insetting of the flap.

Three-staged forehead flap: In some cases of complex reconstruction, better contouring and definition of the nasal contour is required. In these cases, the flap is re-elevated one month after the first stage from distal upwards. Thinning is done keeping 2–3 mm of subcutaneous tissue with the flap with pedicle intact, and re-insetting is done. After the flap is settled, the division of the flap is planned after one month.

Indications

1. Forehead flap (midline, paramedian, or its variations) is used for total nasal or subunit nasal reconstruction.

2. Forehead flap can also be used to reconstruct lamellar defect of upper eyelid or lower eyelid, medial canthal region or small defects of cheek.

Advantages and Disadvantages

Forehead provides ideal tissue for the nasal reconstruction in terms of colour and texture match. The disadvantage of using forehead flap is leaving a midline scar in the forehead. Sometimes, a small gap left to heal by secondary intention leaves a scab and a scar which is unacceptable to the patient.

Contraindications

1. The only absolute contraindication is a full thickness cut injury in the glabella to the forehead region.
2. Other conditions, like orbital exenteration or craniofacial surgery such as fronto-orbital advancement in which the supratrochlear artery is damaged, can be considered as relative contraindications. Plexus around glabella and longitudinal branches from the dorsal nasal artery can support the flap in such cases.

Planning

The frontal notch can be located on deep palpation. The supratrochlear artery and its axis can be Doppler marked along the line of medial eyebrow. A pre-operative template of the flap is made with the approximate size of the defect, and planning in reverse with the template is to be done (Figure 22.13). Old literature suggests shaving a forehead of approximately three inches from the browline for total nasal reconstruction. For better estimation, one should match the distance from glabella to the frontal hairline and compare with a template of the defect. To increase the length of the flap, sometimes a more oblique flap may need to be planned, or else Gillies' up-and-down flap can be done if more length is required (Figure 22.14).

Pre-Operative Preparation

For easy post-operative care and dressing, the hair can be trimmed. Also, if extension of the flap to the forehead hair is planned, the epilation or removal of the forehead hair is required.

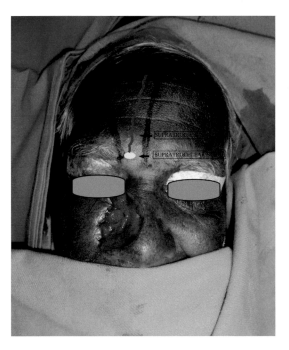

Figure.22.13 Planning and marking of paramedian forehead flap.

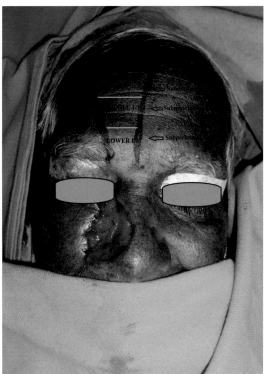

Figure. 22.15 Plane of elevation of forehead flap.

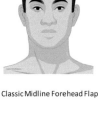

Classic Midline Forehead Flap

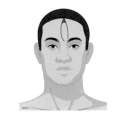

Paramedian Forehead Flap

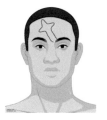

Seagull Forehead Flap

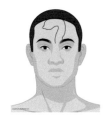

Gillies' Forehead Flap

Figure.22.14 Types of forehead flap.

Anaesthesia Concerns

Oral intubation is required. After elevation of the flap, the nasal intubation may interfere with the insetting of the flap. After intubation, the oropharyngeal passage is packed with reel gauze as there is a chance of blood trickling into the throat while insetting over the nose.

Operative Steps Including Position

The patient is kept in supine position. The surgeon stands at the head end of the table. Neck requires slight extension with a small support kept between the shoulders. Head is stabilised in the head ring.

The supratrochlear artery after its origin is sub-periosteal below the orbital septum. After piercing the orbital septum in the superomedial angle of the orbit, it runs in the sub-muscular plane in the lower one-third of the flap. At a variable distance of 10–25 mm (mean 20 mm), the artery pierces the frontalis muscle and runs superficial to the muscle in the middle one-third of the flap. Lastly, at the termination, the artery is sub-dermal (Figure 22.15).

After painting and draping, the template of the flap is made as per size of the defect. Accurate size of the flap is confirmed by planning in reverse. Using the template, marking of the flap is done over the forehead.

Steps

1. The flap is elevated distal to proximal.
2. Dermis deep, skin incision is made with a no. 15 surgical blade. The upper one-third of the flap is elevated in subdermal plane.
3. As the dissection reaches the junction of upper and middle thirds, the frontalis muscle is cut, taken with the flap, and now the flap is elevated in submuscular plane in the middle one-third of flap.
4. As the lower one-third of the flap is reached, the periosteum is cut and the flap is elevated in the subperiosteal plane.
5. When supraorbital margin is reached, gentle dissection is done to release the tethering effect of the periosteum to free the pedicle. It also increases the length of the flap, helps in easy rotation of the flap and prevents twisting of the pedicle.

Management of the Donor Site

The forehead flap is unique in that the donor and recipient area stand in the most aesthetically prominent part of the face.

Attempts should be made to primarily close the donor area in single layer with slight undermining of the margins (Figure 22.16).

- Triangulating sutures or approximating sutures should not be applied at the base of the flap because this will compromise the vascularity.
- A small gap left after the approximating sutures should heal by secondary intention. Split skin grafting should always be kept as last option.

Division and Insetting

See Figure 22.17.

- It is planned for 10 days–14 days.
- At the time of insetting, if the distal portion of the flap is taken well, then 50% of the flap is elevated for thinning if required.

Post-Operative Care

Post-operatively, minimal care is required. Any compressive and bulky dressing is avoided. Pedicle is covered with paraffin gauze with antibiotic

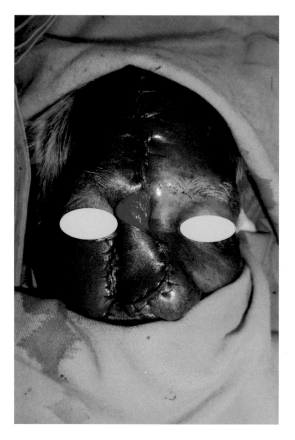

Figure.22.16 Elevation and insetting of flap.

ointment to prevent it from desiccation. The rest of the flap and suture line is covered with paraffin gauze with a small surgical soft pad. The dressing over the donor area, if closed under tension, may be reinforced by Dynaplast dressing. The dressing can be changed on the first or second postoperative day if it gets soaked. After a few days, the flap dressing can be left open and patient can be advised to apply antibiotic ointment only. The donor site sutures are to be removed after one week.

Complications and Management

1. Total flap failure is usually not a complication unless the pedicle is damaged or inadvertently not included in the flap.
2. Flap necrosis is a major complication. If the procedure performed is technically correct, full thickness flap necrosis has been reported with smoking and very rarely with diabetes and vascular disorders.
3. Minor complications are common, like epidermolysis, tip necrosis and growth of hair at the

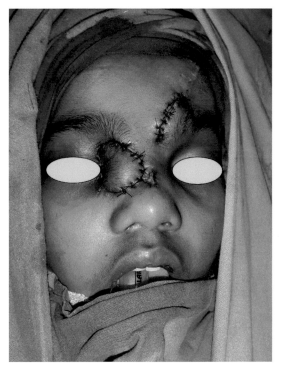

Figure 22.17 Division and insetting of forehead flap for basal cell carcinoma around medial canthus of right eye.

tip of the flap if long flap is elevated from the hair-bearing area. Depilation of the visible hair of the flap should be done before insetting. Still, it may require laser or chemical depilation if the hair growth becomes annoying to the patient.

4. Brow elevation of the ipsilateral side.

For a complete loss of the flap, paramedian forehead flap from the spared supratrochlear artery, nasolabial flap or other local flap is required.

Partial necrosis of the flap and tip necrosis can be managed by repeated dressing and healing by secondary intention, or if defect is greater, then debridement followed by graft or a small local flap. If the flap is long and there is play in the pedicle, then the flap can be re-elevated and advanced into the defect.

LATERAL FOREHEAD FLAP

Introduction

The name "lateral forehead flap" is a misnomer. The lateral forehead tissue used in this flap is based on the superficial temporal artery. This flap is used conventionally for the reconstruction of the cheek defects after carcinoma excision.

The usefulness of the lateral forehead flap was reported by Blair et al. and popularised by McGregor in the 1960s. McGregor named it a temporal flap as it was not a classical forehead flap. Forehead flap gained its popularity for reconstruction due to its robust and consistent blood supply, plus its length and thus greater amount of tissue available for reconstruction, proximity of the donor area and hairless tissue. As well, elevation is technically easy.

In the early 19th century, for a full thickness cheek defect two flaps were planned, one forehead flap and the other a cervical or a deltopectoral flap. Later, after detailed knowledge was gained of the flap's vascular supply, various modifications of the forehead flap were used, like the axial folded flap and the contra-axial folded flap in which a single large flap would suffice for coverage of the entire defect.

Vascular Anatomy

The lateral forehead flap is an axial pattern flap based on the frontal branch of superficial temporal artery. The superficial temporal artery is the terminal division of the external carotid artery. Initially it lies in the deep tissue of the parotid gland; it then pierces the deep fascia and becomes superficial in front of the tragus, where it is easily palpable. Running about 5 mm anterior to the tragus, it crosses the zygomatic arch, remaining anterior to the anterior temporal nerve and superficial temporal vein. The artery terminates about 2–4 cm above the zygomatic arch by dividing into frontal (anterior) and posterior (parietal) branch (Figure 22.18).

Another prominent zygomatic branch (Figure 22.19) arises from the stem in 80% of cases and from the frontal branch in 20% of cases. The level of branching of the zygomatic branch is not constant and it branches above the zygomatic arch in only 60% of cases. Likewise, the origin and course of the frontal branch depends upon the origin of the zygomatic branch.

The central forehead is supplied by both supratrochlear and supraorbital artery. Temporal region on each side is supplied by superficial temporal artery. The anatomical territory of superficial temporal artery on each side finishes at the ipsilateral supraorbital region, which supplies the proximal third part of this flap. So, in a classic

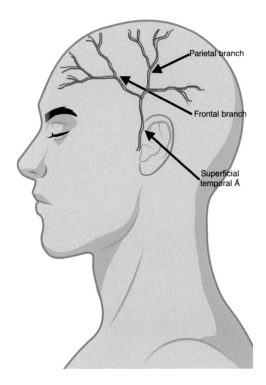

Figure.22.18 Course of superficial temporal artery.

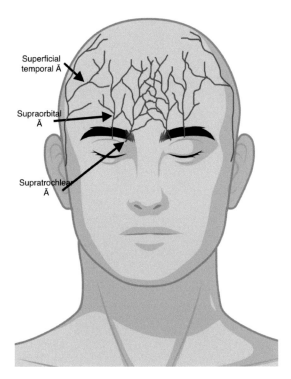

Figure.22.20 Arterial anastomosis of major vessels in forehead.

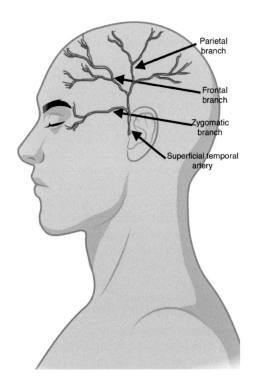

Figure.22.19 Branching of superficial temporal artery.

lateral forehead flap, the frontal and the zygomatic branches of superficial temporal artery supplying the forehead are better addressed as feeders to the flap and the rest of the forehead, and the extended forehead flap is actually supplied by rich anastomosis between these vessels with supratrochlear and supraorbital artery of ipsilateral and contralateral side (Figure 22.20).

While elevating the forehead flap, the zygomatic artery should be included because it will increase the flap's perfusion pressure and the blood supply.

Staged Procedure

Lateral forehead flap is a two-stage procedure. Stage 1 is transfer of the flap and stage 2 is division of pedicle and insetting of the flap.

Indications

- Most commonly used for defect following excision of benign tumour and carcinoma in tongue, check, base of tongue.
- Patient with hemi-mandibulectomy.

- Earlier used for reconstruction of oesophagus following excision of tumour from cervical oesophagus.
- Post-traumatic soft tissue defect in face.
- Sometimes used for neck reconstruction to cover the exposed carotid artery.

Advantages

- It provides a wide and long flap. It has wide arc of rotation so that it can reach the lower border of the mandible. It can be used as a folded flap to provide inner mucosal lining and outer skin cover. Technically it is easy and less time is required for reconstruction as compared to free flaps.

Disadvantages

- Staged procedure.
- Facial disfigurement.
- Loss of facial expression of the donor area (forehead).
- Visible forehead scarring due to split skin grafting at flap donor site.
- Prolonged stay in hospital due to staged procedure.
- May result in trismus if small flap is used for angle of mouth or cheek.

Contraindications

Previous trauma, surgery or radiation therapy to forehead.

Subunit Principle

The face is subdivided into several aesthetic sub-units. It helps to plan a surgical procedure which results in less visible scars. It is known that scars within a subunit are noticeable, so it is better to plan a surgical procedure which leaves a scar in the borders of a subunit rather than in the middle of a subunit. It is always advisable to use a whole central subunit as a flap when total forehead flap is planned. When extended forehead flap is planned, the whole contralateral superficial temporal artery territory is used for better cosmetic appearance after skin grafting with less visible scars.

Pre-Operative Preparation

Usually, only palpation is required to assess the superficial temporal vessels. If there is previous history of trauma or a surgical scar over the forehead or over the course of the artery, then Doppler study can be done. To maintain hygiene and for ease of dressing in the post-operative period, it is preferable to have the head shaved completely.

Position

Supine with slight neck extension. After excision of the defect, the head is kept in straight position for elevation of the flap.

Anaesthesia Concerns

Nasal intubation is required in such cases. After elevation of the flap, oral intubation may interfere with the insetting of the flap if reconstruction is done in the oral cavity.

Flap Markings

See Figure 22.21.

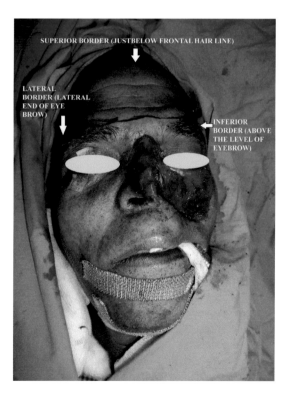

Figure 22.21 Flap markings showing superior, inferior and lateral border.

For a Complete Lateral Forehead Flap

- Pivot point: Anterior to tragus where the artery comes to lie in the superficial plane
- Upper border: Just below hairline
- Lower border: Just above eyebrow
- Lateral border: Coincides with the lateral end of the eyebrow, preserving the temporal hairline

For an Extended Lateral Forehead Flap

In the extended flap, the lateral forehead subunit is taken up to an imaginary line connecting the inferolateral orbital rim to the sideburns inferolaterally.

Flap Harvest

After induction of general anaesthesia, the oropharyngeal passage is packed with reel gauze because there might be trickling of blood into the throat while insetting. The subcutaneous plane can be saline infiltrated using 10 ml syringe and 24-gauge needle. It causes hydro-dissection and helps in easy flap elevation. At the distal part of the flap skin, incision is directly deepened up to the forehead pericranium. Once the sub-fascial plane is identified, the dissection is done in this plane above the pericranium. Progressively, the skin incision is extended proximally and flap elevation is done in the subfascial plane. When the temporalis fascia is reached on the pedicle side proximally, there is tethering present between the fascia of flap and the temporal fascia. To elevate the flap in the sub-fascial plane from the temporalis, now fine dissection is done till the pivot point of the flap is reached, preferably with scissors. Use of electrosurgery is minimised over the periosteum for better uptake of the split skin graft (Figure 22.22).

Transfer of the Flap

1. For cheek defect: It can be turned down through a tunnel in the cheek or can be interpolated over the skin bridge (Figure 22.23). There remains a fistula in the upper part of the defect, which is repaired in the second stage at the time of division, and insetting of the flap and the stump of the flap can be returned or discarded.

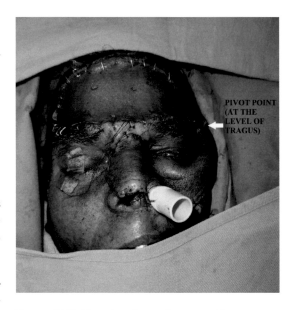

Figure.22.22 Flap elevation and transposition across pivot point to cover soft tissue defect over nose and left malar area.

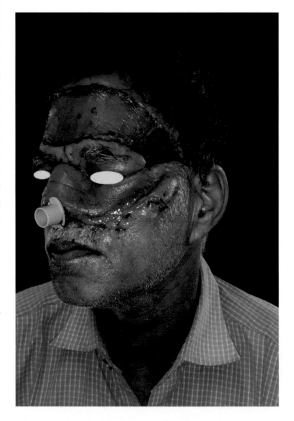

Figure 22.23 Insetting of flap by interpolation of the flap over the skin bridge to reach the defect.

2. For intraoral reconstruction, the flap can be tunneled behind the zygoma. If the tunnel is inadequate, then a part of the zygoma can be fractured or can be taken out to accommodate the pedicle of the flap.

POST-OPERATIVE CARE

Post-operatively, minimal care is required. Any compressive and bulky dressing is avoided. Pedicle is covered with paraffin gauze with antibiotic ointment to prevent desiccation. The rest of the flap and suture line are covered with paraffin gauze and a small surgical soft pad. Donor area is skin grafted and usually a tie-over or bolster dressing is applied, which is removed at 5–7 days post-operatively and graft uptake is assessed. If uptake is good, it can be left open after 2–3 dressing changes.

DIVISION AND INSETTING

It is planned after 14 days. At the time of insetting, the flap is divided at the upper border of the flap, and the fistula is closed at the upper border of the flap from where it is brought down to the cheek. Aesthetically, it is better to trim and close the small remaining stump of the flap than to return it the donor site.

COMPLICATIONS AND MANAGEMENT

Flap failure is usually not a complication unless the pedicle is damaged or inadvertently not included in the flap. Epidermolysis, infection and suture dehiscence are minor complications. Facial disfigurement at the recipient site and scars from split skin grafting are sometimes annoying to the patient.

TRAPEZIUS FLAP

Introduction
The trapezius flap can be used as upper, middle or lower flap based on their respective vascular supply. The trapezius flap was first described in 1984 and called the cervicodorsal flap. Easy surgical steps, large cutaneous paddle and expendable donor site are distinct advantages of this flap.

Surgical Anatomy

Understanding the anatomy of the muscle is important for the safe elevation of this flap.

Origin
The muscle originates from medial one-third of the superior nuchal line of the occipital bone, the ligamentum nuchae, the spine of C7 and all spines of the thoracic vertebrae and the intervening supraspinous ligaments

Insertion
Insertion of the muscle is in three parts (Figure 22.24).

1. Superior part: Muscle originating from skull and upper portion of the vertebral column descends downward and laterally to attach to the lateral third of the clavicle and to the acromion of the scapula.
2. Middle part: Runs horizontally to insert into medial margin of the acromion and upper lip of the crest of the spine of the scapula.
3. Inferior part: Runs upwards and lateral to insert into the deltoid tubercle at the root of spine.

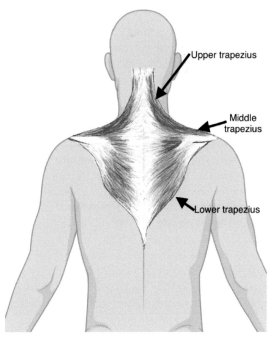

Figure.22.24 Orientation of trapezius muscle fibre.

Clinical Significance of Upper Fibres

Due to the attachment of the upper fibres of trapezius to the shoulder girdle bones (i.e., clavicle and spine of scapula), these fibres provide stability to the shoulder girdle. This function of the muscle is important and cannot be replaced by any other muscle. Therefore, denervation of the muscle or loss of the upper muscle fibres results in shoulder drop.

Vascular Anatomy of Trapezius Muscle

Most inconsistent of this useful flap is its blood supply.

- Classical description: Blood supply of the trapezius is from transverse cervical artery. The transverse cervical artery at the upper border of the trapezius divides into ascending and descending branches. The ascending branch (superficial branch) supplies the middle portion of the muscle. The descending branch (deep branch/dorsal scapular) runs deep to the trapezius and supplies the lower third of the muscle.
- More commonly accepted: The dorsal scapular artery, also called the descending/deep branch of transverse cervical artery, which supplies the lower trapezius muscle, arises separately from the transverse cervical artery just after its origin from subclavian artery (66%). In 26% of cases, it is a branch of the transverse cervical artery.
- It then passes in between the trunks of the brachial plexus, takes a sharp turn and goes deep to the levator scapulae muscle, comes out between rhomboidus major and minor muscles and runs on the deep surface of the trapezius between the scapula and vertebral column. This predominantly supplies the lower one-third of the muscle.

The course and anatomy of the vessels are variable proximal to levator, but distal to levator they are fixed. Proximally, the transverse cervical artery and the dorsal scapular artery may have separate origin, or the dorsal scapular artery may originate at the transverse cervical artery (named the descending branch of the transverse cervical artery). Distal to the levator, the anatomy is fixed; the transverse cervical artery passes over the levator muscle and the dorsal scapular artery passes below the levator muscle.

The vascularity of the trapezius muscle thus can be summarised as:

- Upper part/superomedial part: Occipital artery
- Middle part: Transverse cervical artery/ ascending branch of transverse cervical artery
- Lower part: Dorsal scapular artery/descending branch of transverse cervical artery
- Paraspinal part: Perforating branches of posterior intercostal arteries and veins

Three clinically useful flaps can be planned based on the arterial axes of trapezius flap:

1. Upper trapezius flap
2. Middle trapezius flap
3. Lower trapezius/classical trapezius flap

UPPER TRAPEZIUS FLAP

Upper trapezius flap includes the superior descending part of the muscle (the part of the muscle originating from occipital and upper cervical vertebrae).

Position: Supine or modified lateral decubitus.

Blood supply: Occipital artery and paraspinal perforators.

Marking: See Figure 22.25.

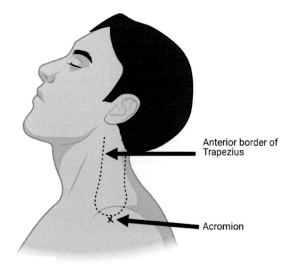

Figure 22.25 Marking of upper trapezius flap.

- Anterior border: Along anterior edge of trapezius.
- Posterior border: Parallel to the anterior border.
- Width of the flap: Can be assessed by the pinch test. The amount of skin that can be closed primarily is taken as skin paddle.
- Lateral extent: Up to the acromion, as the upper muscle fibre attachment of trapezius is up to the acromion. The lateral extent can be elongated if required, but it is a random skin flap and elevated at 1:1 ratio.

Flap Elevation

Anterior incision is made first. Skin incision is deepened to fat and fascia to identify the anterior edge of trapezius.

Once the trapezius is identified and location of the remaining skin paddle over the muscle is confirmed, the rest of the skin incision is completed. Flap is elevated from lateral to medial.

Up to the acromion, the flap is elevated to include the deltoid fascia.

When the dissection reaches the acromion, the trapezius is then sharply elevated off its bony insertion to spine.

During the elevation from lateral to medial, the transverse cervical artery (TCA) and veins are ligated in the anterior margin for proximal elevation of flap.

Medially, blunt dissection between the trapezius and supraspinatus is done up to the origin of the trapezius from the cervical spine and midline to complete the elevation of flap.

The flap is then transposed into the defect.

Post-Operative Care

A suction drain can be inserted in the donor area to prevent haematoma. Patient should be in prone or lateral position to prevent pressure on the flap pedicle and the suture line.

Complications

Flap necrosis can occur if the flap is elevated in the wrong plane and the pedicle is accidentally left. The surgeon should attempt to close the donor site primarily.

MIDDLE TRANSVERSE TRAPEZIUS MYOCUTANEOUS FLAP

The use of middle transverse trapezius muscle flap may cause drooping of shoulder as the middle trapezius fibers holding the acromioclavicular joint are cut. Also, if the donor area is not closed primarily, it leaves an unsightly, painful scar over the shoulder joint. Both these reasons limit the use of this flap. More reliable options with larger skin paddle are available for reconstruction.

Indications

1. Lining of intraoral defect.
2. Coverage of the neck defect.
3. Coverage of the carotid vessels.

Blood Supply

Transverse cervical artery.

Position

Supine position with neck turned to the other side.

Marking

Skin island is marked over the acromioclavicular area with more of the skin element towards the spine of scapula, as the bulk of muscle is posteriorly towards the spine of scapula. Marking is done as shown in Figure 22.26.

Flap Elevation

Anterior incision is made along the anterior border of trapezius and subplatysmal skin flaps are elevated anteriorly and posteriorly. Posterior belly of omohyoid is identified. The transverse cervical artery is identified below the posterior belly of the omohyoid and is traced laterally as it goes below the trapezius muscle.

After the transverse cervical vessel identification, the location of skin paddle is verified again. Keeping 2–3 cm excess skin distal to the muscle margin, skin incision of the flap is now completed laterally, posteriorly and medially over the acromioclavicular area.

Once the trapezius is identified and location of the remaining skin paddle over the muscle is

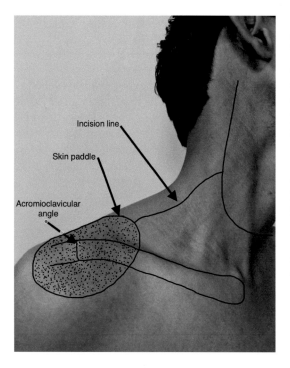

Incision line

Skin paddle

Acromioclavicular angle

Figure.22.26 Marking of middle trapezius flap.

confirmed, the rest of the skin incision is completed and tacking sutures are applied between the muscle and the skin.

Now the flap is elevated from lateral to medial, cutting the trapezius muscle from the acromioclavicular area and going deep to it.

Careful blunt dissection is done medially below the muscle taking the vascular pedicle with the flap.

The following two structures may need to be cut if they prevent the arc of rotation of the flap:

1. Dorsal scapular branch if it arises from the transverse cervical vessels.
2. Spinal accessory nerve or its branches.

Medially, part of the trapezius muscle can be taken as a carrier of vascular pedicle. At the medial-most end, only fat fascia layer is available as carrier of the vascular pedicle because the transverse cervical vessel diverges from the trapezius muscle medially. The flap is then transposed into the defect.

Post-Operative Care

A suction drain can be inserted in the donor area to prevent haematoma. Patient should be placed in supine position.

Complications

The course of the transverse cervical vessels diverges from the trapezius medially, so flap necrosis can occur if the island of the flap is accidentally elevated without the vascular pedicle at the medial part of the flap elevation. The surgeon should attempt to close the donor site primarily.

LOWER TRAPEZIUS FLAP

Blood supply: Dorsal scapular artery/Descending branch of transverse cervical artery

Indications

- Soft tissue defect after excision malignant and benign tumour from the following:
  1. Posterior scalp region, posterior cranial fossa.
  2. Larynx.
  3. Rarely lip, oral cavity and mandible.
- For coverage of the exposed implant over cervical or thoracic region.

Advantages

- Located far from the previously operated area.
- Away from possible area for irradiation.

Modifications

1. Vertical trapezius myocutaneous flap
2. Vertical trapezius islanded flap
3. Extended vertical trapezius myocutaneous flap

Position: Prone or lateral decubitus position

Marking: Pre-operative marking is done in sitting position.

The trapezius cannot be palpated in the back, so for marking of the flap, the trapezius muscle margins, medial border of scapula and inferior angel of scapula are marked to plan the skin paddle, as shown in Figure 22.27.

The lower musculocutaneous or muscle flap is based on the vessels of the middle and lower third of the trapezius muscle. The skin island is marked between the medial margin of scapula and dorsal spine. The width of the flap can be decided by the skin pinch test for the primary closure of the donor site. Inferiorly the flap can be extended about 5 cm

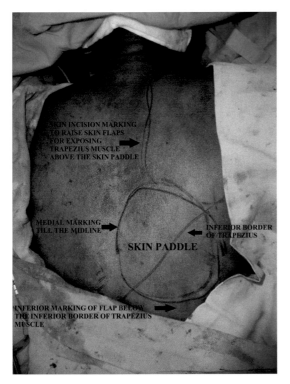

Figure.22.27 Marking of the skin paddle of lower trapezius flap.

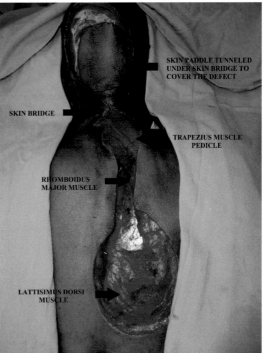

Figure.22.28 Elevation of the lower trapezius flap.

beyond the lower margin of muscle that is below the inferior border of scapula. An extra island of skin can be taken if required, but may need trimming if bleeding is unsatisfactory from the extra skin.

The distal part of the flap is the extension of the skin beyond the trapezius muscle. Distally, the flap contains only skin and subcutaneous tissue.

Flap Elevation

Flap elevation begins inferolaterally. Skin incision is deepened down to fascia and fat to clearly expose the latissimus dorsi muscle. Continuing proximally and medially, the dissection is done just superficial to the latissimus dorsi muscle. In this way, the trapezius automatically gets incorporated in the skin flap.

The medial skin incision is completed and the trapezius muscle is cut from its origin from the dorsal spines to complete the distal elevation of the flap.

The flap can now be upturned to confirm the dorsal scapular pedicle of the flap. After confirmation of the pedicle and skin paddle over the muscle, the superior skin incision is completed. Proximal to the proximal margin of the skin island, a skin incision is made to raise skin flaps and expose trapezius. For proximal part of flap elevation, blunt dissection is performed slowly below, toward the trapezius, to expose the rhomboidus major.

To complete the flap elevation, medial and lateral vertical cuts are made on the trapezius muscle proximal to the skin paddle, taking 3–4 cm of the trapezius muscle containing vascular pedicle. Flap elevation stops at the level of scapular spine (Figure 22.28).

The upper one-third of muscle is not taken with the flap to prevent the complication of shoulder drooping. The musculocutaneous flap with muscle pedicle is then interpolated or tunnelled under the skin of the neck to the recipient site (Figure 22.29).

Post-Operative Care

A suction drain can be inserted in the donor area to prevent haematoma. Patient should be in prone or lateral position to prevent pressure on the flap pedicle and the suture line.

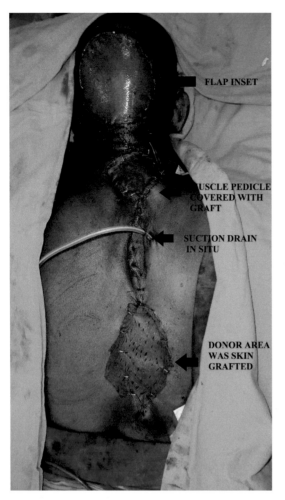

Figure.22.29 Tunnelling and inset of lower trapezius flap.

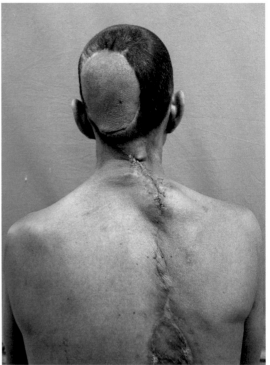

Figure 22.30 Well-settled lower trapezius flap with donor site skin grafted.

Complications

Flap necrosis can occur if flap is elevated in the wrong plane and the pedicle is left accidentally. The surgeon should try to close the donor site primarily. If the donor site is managed with skin graft, there are chances of graft loss, so pressure over the grafted area should be avoided (Figure 22.30).

Elevation in the wrong flap may lead to flap necrosis.

If donor area is not closed primarily and skin grafted, the patient may complain of discomfort and pain on supine position. Patient may develop an unstable scar if grafted area is not taken care of.

If the flap is used for head, patient may complain of dull aching pain due to constant band of the muscle pedicle in the neck. Patient will keep the head in extension and find it difficult to flex the head, so sometimes the subcutaneous muscle pedicles need to be divided when the flap settles after few months.

BUCCAL MUCOSAL FLAP

Introduction

Intraoral defect reconstruction has many options. Deltopectoral flap, pectoralis major myocutaneous flap and free flaps are workhorse flaps. In cases of premalignant lesions and early-stage carcinoma, usually the defect is small. Small defects can be managed by split skin grafting, random buccal flaps or facial artery myomucosal flap. Small defects are traditionally left open for secondary healing by granulation and epithelisation, but it is always better not to leave a raw area if possible. Buccal mucosa has rich vascular supply, giving the opportunity to use buccal tissue as a random tissue.

General Consideration for Elevation of Buccal Flap

Buccal mucosal flap is a random pattern flap based on the rich blood supply of the oral mucosa. Usually, it is composed of mucosa and 1–2 mm of sub-mucosa. The preferred width of the flap is 1–1.5 cm, so that the donor site can be closed primarily. The buccal mucosal flap, when elevated with a thin layer of buccinators muscle, is called a buccal myomucosal flap. Inclusion of a thin layer of the muscle improves the blood supply of the flap.

For tonsillo-lingual defect, posterior palate defect/fistula or small defect in the posterior floor of mouth, a posterior-based flap is used. The flap is usually tunnelled from behind the molar tooth.

For nasal reconstruction or lip reconstruction, if required, an anteriorly based flap is used.

For Palatal Defect

The base of the flap is designed in the retromolar trigone and is directed towards oral commissure (Figure 22.31). The anterior incision is planned 2–3 mm away from the parotid duct orifice. The flap is turned inside the mouth to cover the defect

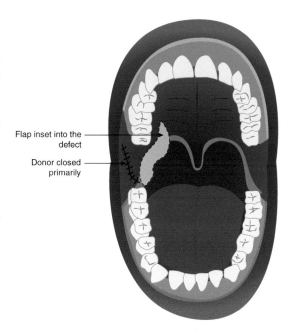

Figure 22.32 Posteriorly based flap to cover the palatal defect.

(Figure 22.32). Avoid the opening of the buccal fat pad fascia. The flap needs division and insetting after two weeks. If the flap crosses the molars, a temporary bite block can be used to protect the pedicle. The block can be removed and oral cavity can be rinsed regularly.

For Lip/Vermilion Reconstruction

Unilateral or bilateral mucosal/musculomucosal flap based on angle of mouth can be elevated to cover the lip or vermilion defect. The distal end of the flap lies just up to or beneath the opening of the parotid duct (Figures 22.33 and 22.34).

Oropharyngeal Defect

For covering a defect in the tonsillo-lingual/posterior pharyngeal wall region, a posterior based mucosal/musculomucosal flap extending from cheek to the angle of mouth just below the parotid region can be planned. The flap is planned adjacent to the defect and transposed to the defect.

Indication

As the donor area is limited, this flap can only be used only for lining of small 1–2 cm defects of

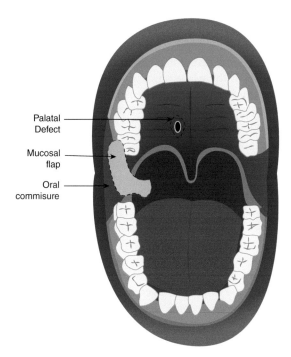

Figure 22.31 Planning of buccal flap based on retromolar trigone.

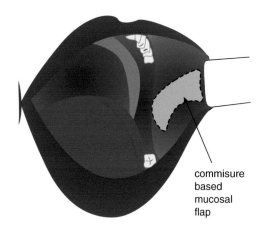

Figure 22.33 Planning of anterior buccal flap based on oral commisure.

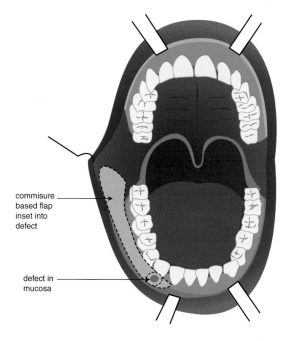

Figure 22.34 Anteriorly based buccal flap to cover lip mucosal defect.

post-pharyngeal wall, tonsillar region, lateral part of floor of mouth, cheek, vermilion and lip.

Contraindication

Patients of submucosal fibrosis in which there is already a decreased mouth opening.

Advantages

Proximity of the donor area and technically easy steps are the prominent advantages of the buccal flap.

Disadvantages

As the donor area is intraoral, the mouth opening may be decreased when the donor area is healed. This may cause significant problem in patients with submucosal fibrosis in which there is already restriction of mouth opening.

If there is interpolation of the flap when the defect is not adjacent, then the pedicle will need one more surgery under general anaesthesia for division and insetting after two weeks.

Anaesthesia Concerns

Patient requires nasal intubation if a buccal flap is planned pre-operatively.

Post-Operative Care

Gentle lavage with betadine saline should be done daily to keep the oral cavity clean. Patient to be kept nil by mouth for 2–3 days till the suture line shows signs of healing. After a few days, patient should be kept on clear fluids for two weeks.

Complications and Management

There are always chances of infection and dehiscence if the flap is sutured under tension. If there is dehiscence, wound care is done daily till the margins and bed of the wound are ready for re-do surgery. If there is adequate granulation tissue, the area can be grafted or a regional flap like pectoralis major or deltopectoral flap can be planned if any critical area is exposed.

RADIAL FOREARM FLAP

Introduction

Radial forearm flap, also known as the Chinese flap, was first described by Yang et al. in 1981. It is a workhorse flap for reconstruction in the head and neck region. It is a fasciocutaneous flap based on radial artery and its venae comitantes along with the subcutaneous cephalic vein. Because of this alternate venous drainage system, either the superficial or the deep veins can be used for venous drainage or both can be used together (Figure 22.35). The radial forearm flap has the unique characteristic of thin, pliable soft tissue components with minimal bulk, and it can be easily moulded and adapted to

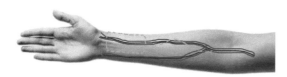

Figure 22.35 Vascular anatomy and flap marking of radial forearm flap.

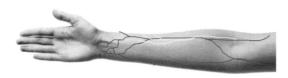

Figure 22.36 Anatomy of superficial venous system and relationship with lateral antebrachial cutaneous nerve.

resurface oral soft tissue defects. This flap can be utilised as an innervated or sensate flap or it can be raised with a bone segment of the radius as an osteocutaneous flap. The sensory recovery in the radial forearm skin paddle can be facilitated by anastomosing the antebrachial cutaneous nerve to a sensory nerve at recipient site (Figure 22.36).

Indications and Advantages

The radial forearm flap, due to its thin pliable soft tissue component, is widely used for head and neck soft tissue reconstruction in both intraoral soft tissue defects after excision of carcinoma cheek, tongue and palate and for extraoral defects like lip, perforating defects of cheek and carcinoma of the oesophagus. Any post-traumatic small to medium soft tissue defect can be resurfaced with this flap.

The anatomical advantage of this flap is its high-calibre vessels (artery 2–3 mm, cephalic vein 3–4 mm, deep veins 1–2 mm) and long vascular pedicle. Simultaneous flap raising is possible in the forearm with resection in the head and neck region. Because of its reliable and constant anatomy of vessels, it is easy to harvest, thus recommended for beginners. Multiple skin paddles can be harvested.

Contraindications and Disadvantages

Despite its many indications and advantages, this flap has its disadvantages related to the donor site and the complete interruption of radial artery flow to hand and forearm, as the radial artery is a major dominant vessel of the forearm and hand. In pre-operative planning, an Allen test should be performed to rule out radial artery dominant hand and check the integrity of the palmar arch. If doubt exists after the Allen test, pre-operative angiography is ordered. Donor site complications like problems in graft take and visibility of the grafted area are added to the disadvantages. Oedema of hand, reduced extension, loss of sensation over the anatomical snuff box due to damage to the superficial branch of radial nerve and cold intolerance have been reported.

The contraindications are due to anatomical dominance of the radial artery over the ulnar artery (though the ulnar artery is the dominant artery in regular findings) and lack of communication between the deep and superficial palmar arch.

Investigations

In a doubtful Allen test, pre-operative angiography is advised to reveal the dominant blood supply of the hand and to establish the integrity of the palmar arch.

Pre-Operative Preparations

The flap donor forearm should be shaved. Thighs should be shaved for preparation as skin graft donor site. No cannulation or venipuncture should be done on the forearm and hand of the left or non-dominant site.

Patient Positioning

Patient is positioned supine with arm abducted and supine exposing the volar aspect of the forearm. Scrubbing of the non-dominant upper extremity is required from nail to axilla. The flap can be harvested with or without tourniquet, but it is desirable to have a bloodless field during dissection flap raising under tourniquet control.

Anaesthesia Concerns

Flap harvesting is usually done under general anaesthesia, as in head and neck reconstruction, in case of carcinomas or under brachial plexus block. When the flap is harvested under tourniquet control, tourniquet time should be noted and should not exceed 1.5 hours.

Operative Steps

A pattern of the defect is transferred to a piece of cloth or towel and the required length of the pedicle is measured. The outline of the flap dimension is marked over the forearm, leaving the distal one inch from the distal wrist crease.

The marking is done over the volar aspect, leaving the ulnar border and the territory of the ulnar neurovascular bundle untouched. Medially the flap margin should be planned lateral to the flexor carpi ulnaris (FCU) tendon; laterally the flap margin can be extended to the dorsolateral aspect of the forearm (Figure 22.37).

Under tourniquet control, the incision is made over the skin on the course of the radial artery and exposure of the radial artery with venae comitantes, cephalic vein and antebrachial cutaneous nerve is done. The margins of the flap are incised first over the ulnar border of the flap and deepened till the forearm fascia is reached. The deep fascia is incised till the paratenon of the FCU tendon is exposed. The paratenon is left untouched.

The distal margin of the flap is incised through the skin and fascia. The flap is now elevated from the medial border and inferior border transecting the fibrous attachments between the forearm fascia and paratenon of the flexor digitorum superficialis and palmaris longus muscle. As the flap elevation proceeds, the paratenon of the strong flexor carpi radialis tendon is reached and is freed distally. Radial to the FCR tendon lies the radial artery which runs in the intermuscular septum between FCR and brachioradialis tendons. At the most distal point of the septum, at the distal incision site, the septum is opened and a short segment of the

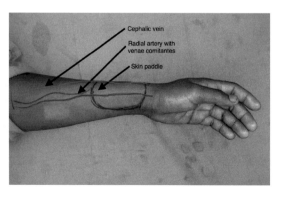

Figure 22.37 Skin marking of radial forearm flap showing main vessels of the flap.

radial artery is exposed. The superficial branch of the radial nerve which ramifies distally into two to three branches is identified and preserved.

The radial artery is ligated and divided between ligatures at the distal end of the flap. Now the lateral border of the flap is incised. The cephalic vein usually lies subcutaneously above the fascia and it is included in the flap. During its dissection, the superficial branch of the radial nerve is freed and the distal cephalic vein is ligated. No attempt should be made to separate the cephalic vein from the skin paddle.

Attention should be paid here to the difference between the plane in which the cephalic vein lies and in which the radial artery with its two venae comitantes lie. In fact, the cephalic vein lies more superficial. The fascia over the brachioradialis tendon and muscle is incised and the intermuscular septum containing the vascular pedicle is reached. The superficial branch of the radial nerve is now completely freed distally from the skin paddle and is retracted away from the field by skin hooks.

Now the flap is raised from distal to proximal dissection including the intermuscular septum and the fascia. Care should be taken not to separate the arterial pedicle from the flap skin paddle. The distal portion of the flap is rich in septal perforators arising from the pedicle as there is only a tendinous part of the muscle. Also, centering the flap on the distal part of the forearm has the advantage of obtaining a long vascular pedicle, which is very much desirable in head and neck reconstruction.

At the medial border of the brachioradialis muscle and tendon, the surgeon should dip down to include the intermuscular septum with the flap. The fascia of the flap with the intermuscular septum is separated from the brachioradialis muscle.

As the pedicle dissection proceeds proximally, one must be careful to separate the pedicle from the belly of brachioradialis by retracting the muscle. It is often found to be tethered to the muscle, so in this way injury to the pedicle is avoided. During the dissection of the pedicle, the perforators supplying the flexor policis longus muscle and the underlying tissue are often found arising from the inferior aspect of the pedicle. These are to be carefully cauterised or clipped.

Now the proximal pedicle is dissected from its bed and also the cephalic vein, which is taken when the flap is dissected proximally in the suprafascial

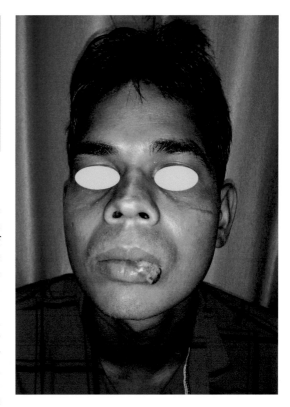

Figure 22.38 Elevated flap with components.

plane (Figure 22.38). If the cephalic vein is to be used as a draining vein of the flap, the venous return of the flap through the proximal cut end of the cephalic vein should be confirmed before the flap pedicle is divided and after deflation of the cuff. If there is any doubt, a deep vein must be chosen for anastomosis.

The radial artery with venae comitantes can be dissected up to the bifurcation from the ulnar artery. The venae comitantes of the radial artery should be carefully separated from the artery and from one another for a few centimetres by meticulous dissection under magnification. The cephalic vein can be taken longer than the arterial pedicle. The flap pedicle ligation is done only when the recipient vessels are ready.

After flap transfer the flap donor site in the forearm is skin grafted after meticulous haemostasis. The forearm and wrist is splinted in neutral position of the wrist.

Figures 22.39 through 22.42 show a patient with carcinoma of the lower lip with post-excision defect and subsequent reconstruction with radial forearm free flap. Figures 22.43 and 22.44 show long-term follow-up with adequate mouth opening.

Post-Operative Care, Complications and Management

The flap needs to be clinically monitored frequently for the first three days post-operatively to rule out any vascular compromise. The skin-grafted area of the flap donor site usually heals nicely and dressing is changed at 4–5 days post-surgery. Skin graft uptake and satisfactory wound healing occurs around 7–15 days post-operatively.

Any kind of post-operative vascular compromise should be aggressively dealt with by exploration of the anastomosis site and by performing

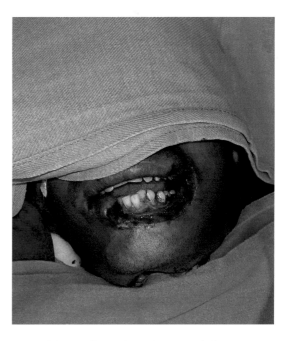

Figure 22.39 Carcinoma of the lower lip.

Figure 22.40 Defect in lower lip created after resection of tumour.

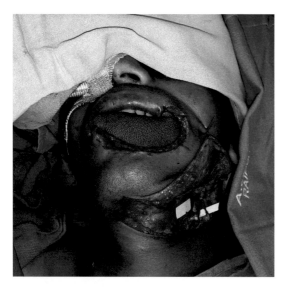

Figure 22.41 Radial forearm flap after transfer and vascular anastomosis.

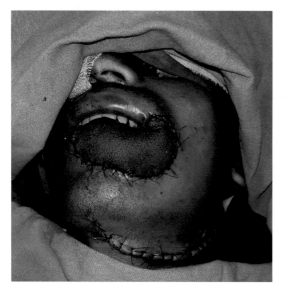

Figure 22.42 Radial forearm flap after inset.

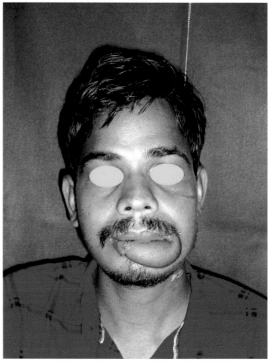

Figure 22.43 Post-operative picture.

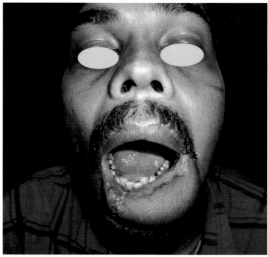

Figure 22.44 Adequate mouth opening at follow-up.

re-do anastomosis. In cases of delay in healing of the flap donor area, primary wound care with regular dressing is all that is required.

Rehabilitation

The flap donor upper limb usually has less functional deformity. Finger movement can be started in the immediate post-operative period and wrist movement can be started after 10 days when there is satisfactory graft take.

FREE FIBULA FLAP

Introduction

The search for ideal bone flap for reconstruction of the bony defects in the head and neck region like jaws and in the long bones came to an end when Taylor performed free fibula myo-osseous flap for post-traumatic defect of the tibia in 1975. Subsequently, in 1983, Chen and Yan first performed a free fibula flap with a skin paddle and confirmed the viability of a skin paddle attached to the fibula flap based on the perforators of the peroneal artery in the posterior peroneal septum. The spectrum of use of the fibula flap was expanded when Hidalgo performed first lower jaw reconstruction using osteotomy of the fibula to mimic the shape of the mandible. Then many surgeons described multiple modifications, like folding of the fibula to make it double barrel, double skin paddle for through-and-through defects of the cheek or making the skin paddle sensate by incorporating the sural nerve and making a neuronal anastomosis.

Indications

Free fibula flap is the most widely used bone flap, finding its application in the jaw, mandible or maxillary defects. It is also the bone flap of choice in extremity long bone defects of more than 6 cm, i.e., tibial defect in the lower extremity or long bone defect in the upper extremity.

In cases of mandible reconstruction for malignant cases where a soft tissue defect is the result along with the bone defect in the submandibular region, the flexor hallucis longus muscle or a part of the soleus muscle can be taken with the bone to fill the soft tissue defect.

Advantages

The fibula flap has many advantages. This is the longest bone flap available with good cortical bone density. It can be used as bone flap only or bone flap with skin paddle. Flap raising can be carried out via the two team approach, especially in head and neck reconstruction. As long as 25 cm bone can be harvested, thus entire mandible can be replaced. Multiple/segmental periosteal blood supply from the peroneal artery allows multiple osteotomies even at 2 cm interval without affecting the vascularity of the segment, so that a perfect shape mimicking the native mandible can be given.

Following the principles of reconstruction, free fibula flap with skin paddle serves for reconstruction of bony defect of mandible with mucosal lining or outer skin coverage in composite defects of the mandible. The flap possesses a vascular pedicle of good calibre peroneal artery and two venae comitantes and is of adequate length.

The skin paddle harvested with bone is pliable and attached with the bone by long posterior peroneal septum, allowing for its movement for intra-oral lining or extra-oral coverage.

Disadvantages

- In elderly individuals there are atherosclerotic changes of the lower limb vessels, often involvement of the peroneal artery, which poses problems in anastomosis and patency of the vessels.
- Sometimes the peroneal artery is the dominant blood supply (peronea magna) and thus sacrificing the peroneal artery during the harvest of the flap jeopardises the survival of the limb.
- Survival of the large skin paddle is sometimes questionable.
- Sometimes the perforators supplying the flap skin paddle arise from posterior tibial vessels, which warrants harvesting the skin paddle separately and anastomosing the perforators with peroneal vessels, further complicating the procedure.

Anatomy of Fibula Flap

Fibula bone is surrounded by many important anatomical structures. Along the long axis of the fibula bone run the axial vessels of the leg: the peroneal vessels. The peroneal artery, which is the dominant blood supply of the fibula flap, is accompanied by two venae comitantes. The peroneal artery originates from the posterior tibial artery a few centimetres from the origin of the anterior tibial artery at the popliteal artery.

The peroneal artery gives rise to multiple periosteal supplies. The medullary supply of the fibula bone is through the nutrient artery. Along with this, several cutaneous perforators arise from this artery and run through the posterior peroneal septum to supply the lateral calf. These are the basis of blood supply of the skin paddle of the flap.

The peroneal artery is usually accompanied by two venae comitantes and forms the pedicle of the flap. The vessels run along the medial border of the fibula.

Pre-Operative Investigations

There may be variations in the calibre and the possibility of atherosclerotic changes in the anterior and posterior tibial arteries in the lower limb. Conventional angiography or the less invasive magnetic resonance angiography is indicated before raising the fibula flap, particularly in individuals having clinically absent pulses in anterior and posterior tibial vessels. If any abnormality is detected, then sacrificing the peroneal artery with the fibula flap may be abandoned and other options should be considered.

Marking the cutaneous perforators along the posterior intermuscular septum pre-operatively helps in locating them intraoperatively and avoids injury to the same during flap harvesting.

Pre-Operative Preparation

Location of the perforators supplying the skin paddle of fibula flap should be determined with hand-held Doppler probe and marked. Pulsation of the anterior tibial artery and posterior tibial artery should be clinically assessed. If one of these vessels is found to be non-pulsatile, then magnetic resonance angiography should be ordered to rule out any anatomic anomaly, namely, dominant peroneal artery. Arteria peronea magna, clinical signs of missing foot pulses and deep vein thrombosis should be looked for. Presence of these clinical parameters provokes more investigations or suggests choosing the other leg as flap donor. Also, history of any trauma or fracture, if present, should be investigated properly.

Patient Positioning

The flap harvest is done in supine or lateral decubitus position with the donor leg flexed up to 135 degrees at knee. For better access, the ipsilateral hip is elevated with a beanbag or folded sheet or towel. By maintaining this position, the posterolateral aspect of the leg is exposed and muscles like the inverters and everters of the foot are disengaged or relaxed by elevating the foot. The surgeon can harvest the flap in sitting position. The foot should be padded in dorsiflexed position. The entire lower limb is prepped circumferentially and the foot is draped. Flap raising is usually done under tourniquet control. Tourniquet cuff should be applied prior to painting and draping of the limb. Some

surgeons prefer flap harvesting without tourniquet inflation.

Operative Steps

Usually, the skin paddle is centred vertically along the septum and centred at the junction between middle and lower third of the fibula. The skin paddle should be designed as per the requirements for mucosal defect or skin defect to be reconstructed after locating the perforator in the septum.

The lower osteotomy sites should be marked at a distance of at least 6 cm from the lateral malleolus for the stability of the ankle joint and the proximal osteotomy site should be marked at 6 cm from fibular head to protect the peroneal nerve (Figure 22.45).

1. Skin incision is made along the peroneus longus muscle, keeping a distance of 2 cm from the posterior intermuscular septum. The incision is slightly curved anteriorly according

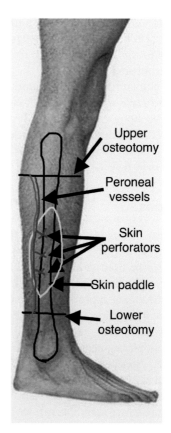

Figure 22.45 Flap marking of free fibula osteocutaneous flap.

to the location of the perforator (marked pre-operatively).

2. The peroneus longus and brevis muscles are separated from the fibula periosteum with sharp dissection.

3. Anterior peroneal septum is incised with utmost care not to injure the anterior tibial vessels and deep peroneal nerve, reflecting the anterior compartment muscles from the interosseous membrane.

4. The proximal and distal osteotomy sites are marked. Usually the distal osteotomy site is marked 8 cm above the ankle and the proximal osteotomy site is marked 6 cm below the fibular head. It is to be noted that the peroneal pedicle is a few centimetres away from the bone in the both the proximal and distal. After osteotomy is performed, two bone-holding forceps or skin hooks are used to retract the segment of fibula to be harvested.

5. The interosseous membrane is incised 1 cm from the fibula border. Making the fibula bone retracted more outwardly and dividing the interosseous membrane after osteotomy makes a space for dissection at the lower end. The distal peroneal pedicle is dissected and divided between ligatures.

6. The surgeon now divides the tibialis posterior muscle, which is found next to the interosseous membrane, the muscle fibres shaped like an inverted V. This makes the peroneal artery pedicle visible.

7. Posterior dissection is done separating the soleus muscle from the upper end of the fibula. Incision is made at the posterior marking of skin paddle. The skin paddle should be separated posteriorly from the soleus and flexor hallucis longus muscles, taking due care not to damage the sural nerve and short saphenous vein. The crural fascia should be included while making the posterior incision to safely protect the perforators.

8. The peroneal artery perforators supplying the skin paddle should be carefully preserved. If no septal perforators are found, then a chunk of soleus muscle should be taken with the bone for preserving musculocutaneous perforators. The posterior intermuscular septum should be preserved during harvest of the flap skin paddle.

9. The surgeon elevates the fibula bone, along with the skin paddle and, if needed, cuffs of soleus muscle at the perforators.

10.

11. Now the flap is elevated from distal to proximal direction by dividing the flexor hallucis muscle, and the posterior intermuscular septum is divided at sites other than its attachment at the skin paddle.

12. During the medial dissection, the tibial nerve and the posterior tibial vessels should be identified and retracted medially.

13. Perforators supplying the soleus muscle are clipped or ligated and divided. Care must be taken not to strip the pedicle from fibula or injure it.

14. The fibula is now 360 degrees free from its muscular attachment, except at the peroneal pedicle and the flap skin paddle, with or without a cuff of muscle.

15. The proximal pedicle dissection is carried out and the peroneal pedicle is separated from the posterior tibial pedicle, carefully protecting the important blood vessels.

16. Before the tourniquet is deflated, the flap pedicle dissection is done at the proximal end, separating the peroneal artery from both of its venae comitantes.

17. Tourniquet is deflated and the surgeon checks for bleeding from the flap skin paddle.

Post-Operative Care, Complication and Management

Post-operatively the flap is to be monitored clinically for detection of any early vascular compromise. Vascular compromise, if detected, should be managed at the earliest by re-exploration of the anastomosis site and re-doing anastomosis, if needed. The neck should be examined regularly for any collection or haematoma. Drains should be regularly inspected for any blockage. Neck position should be maintained so that there is no unnecessary stretch or any kinking of the pedicle.

The donor site is usually skin-grafted and splinted with the foot in dorsiflexion. This dressing is removed 5–7 days post-operatively and graft uptake is assessed. Leg drain can be removed at the first dressing.

Complications in a free fibula flap can be categorised as recipient site complications and donor site complications. Recipient site complications include vascular compromise in the flap, which must be dealt with urgently, as soon as it is detected. A low threshold should be kept for exploration and re-anastomosis in order to salvage the flap. Hematoma or collection in the neck can be prevented by meticulous haemostasis. In the post-operative period, it has to be managed with care. The haematoma should be evacuated with care not to disturb the vascular anastomosis site. Vascular complications are significantly more common in smokers. Therefore, cessation of smoking is of paramount importance in all head and neck reconstruction.

Other complications, like suture dehiscence, infection or partial flap skin loss, can happen. Post-radiotherapy, the unique complication of osteoradionecrosis can occur in the transferred fibula. It may give rise to implant failure and exposure, osteomyelitis or pathological fracture.

Donor site complications include graft loss, especially over the lower end if the tendon of peroneus longus was stripped off its paratenon. It is usually managed by dressing and secondary healing. Sensory loss to the foot can occur if the superficial peroneal nerve was inadvertently injured. If tibial nerve is damaged inadvertently, post-operative foot drop can happen. Fibrosis of the flexor hallucis longus muscle can cause flexion contracture of the great toe in some patients, which may require release.

Figures 22.46 and 22.47 show a case of carcinoma lower alveolus with post-mandibulectomy defect. Figures 22.48 and 22.49 show the harvested fibula bone and its fixation to the native bone with miniplates after osteotomy. Figures 22.50 and 22.51 show the long-term follow-up of the same patient with maintained jaw outline and adequate mouth opening.

PROSTHESIS IN HEAD AND NECK RECONSTRUCTION

Head and neck carcinoma is a debilitating illness. Surgical reconstruction is always a favoured option. Maxillofacial prosthetic treatment is not an alternative to reconstructive surgery, but prosthetic rehabilitation is required when surgical reconstruction is not possible in some circumstances, like patients of advanced age, poor health, irradiated tissue, certain complex deformity and

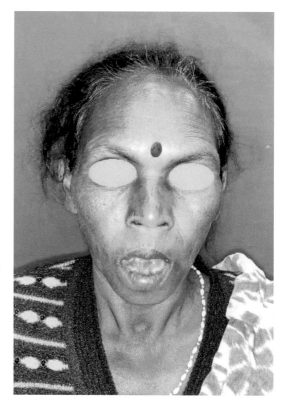

Figure 22.46 Carcinoma lower alveolus.

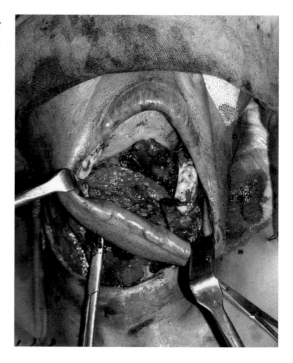

Figure 22.47 Segmental mandibular defect after resection.

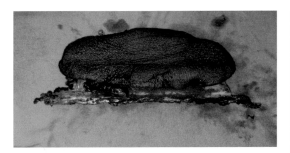

Figure.22.48 Harvested osteocutaneous free fibula flap.

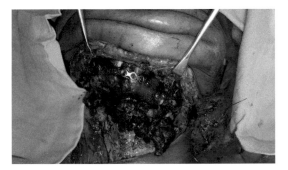

Figure 22.49 Flap after inset and fixation.

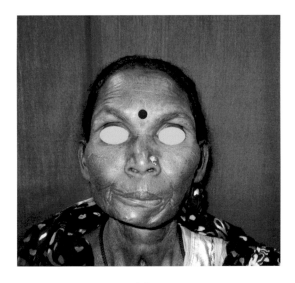

Figure 22.50 Long-term follow-up.

where repeated tumour surveillance is required in advanced disease.

Apart from patient factors, high chances of recurrence and loss of anatomical parts not replaceable by reconstructive methods are other

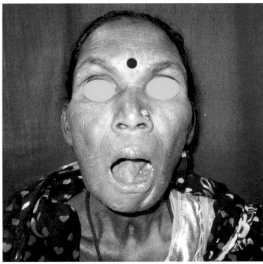

Figure 22.51 Adequate mouth opening at follow-up.

indications for prosthetic management. The detailed description of each prosthetic option is beyond the scope of this book, which gives only an overview of various options available for prosthetic management.

Post-Maxillectomy Defects

Patients requiring maxillectomy will have facial disfigurement with speech problems, difficulty in chewing and deglutition and nasal regurgitation of food and liquid, so the primary goal is to separate oral cavity and nasal cavity.

Small defects and defects without alveolar involvement are suitable candidates for a prosthetic obturator. Retention of the prosthetics depends on the ability to counter various forces like gravitational force, occlusive force, rotational force generated during speech, mastication and swallowing, and so the integrity of the canine and molar teeth is critical for retention. The amount of hard palate left after resection also determines the stability of the obturator. Based on the use, obturator can be divided into the following.

- Immediate/Surgical type: A temporary simple model used immediately after surgery, it acts as new palate to separate oral and nasal cavities, prevent contamination and rehabilitate speech and swallowing just after surgery.
- Interim Type: A more refined model made of softer material. It is used when surgical

obturator and dressing/packing are removed in post-operative period. The interim type is contoured at each visit to fit into the healing defect during the recovery period.

- Definitive Type: Permanent model. The mould is fabricated when surgical site is healed and stable after 8–10 weeks.

Obturators for rehabilitation of maxillectomy defects are made of poly methyl methacrylate (PMMA). There are chances of local or systemic infection following use of PMMA obturators, and consequently they require regular long-term follow-up. Presently, the use of titanium obturators has shown reduced chances of infection.

Segmental Mandibular and Maxillary Defects

Ideal management of the segmental mandibular defects is vascularised bony reconstruction. Apart from providing a bony base for applying teeth implants, the purpose of a bony reconstruction is to prevent deviation of the remaining mandibular segment to preserve aesthetics and to provide support so that remaining swallowing and speech functions can be preserved.

Patients not suitable for vascularised bone transfer due to patient factor or surgeon's lack of technical expertise can benefit from mandibular guide appliances. Similarly, maxillary prosthesis with palatal ramp can take care of the maxillary defect and can be used simultaneously for better rehabilitation.

Velopharyngeal Inadequacy

Velopharyngeal insufficiency results from surgical excision to remove cancer. Few speech appliances are available that can be used for rehabilitation.

Palatal lift prosthesis (PLP) is commonly used to manage VPI due to scarring of the remaining velar tissue. Discomfort, swallowing difficulty and vomiting reflex are common problems of PLP use. Adjustments are required to manage these difficulties as per the requirement of the patient.

A nasal speaking valve (NSV) inserted through nostrils can also be used. Tolerability and effectiveness of the NSV is reported to be better than PLP. Another advantage is that it can be used in edentulous patients.

Extraoral Facial Defects

Prosthetic reconstruction of lost nose, eye and ear is an important aspect of rehabilitation for building up confidence of the patients. These prosthetics must be customised as per the need of the patient, and they require retention systems. The prosthetics are either anchored to spectacles or retained by anatomical undercuts. Recently adhesives have been used for retention of the prosthesis, but patients with an active lifestyle are poor candidates for adhesives. Also, adhesives may result in skin irritation and atopy.

The implant-based anchorage system and prosthesis has now become popular. The implant (anchor) is osteo-integrated to the bone. With the help of abutment/attachment of the bone-integrated implant, the external prosthetic is attached. Ease of use, comfort and maintenance of hygiene are its advantages. Although there are chances of traumatic failure and infection, it is still one of the preferred options.

Facial Prosthetic Material

Leather, porcelain, silver, gelatine and latex are materials that have been used in the past. Acrylic is still used widely, as it is cheap and easily available. Currently, methacrylates, polyurethane and silicon are in use. They are soft, durable, flexible and inert. When moulded, they provide excellent colour and texture match to the surrounding tissues.

Auricular Prostheses

Conventionally, cartilage-based reconstruction is the ideal technique for reconstruction of the ear framework, but multi-stage surgery and inconsistent results with cartilage reconstruction are major drawbacks. Auricular prosthetics has emerged as a good alternative for rehabilitation of the patients.

Auricular prosthetics not only improve aesthetics but in patients with intact ear canal and hearing, they also improve speech recognition by acoustic gain and sound amplification. In patients with obliterated canal but intact conductive hearing, prosthetics are used solely for aesthetic purposes and a bone-anchored hearing aid can be used to rehabilitate hearing. Auricular prostheses can be adhesive-based or implant-based. Implant-based prosthetics are costly but are better tolerated and user friendly.

The major complication is skin reaction at the site of the implants. Higher failure rates occur in cases where an implant is used in irradiated bones.

Orbital Prosthesis

Planning and placement of suitable ocular or orbital prosthesis is a difficult procedure. It depends upon the type of the surgical procedure undertaken, i.e., evisceration, enucleation or exenteration.

After evisceration, when the tenon's capsule and extraocular muscles are intact, rehabilitation is done using a prosthetic eye. The prosthetic eye moves almost like a normal eye. After enucleation, rehabilitation is done with an orbital implant and the cut extraocular muscles are retracted to attach to the implant.

Following exenteration surgery, the orbital cavity is prepared, usually with split skin graft or soft tissue flap if required. The orbital prosthesis is then fabricated, covering the whole orbital cavity with the impression taken from the opposite eye. It is then painted to optimise the colour match.

The planning also depends upon the bony stability and contour of orbital boundaries, particularly inferior margin and closure of sinus cavities.

Nasal Prosthesis

Reconstruction of the nasal unit is of paramount importance as nasal deformity is visibly unacceptable to the patient. Choice of reconstruction for nose is forehead flap. But prosthetic reconstruction is required if there is flap failure or if patients opt for prosthetics primarily. In the past, adhesive-based prosthetics had high failure rates caused by moisture and humidification due to repeated air changes in the nasal cavity.

A better alternative to the adhesive system is the implant-based prosthetic. The anchors can be placed in the nasal cavity or glabella. The placement depends upon the amount of bony support available. Zygoma is also used if the bone of the nasal cavity or glabella does not support the implant.

While fabricating nasal prosthetics, care should be given to limit the disruption of the nasolabial crease. There should be a smooth transition of the prosthesis to the native facial issue.

Dental Implants and Prosthetic Rehabilitation

For dental rehabilitation, conventional prosthesis, tissue-supported prosthesis and implant-based prosthesis are the available options. It is also the choice for bony reconstruction of maxillary/mandibular defect. Interdisciplinary planning is required for planning of dental prosthetic placement. With the advancement in microsurgery and availability of osteocutaneous fibula and iliac crest for bony reconstruction, osteo-integrated implants are being increasingly used for dental rehabilitation.

Advantages of Using Prosthodontic Rehabilitation

1. It provides early non-surgical option for rehabilitation.
2. Results are aesthetically satisfying.

The need for maintaining oral hygiene, chances of infection and necessity of regular long-term follow-up should be explained to the patient before taking up maxillofacial prosthetic management.

Index

Note: Page numbers in *italics* indicate figures and in **bold** indicate tables on the corresponding pages.

For Product Safety Concerns and Information please contact our
EU representative GPSR@taylorandfrancis.com Taylor & Francis
Verlag GmbH, Kaufingerstraße 24, 80331 München, Germany